About Island Press

Island Press, a nonprofit organization, publishes, markets, and distributes the most advanced thinking on the conservation of our natural resources—books about soil, land, water, forests, wildlife, and hazardous and toxic wastes. These books are practical tools used by public officials, business and industry leaders, natural resource managers, and concerned citizens working to solve both local and global resource problems.

Founded in 1978, Island Press reorganized in 1984 to meet the increasing demand for substantive books on all resource-related issues. Island Press publishes and distributes under its own imprint and offers these services to other nonprofit organizations.

Support for Island Press is provided by Apple Computers, Inc., Mary Reynolds Babcock Foundation, Geraldine R. Dodge Foundation, The Educational Foundation of America, The Charles Engelhard Foundation, The Ford Foundation, Glen Eagles Foundation, The George Gund Foundation, William and Flora Hewlett Foundation, The Joyce Foundation, The J. M. Kaplan Fund, The John D. and Catherine T. MacArthur Foundation, The Andrew W. Mellon Foundation, The Joyce Mertz-Gilmore Foundation, The New-Land Foundation, The Jessie Smith Noyes Foundation, The J. N. Pew, Jr., Charitable Trust, Alida Rockefeller, The Rockefeller Brothers Fund, The Florence and John Schumann Foundation, The Tides Foundation, and individual donors.

Fighting Toxics

Fighting Toxics

A MANUAL FOR PROTECTING YOUR FAMILY, COMMUNITY, AND WORKPLACE

EDITED BY
Gary Cohen and John O'Connor

National Toxics Campaign

FOREWORD BY
Barry Commoner

ISLAND PRESS

Washington, D.C. □ *Covelo, California*

Library of Congress Cataloging-in-Publication Data
Fighting toxics : a manual for protecting your family, community, and workplace / edited by
    Gary Cohen and John O'Connor ; foreword by Barry Commoner.
        p.   cm.
    Includes bibliographical references.
    ISBN 1-55963-013-2 (alk. paper). — ISBN 1-55963-012-4 (pbk.)
    1. Environmental health—Citizen participation.   2. Environmental health—
Political aspects.   3. Environmentally induced diseases—Prevention—Citizen
participation.   4. Pollution—Environmental aspects.   5. Toxicology—Political
aspects.   I. Cohen, Gary, 1956–   . II. O'Connor, John, 1954–   .
RA566.F54   1990
363.73'84—dc20   90-4064
                                                                                                        CIP

Printed on recycled, acid-free paper

Manufactured in the United States of America

10   9   8   7   6   5   4   3   2

To
the children of the world
and
Katie O'Connor,
an NTC organizer
who died on the way
to the next campaign

Acknowledgments

This book has been more than eight years in the making. John O'Connor, working for Massachusetts Fair Share in 1981, originally wrote the first "Neighborhood Health and Safety Guide." His manual was the original seed that became this book. Since early 1985, Gary Cohen and John O'Connor have worked on this book—changing and expanding and drawing upon their experiences with the National Toxics Campaign to tailor the book to the needs of local environmental activists.

This book is a tribute to the citizens around the country who have been fighting to defend their families and their communities against toxic poisoning. Their courage, their humility, and their love is the very fabric of the nation's grassroots toxics movement. Their experiences are reflected in these pages. The strategies outlined throughout the book are their strategies, the result of endless hours in meetings and protests and struggles.

Although there are too many citizen leaders around the country to recognize all of them, we must at least salute Adrienne Anderson, Cathy Hinds, Lois Gibbs, Cathy Renaud, Cora Tucker, Larry and Sheila Wilson, Ethel Dotson, Marilyn Ayers, Ted Smith, Rick Abraham, Joyce Johnston, Irene Gillis, Patty Frase, Linda Wallace Campbell, Kaye Kiker, Martha Bailey, Anna Sue Rafferty, Norine Routhier, Dave Shade, Cathy Burd, Rita Carlson, Ernie Witt, Henry Clark, Greg Schirm, Jean Siri, Phyllis Robey, Janice Nadeau, Penny Newman, Becky Leighton, Dianne Takvorian, Linda Burkhardt, Daryl Malek-Wiley, Dolly Lymburner, Mike Belliveau, Larry Rose, Pamela Swift, Grant Smith, Don Weiner, Jesse Deer in Water, Pat Moss, Sandy Buchanon, Bill Ryan, Hank Cole, Eric Draper, Dave Zwick,

Gene Karpinski, Amy Goldsmith, Tony Mazzocchi, Tommy Simms, Michael Picker, Esla Byroe-Andreola, Frank Carsner, Mary Edgerton, George and Wendall Paris, Mae Morgan, Rob Sargeant, Cindy Phillips, Linda King, Linda Meade, Lark Hayes, Rich Gatto, Laurie Maddy, Mike Lux, Mark Ritchie, Carolyn Mugar, Ken St. George, Charlie Rose, Tommy Wolfe, Dick Russell, Susan Dewan, Dave Rappaport, Sheila Robinson, Bonnie Titcomb, Mike Rosselle, Harriet Barlow, Richard Grossman, Richard Regan, Cathy Garulo, Corinne Whitehead, and all the people who worked with them and supported them.

Contents

Foreword

Remember all those environmental laws passed in the 1970s: Clean Air Act, Clean Water Act, Safe Drinking Water Act, Resource Conservation and Recovery Act, Superfund? For the most part, those laws haven't worked. After twenty years of environmental regulation, our environment has never been at greater risk. Why haven't the laws protected us?

The reason is clear. Over the past twenty years, the Environmental Protection Agency and Congress have tried to "control" pollution after it is created, rather than to prevent it. But the controls cannot do the job, often only shifting the pollution problem from one route of exposure to the next. Emissions of pollutants into the air and water have declined by an average of only 10 to 20 percent in the last fifteen years instead of the 90 percent called for in environmental laws, and many emissions—especially of toxic compounds—have increased.

There are some environmental successes, however. Pollution levels of a few chemicals—levels of lead in the air, DDT and PCBs in wildlife and people, mercury in fish, strontium 90 in the food chain, and phosphates in some rivers—have been reduced by 80 to 90 percent. The successes explain what works and what doesn't. Every success on this short list of improvements reflects the same action: production of the pollutant has been stopped.

DDT and PCB levels have dropped because their production and use have been banned. Mercury is much less prevalent because it is no longer used to manufacture chlorine. Lead has been taken out of gasoline. And strontium 90 has decayed to low levels because the United States and the Soviet Union stopped the atmospheric nuclear bomb tests that produced it.

The lesson is plain: pollution prevention works; pollution control does not. Where production technology has been changed to eliminate pollutants, the environment has improved. Where an attempt is made to trap the pollutant in a control device—the automobile's catalytic converter or the incinerator's scrubber—environmental improvements are modest or nil. Once toxic chemicals are created, efforts to control their effects have nearly always failed. However, when a pollutant is stopped at the point of production, it can be eliminated. Once it is produced, it is too late. Pollution is like an incurable disease; it can only be prevented.

We seem to be learning this lesson, but not acting on it. On January 19, 1989, former EPA administrator Lee Thomas acknowledged that much of the EPA's past effort "has been on pollution control rather than pollution prevention" and that "EPA realizes there are limits on how much environmental improvement can be achieved under these [control] programs, which emphasize management after pollutants have been generated." This statement actually calls for a major overhaul of the nation's environmental programs, which are based on laws that trigger regulation only after pollutants are created.

Despite these occasional bursts of insight, the federal government continues to pursue its failed policies of pollution control. It continues to permit incinerators; it continues to give polluters permits to discharge into our rivers; it continues to allow companies to use ozone-destroying chemicals; it continues to allow cancer-causing pesticides in food.

President Bush has cast himself as an "environmentalist." Yet his answer to air pollution is to encourage polluters to buy and sell their "right" to pollute. Rather than preventing pollution, Mr. Bush wants to legalize it.

Most of our environmental problems result from the sweeping technological changes that transformed the global economic system after World War II: the shift from fuel-efficient railroads to gas-guzzling cars and trucks; the substitution of synthetic fertilizers and pesticides for crop rotation, ladybugs, and birds; the replacement of natural materials like cotton, wood, and rubber with plastics and synthetic building materials; the use of chlorinated solvents instead of soap and water to clean machines. These changes in production technology have brought on the environmental crisis.

To end the environmental crisis we must introduce environmentally sound technologies of production. If railroads and mass transit were expanded, if electric power were decentralized and based on renewable sources, if we used organic cleaners instead of chemical solvents, if we stopped growing food with dangerous pesticides, if homes were weatherized, if brewers were forbidden to put plastic nooses on six-packs of beer, if supermarkets were not allowed to wrap polyvinyl chloride plastic around everything in sight, if we banned Styrofoam, if the government became the major market for recycled goods, then we could push back the toxic invasion of our planet.

To create an ecologically sound, sustainable economy will require sweeping changes in the major systems of production—agriculture, industry, energy, and transportation. This will cost us perhaps $100 billion annually for the next ten years or more. Where can that much money be found? It can be found in the military budget, which, in the world of *glasnost,* is bloated beyond reason. But the government is failing to act on these solutions, which industry will resist. The question is: What are *we* going to do? Only well-informed citizens can meet this challenge. In communities around the world we must learn how to pressure polluters and municipalities to take the right actions to protect the environment and public health.

That is why this book is so essential. The National Toxics Campaign has put together a blueprint that shows how citizens can prevent pollution in their communities. *Fighting Toxics* provides the background to our environmental crisis and outlines a step-by-step approach to address it at the local level. *Fighting Toxics* is a primer on environmental democracy. It offers a cohesive strategy for teaching citizens how they can gain control over decisions that affect the economic and environmental health of their communities.

I hope that all who care for the planet and their community read this book and take action to defend them both from the growing environmental assault.

BARRY COMMONER

Fighting Toxics

Introduction

GARY COHEN

When Cathy Hinds and her family moved to rural Maine, she envisioned clean air, clean water, and a large backyard for her children to raise animals. What she found was very different. They couldn't drink the water because it was contaminated with more than twenty-seven chemicals from a nearby toxic waste site. Her children couldn't play in the neighborhood because poisonous chemicals were evaporating out of the ground. The children tried to raise pets, but their cat gave birth to a litter of deformed kittens. Cathy had one miscarriage; a year later she got pregnant again and on December 22, 1984, she gave birth to her first son. Three days later, on Christmas Day, when most parents were opening gifts with their children, Cathy and her husband were explaining to their daughters that their three-day-old baby brother had died.

This is not an isolated incident. Every day a new community learns that its drinking water is contaminated. Every day a new community discovers that it is living next to a toxic waste dump. Every day a new community finds out that the industrial facility down the street is poisoning them by spewing toxic chemicals into the air, water, and land.

The Environmental Protection Agency (EPA) has identified over 30,000 uncontrolled toxic waste sites in the United States. That list continues to grow. According to a General Accounting Office report issued in December 1986, the EPA "does not know if it has identified 90 percent of the potentially hazardous sites or only 10 percent." By one estimate there may be as many as 370,000 toxic waste sites in the nation. These statistics do not include the dangers posed by chemical producers and chemical users in thousands of plants nationwide.

Toxic chemicals have invaded almost every aspect of our lives. Pesticide residues are in the food we eat; heavy metals and synthetic chemicals are in the water we drink; and hundreds of chemicals are in the air we breathe daily.

Cathy Hinds didn't suffer quietly. She also found out she wasn't alone. Other women in the neighborhood had miscarriages and their families suffered from a variety of illnesses. Cathy organized her neighbors and together they pressured the state to clean up the site. She also received help from the National Toxics Campaign and discovered that thousands of women nationwide were also organizing to protect their families. Cathy has been organizing ever since.

Across America, there is a growing grassroots movement that is demanding the right to live in a community free of environmental threats. People are demanding the right to know about the hazards in their communities and the right to be protected from them. In every state, citizens are involved in campaigns to clean up Superfund sites, stop the siting of hazardous waste facilities or incinerators, prevent Bhopal-like chemical disasters, and pressure industry to reduce its hazardous waste generation and emission.

HOW THIS MANUAL CAN HELP

Fighting Toxics is written for people dealing with toxic threats in their communities. It provides information and guidance on the complex issues involved in all toxics problems. It also seeks to encourage citizens to take greater control over their neighborhoods and win solutions to the toxic threats facing them. It is a how-to book for reestablishing local democracy in your community.

The Guidelines for Action described in these pages are derived in large part from local citizen campaigns around the country. People are already taking a lot of the steps outlined in the book. Some strategies, such as the inspection and negotiation models described in Chapters 5 and 8, are relatively new concepts developed by the National Toxics Campaign. But even these innovative approaches have proved successful in many local campaigns around the country.

We would like local activists to experiment with the strategies described in these pages and let us know which ones worked and which didn't. We plan to revise and expand this book over the coming years and will be including many new anecdotes and case examples based on what you tell us. Since this is a citizens' manual, we hope you will get involved in making this a resource for citizens everywhere in America.

There are ten chapters in the manual plus a resource section at the end. Each chapter focuses on a particular aspect of toxic problems in communities. Together they form a blueprint for action for citizen campaigns to gain:

- Organizational strength and bargaining power
- Access to the government's computer databases on toxics
- Citizen inspections of polluting factories
- Toxic waste reduction and toxic use reduction by industry
- Media coverage
- Pollution prevention in local communities

Part I, Turning the Toxic Tide, comprises six chapters. Chapter 1 offers a broad overview of the problem. The chapter provides a conceptual background to the rest of the book. It describes the scope of the toxics crisis, the problems of the petrochemical industry, and a way to change the way goods are produced in this country to reduce the toxic threat.

Chapter 2 explains how to organize in your community: nuts and bolts information on how to do doorknocking, how to build your organization, how to recruit people, and how to develop a campaign strategy. There is also a practical list of thirty-five different actions that citizens can use in their local campaigns.

Chapter 3 is a primer for citizen campaigns that aim to influence the way corporations do business. It discusses the basic concepts of the "corporate campaign." There is also a case study of a campaign that succeeded in moving a bank to put up money for a Superfund site cleanup.

Chapter 4 tells you how to do research and obtain information. It offers hints on using the Freedom of Information Act and dealing with government workers. The chapter explains the different sources of information about toxics: government, industry, and libraries. It also explains how to use the national right-to-know law, which can provide citizens with information about what chemicals a company dumps into the community's air, water, and land.

Chapter 5 is about the neighborhood inspection—a new strategy that the National Toxics Campaign and its affiliates are using in many efforts nationwide. The neighborhood inspection involves citizens in actual in-plant visits to polluting facilities to evaluate their chemical management practices and make recommendations for needed improvements. Moreover, citizens inspect the plants with their own industrial engineer, who trains them beforehand in what to look for and what kind of questions to ask. This chapter is an essential primer for this innovative strategy.

Chapter 6 is all about the media: how to get its attention, how to relate to reporters, how to design and write a press release. There are also tips on holding a press conference and creating a message that the media will understand.

Part II, Toxics and the Law, could be a book in itself. It is certainly the most comprehensive guide to using the law to win local toxics campaigns that we have ever seen. Chapter 7 presents a brief overview of current environmental legislation and comments on the progress of its enforcement. Chapter 8 focuses on your recourse under the law: how citizens can use the law to force action at a site or prevent unwanted toxics there. It tells you when it's appropriate to sue, when you need a lawyer, and when you're better off *without* a lawyer. Chapter 9 explains the legal aspects of running a local toxics campaign. It suggests imaginative ways to make the laws work for you as you wage a local campaign against hazardous chemicals.

Part III, The Ultimate Solution, looks to the future. Chapter 10 advances a new approach to the toxics crisis: reducing the use of toxic materials. For the past twenty years the debate around toxics has focused on controlling toxics once they are created. Policymakers have been concerned with managing toxics, rather than preventing them. In this chapter, an innovative way of thinking about the problem is addressed. Essentially we need to begin focusing on the industrial processes themselves and reduce the front-end use of the most dangerous toxic chemicals.

Finally, there's a Resources section at the end of the book that includes reading lists and contacts for getting information and getting involved in the fight to secure a toxics-free future for all of us.

THE NATIONAL TOXICS CAMPAIGN

The National Toxics Campaign (NTC) is a coalition of thousands of ordinary citizens, environmental groups, statewide consumer organizations, family farmers, lawyers, educators, public health experts, scientists, and business people working together to solve the nation's toxics crisis. NTC brings together a unique blend of local energy and national experts—with the political sophistication to have a real impact on local, state, and national policy. The National Toxics Campaign is also the only national environmental organization with a board of directors made up exclusively of "toxics survivors," people who daily face the toxics threat and who have devoted their lives to fighting to protect their communities.

Since 1983, NTC has supported citizens across the country in many capacities. It has assisted local efforts to clean up hazardous waste sites. It has helped coordinate efforts to establish strong state toxic waste cleanup. It has pushed for right-to-know legislation. Its work in over a thousand communities since the campaign's inception has helped strengthen state and local toxics organizations and win many local toxics issues. The NTC staff provides technical assistance and environmental testing for grassroots groups nationwide. NTC is the nation's only environmental organization with a complete testing laboratory to analyze the full range of toxic chemicals. The NTC's staff has also participated as expert witnesses and presented groups with model tactics and policies for pollution prevention in thirty-five states.

On the national level, NTC spearheaded the fight to win the new $9 billion Superfund reauthorization—the program designed to clean up the nation's worst toxic waste sites. As part of this effort, NTC orchestrated the highly acclaimed "Superdrive for Superfund," in which four trucks criss-crossed the country, stopping at 200 toxic waste sites to collect toxic samples and petitions to bring to Congress. This campaign yielded two million signatures from Americans demanding a strong Superfund cleanup program. NTC also brought toxics victims to Washington for key votes in Congress. This campaign culminated in October 1986 with the passage of a much strengthened Superfund and the first national right-to-know law.

But the Superfund law, and other laws, do not address the billions of tons of emissions from industrial production each year, or the manufacture of hazardous products, or the continued use of dangerous chemicals when safer alternatives exist. Even though toxic waste reduction is generally recognized as the safest and sanest hazardous waste management practice, numerous studies have shown that reduction methods are rarely used by industry. More often, wastes are either injected into the ground or released to the air, water, and land. Industry is not doing enough to reduce its toxic waste and prevent toxic threats, and government is doing very little to protect the public's health.

To address these environmental threats, NTC launched a toxics prevention campaign to work on the local, state, and national levels to implement programs that will help prevent toxic hazards and encourage industry to reduce its use of toxic chemicals and cut down on its generation of toxic waste. NTC views the coming years as the time to build a base of citizen support and proper policy options to make pollution prevention a national priority for citizen groups and policymakers alike.

Through local prevention projects and statewide legislative and policy efforts, NTC is developing a comprehensive toxics prevention strategy to encourage chemical industries and other toxics users to substantially reduce the manufacture, use, emission, and disposal of the most dangerous toxic chemicals. Recently, the NTC worked with 1,200 supermarkets in North America to get them to sign "Pesticide Reduction Agreements" promising to stop selling produce containing residues of cancer-causing pesticides by 1995. NTC's Consumer Pesticide Project is a good example of how citizens working directly with industry can stop dangerous chemicals from invading our lives. Although there are laws on the books that are supposed to protect America's food supply, the EPA continues to allow sixty-nine different cancer-causing pesticides and fungicides to be used on our fruits and vegetables. Where government has failed, organized citizens can be successful.

NTC wants to help citizens defend their families and communities. This book, *Fighting Toxics,* is a key component of that effort. It tells how citizens on the local level can win solutions to the environmental crisis that affects us all. The technical, legal, political, media, and policy tools presented here are intended to help citizens build the groundswell of activity into a tidal wave that can force polluters and politicians on all levels to stop the poisoning of our planet.

THE CAMPAIGN FUND

The National Toxics Campaign Fund is the principal research, education, and organizing arm of the National Toxics Campaign. The Campaign Fund is also the principal sponsor of this book. The Campaign Fund's staff works to provide NTC with model policies, organizing assistance, educational outreach, environmental testing, and research materials to strengthen the emerging power of NTC and to help citizens in their campaigns nationwide. The Campaign Fund is a nonprofit organization.

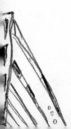

Turning the Toxic Tide

1

The Toxics Crisis

JOHN O'CONNOR

Uncontrolled toxic chemicals and wastes have reached crisis proportions. "Toxics" are perhaps our nation's Number 1 hidden health problem. Each of us now contains dozens of synthetic chemicals in our bodies that can cause cancer and birth defects. Our nation's waters show signs of increases of dangerous solvents, heavy metals, plastic residues, pesticides, and other chemical products from the modern petrochemical age. Acid rain, airborne toxics, and the chlorine-based chlorofluorocarbons (CFCs) are destroying our atmosphere. Asbestos in the nation's schools is poisoning thousands of children. Much of the food we eat contains residues of pesticides and herbicides that can cause long-term health damages. This year, more than a thousand new synthetic chemicals will enter our communities largely untested for their contribution to birth defects, reproductive damage, behavioral effects, and cancer.

The public health, the environment, and even life itself is being threatened because the United States and other nations overproduce and overuse very dangerous, largely untested, synthetic chemicals. Corporate negligence coupled with a weak and ineffective regulatory system is only making the situation worse. At the same time, real solutions are sitting on the shelf waiting to be put into practice. The hard question is not "how do we solve the toxics crisis?" but, rather, "how do we, as organized Americans, reshape corporate behavior and the legal system to get reasonable solutions put into action?" How can we muster the people power and political muscle to get lawmakers to put the available solutions into action?

The rallying cry for solutions to the toxic crisis has in large part emerged

11

from citizen groups across the country who have had to protect their families from local toxic health threats. A set of new ideas and approaches has surfaced that for the first time points a way out of our current predicament. Citizens are taking steps to monitor toxic chemical producers and users as well as toxic waste facilities. The new democratic "citizen-based" regulatory approach—which we term *environmental democracy*—offers a fundamental shift in the way we think about regulating industry.

The basic strategy is quite simple: Since it is the chemical products and processes that have brought about the crisis, the solution lies in changing what is produced and how it is produced. Until recently, most decisions regarding the production and use of toxic substances have been made solely by industry. Now, however, citizens are beginning to pressure industry to reduce its production, use, and disposal of toxic chemicals. They are legitimately demanding to know what is being produced, how it is produced, and how much waste is being created at the same time. They are also asking how much of the toxic chemicals could be reduced or eliminated and replaced with safer substitutes. Citizen groups in countless communities are pushing all levels of government as well as chemical polluters directly to allow involvement in process and product decisions. Citizen groups are saying no to garbage incinerators and dumps and saying yes to waste reduction, recycling, and composting. Up until now government has given industry the privilege to emit deadly chemicals into our communities. In response to this assault, citizens must win the right of home rule—to be empowered to block the siting of dangerous waste facilities in their communities, while also participating in decisions about what is produced within their city limits. This is the basis of environmental democracy. To understand how this change is coming about, let us look deeper into the problem.

THE EXTENT OF THE PROBLEM

Toxic chemicals are in the air we breathe and the water we drink. They are in our workplaces, on our farms, and in our neighborhoods. Government inspections and industry's "self-reporting system" have confirmed over 30,000 hazardous waste sites throughout the country—a list that is growing at the rate of a thousand new sites every few months. This list does not include any of the 300,000 "unofficial" pits, ponds, and lagoons containing suspected hazardous waste. Seventy percent of these unofficial dumping areas are not lined with clay or other materials required at official sites, so contaminants are quickly absorbed into the ground and find their way into groundwater. According to a 1987 EPA report, all landfills, even the lined ones, eventually leak.

Over 560 million tons of hazardous waste is generated by American industry annually—more than 2 tons for every U.S. citizen. Most of our drinking water systems contain at least one and probably several cancer-causing chemicals. One national survey showed the presence of TCE (a toxic solvent) in one-third of the groundwater wells tested. Another authoritative government study identified more than 200 industrial chemicals and pesticides commonly found in the body tissue of 95 percent of Americans tested.

How dangerous are toxic chemicals to humans? The answer has several parts. First, industry, government, and citizens all agree that toxic chemicals pose a significant problem. Moreover, some statistics suggest that the spread of toxic chemicals into the environment is causing a public health crisis of major proportions. Each year 100,000 deaths are attributed to occupational exposure. It has been estimated that each week as many as 500 people in the United States die from diseases related to asbestos exposure alone. The birth defect rate has doubled in the last twenty-five years, and scientists believe that part of this increase is due to exposure to toxic chemicals. The sperm count has declined by roughly 20 percent since the emergence of synthetic petrochemicals in the 1940s.

But these frightening statistics have not been alarming enough to change state and national toxics policies. One reason for this failure is that it's extremely difficult to find evidence linking specific toxic chemicals to specific diseases, and this is where the conflict really begins. Part of the difficulty arises because most of the diseases contracted by people exposed to toxics are relatively common, such as lung cancer, which is believed to be triggered by a variety of factors. There is an abnormally high incidence of leukemia in persons who work regularly with benzene, for example, but companies are quick to point out that leukemia has also been related to other factors. Only a few rare diseases are indisputably caused by exposure to toxic materials: Mesothelioma, a cancer of the lung or abdomen, occurs only in people who have been exposed to asbestos; angiosarcoma, a rare form of liver cancer, results from exposure to vinyl chloride gas. There are others, but cancers don't have labels that specify their cause. But as the scientific community continues to study these toxic chemicals and their interrelationship, they are beginning to understand the connection between toxic exposure of many types and higher rates of illness.

Beyond the threat to human health from chemical products and wastes there is also the threat of planet-wide destruction from certain substances.

Particularly dangerous are the ozone destroyers, which include chlorine-based CFCs, halons, carbon tetrachloride, and methyl chloroform. These chemicals are used to make solvents, foams, refrigerants, and fire extinguishers. EPA studies show that the damage done to the outer atmosphere—the ozone layer—by CFCs and other ozone destroyers is so severe that an ever-growing hole is opening up over the South Pole and threatening the existence of this vital protective layer. The EPA estimates that more than 80 million new skin cancer cases may result over the next eighty years because of the damage done to the ozone layer. This layer, which protects life from the dangerous rays of the sun, has been depleted by 3 percent since 1979. Significant loss of this protective shield will mean the end of life on the planet.

SOCIALLY ACCEPTABLE RISKS?

Chemical manufacturers often confuse the issue of their pollution by insisting that modern life involves "socially acceptable risks" that come with the products that consumers demand. But whoever demanded polyvinyl chloride, DDT, dioxin, synthetic clothes, flammable textiles, and toxic building materials? Rather than "market demand," it is the chemical industry itself that has carefully shaped consumer demand by producing large volumes of toxic materials to replace natural-based products and advertising them to the American public. This major shift in production has been based not on what is necessarily needed by society but on the chemical industry's financial self-interest.

"Risk assessment" is the rage in the parts of the scientific community that are allied with the serious chemical polluters. We now hear arguments like "walking across the street is more dangerous than living next to a toxic dump site" or "eating bean sprouts and peanut butter is more dangerous than the cancer-causing pesticide residue in your food." These analyses distort the truth, however, by comparing similar volumes of natural versus synthetic material in a way that ignores the *total* volume of deadly wastes created when synthetics are made, as well as the effects of the sheer volume of synthetic chemicals produced. In 1980, some 370 billion pounds of synthetic chemicals were produced. When nonsynthetic chemical production is added to the total, the chemical industry's annual production is roughly 500 billion pounds—ten times that of the food industry. In 1987, U.S. industry reported dumping 22 billion pounds of toxic chemicals into the air, water, and land. According to the congressional Office of Technology Assessment, the actual figure may be closer to 400 billion pounds. The annual production of vinyl chloride (6.5 billion pounds) equals the dry weight of all U.S. fruit production in a year. While there are indeed exposures in the natural world that must be guarded against (asbestos, aflotoxins), the dangers of new synthetic materials far outweigh the risks associated with natural ones.

The chemical industry would also like us to believe that cancer and other toxic-related diseases are our own fault—caused by lifestyle choices such as smoking cigarettes. The facts, however, show that while there is a high incidence of lung cancer in cigarette smokers, environmental factors beyond the immediate control of the individual play a key role as well. A recent study of females in New Jersey and Wyoming shows a strong connection between cancer and environment. Although women in New Jersey smoke virtually the same number of cigarettes as those in Wyoming, the women in New Jersey—a chemical manufacturing state—had a cancer death rate 36 percent higher than those in Wyoming. "Cancer maps" of types of cancer show a similar pattern of high risk for urban dwellers. Urban industrial centers as well as rural areas near petrochemical facilities expose residents to a cancer risk that has little or nothing to do with lifestyle.

Again, while we must guard against all health threats, we cannot eliminate naturally occurring materials (such as radon) in some regions of the country. We can, however, exercise control over the toxic synthetic materials that pervade our lives. While the threat posed by asbestos, radiation, and heavy metals has received significant attention under law (with improvements still needed), the synthetic chemical industry—which presents the greatest public health threat—remains largely unregulated.

THE PETROCHEMICAL FOCUS

The petrochemical industry got its start during World War II when the demand for products far outweighed what was available. Rubber, for example, normally supplied from parts of Asia, was not available, so synthetic rubber was developed, marketed, and sold as a substitute. Silk for parachutes as well as shortages in cotton and wool for clothing led to the invention and mass production of synthetic fibers—rayon, Dacron, and nylon. Plastics were used to replace scarce metals unavailable for aircraft production or to replace leather. When soldiers first returned from the South Pacific with malaria, the first mass-produced synthetic pesticide, DDT, ushered in the "pesticide revolution": the great war on the insect kingdom.

Scientists learned how to develop new products by splitting, cracking, distilling, and recombining petrochemical feedstocks into new products never before found on the face of the earth.

Since the 1940s, the chemical industry has expanded at a rate that is twice that of the U.S. economy's growth as a whole. The key to the industry's economic success is that it has been able to mass produce millions of tons of synthetic materials for sale at a relatively low price. Compared to other industries, the chemical industry requires massive capital and little labor. The industry has easily penetrated almost every aspect of the market, replacing wood and paper with plastic, cotton and wool with rayon and nylon, leather with vinyl, glass and steel with plastic, natural farming with chemical-intensive farming, and on and on down the line.

But with these technical innovations have come serious problems. Early pesticide use killed nearly one-half of the U.S. bird population in the 1940s and 1950s by some accounts. Cancer rates around chemical production facilities (even in rural areas) are higher than in the rest of the nation. Streams, rivers, and lakes have been made toxic by chemical discharges. There is a national groundwater crisis and a host of other life-threatening problems that face us today. Thousands of chemical dumps litter the nation and will require expensive cleanups over the coming decades.

The synthetic chemical industry is definitely one of the nation's largest sources of toxic pollution. According to Dr. Barry Commoner, director of the Center for the Biology of Natural Systems, the industry generates two barrels of waste for every barrel of product. A recent review of the German chemical industry showed that in plastics there are four units of waste created for every unit of product; in pesticides, three units of waste for each unit of product; and for synthetic dyes, eight units of waste for every unit of product. Thus the industry accounts for more waste than product in many of its operations! According to several EPA studies, the chemical industry generates 70 to 85 percent of all toxic wastes. In one way or another, the industry is responsible for the vast majority of 30,000 hazardous waste sites recognized by the U.S. government.

Solving the public health crisis posed by widespread chemical production will require transforming an industry that produces too many dangerous synthetic products into one that produces safer and more socially useful materials and products. The solution lies in producing and using much less of the most toxic materials and in finding safe substitutes for high-hazard synthetic materials. This approach not only removes the most dangerous materials from the market, but also reduces the amount of toxic waste that is generated and ultimately released to air, water, and land.

Pesticides provide a perfect example. Before World War II and the use of synthetic pesticides, family farmers were losing about one-third of their crop annually to insects. Today, after the pesticide saturation of our farmland, when more than $15 billion each year passes from the farmer to the chemical industry, the farmers are still losing roughly one-third of their crop to insects. And this is after yields per acre have increased dramatically, due primarily to fertilizers and hybrid seed. In other words, the bugs pound for pound are taking a larger amount of the crop than ever while pesticides are becoming less effective and costly. Since World War II, moreover, the number of insects and mites known to be resistant to one insecticide or another has grown from less than 10 species to more than 447 species. Resistant species of rodents, fungi, and weeds are also on the rise.

To solve the toxic chemical crisis will require pressuring the petrochemical industry to reduce the manufacture, use, transportation, and disposal of the worst toxic substances. It will also require getting consumers to demand safer products in their homes and safer food on their tables. Finally, it will require getting industrial workers and farmers to demand safer working conditions and the right to refuse work that is hazardous to their health. In short, it will take a major reorientation of our society to shift from a toxics-based economy to one that is safe and sustainable. But this transition will happen only if citizens are educated and organized in their own communities.

THE TOXICS CYCLE

The toxic pollution problem is made up of several interrelated parts that we will call the *toxics cycle*. The toxics cycle refers to the production, use, and disposal of chemicals and products considered necessary in our society. It is the process that transforms raw materials in the factories and releases them into the marketplace in the form of products and into our neighborhoods in the form of wastes. Probably at least one aspect of the cycle visibly intrudes upon each of our daily lives: the smelly dump in your neighborhood, the smog in the skyline, the dangerous products under the kitchen sink, the solvents on the job, even the chemical fumes from the railroad accident down the street. But what is not so apparent is the way each aspect of the cycle is part of a larger process.

Imagine, for a moment, what would happen if we tried to isolate and get rid of just one piece of the toxics cycle. Correcting workplace gas and dust problems by ventilating toxics away from workers and into the neighborhood would create a community air pollution problem. Cutting down on surface water discharge of chemicals into rivers by dumping the wastes in landfills would create future groundwater hazards. A lasting solution to the toxic pollution problem must treat each part of the cycle at once, not just shift the pollution from one medium to another.

TECHNOLOGICAL SOLUTIONS

Let's look at some practical applications of these ideas. Remember, the real problem is not the lack of technology to deal with hazardous waste. Executives of American industry could stop producing most of its toxic waste soon if they chose to do so—by using safer substitutes, by producing fewer waste-intensive products, by establishing comprehensive waste reduction plans, by recycling, and by other methods. But most of the business community hasn't yet put comprehensive reduction of toxic use and toxic waste on their list of priorities.

The biggest polluters, such as the synthetic chemical industry, are not in business as charitable organizations nor are they particularly concerned about environmental pollution and the public health. Most synthetic chemical producers make their money by manufacturing products that involve tons of toxic emissions into the environment. After the Bhopal accident that killed 4,000 people and injured perhaps 100,000 others, Union Carbide was more concerned with minimizing the public relations damage than minimizing the human damage. In general, industry's goal is to capture the largest share of the profits in the shortest possible time.

But, curiously, numerous studies have shown that investment in stopping or preventing pollution can actually prove profitable for almost all chemical users. Many chemicals that are treated as waste can be reduced or recycled back into the raw materials industry needs. Setting up a closed-loop system and eliminating all chemical emissions essentially takes what was once waste and turns it into a usable material. This means that fewer chemical inputs are required, less waste is generated, there is less of a regulatory burden, there are fewer future liabilities, and the firm enjoys substantial savings.

If industry were to invest in pollution prevention, these investments would more than pay for themselves in a period of one to three years, according to many case studies. Let's take the case of solvents. These are the chemicals most often found in our landfills and drinking water, since they are used in almost every industry. Solvents are regularly used and disposed of improperly, even though inexpensive recovery systems (starting at $7,000) are available. One dry cleaning business in Ontario reduced the amount of solvent purchased from 700 gallons to 300 gallons a month after installing modern recycling equipment. After this initial investment, they saved $450,000 each year. A substance called 111-trichlorethene, a solvent that can cause birth defects as well as destroy the ozone layer, can be replaced by soap and water or BioAct, a new solvent made by AT&T from citrus or orange peels.

The electroplating industry discards 24,000 tons of metals worth $40 million each year due to the lack of recapturing or prevention equipment. An industry consultant estimated it is technically feasible to recover nearly 95 percent of the metals that are now dumped. Currently they put filters on the end of the pipes (pollution control techniques) that take the metal sludge out of the water and then the sludge is disposed of in landfills.

Pollution prevention is also beneficial in a number of less obvious ways. The job of cleaning up America's thousands of dumpsites and changing processes and products to prevent the pollution of our factories would create hundreds of thousands of new jobs. Pipefitters, carpenters, electricians, chemists, engineers, and laborers are all needed to make the changes shop by shop. Moreover, protecting workers and communities from industrial poisoning in general could save American industry billions of dollars by reducing medical care costs and creating a more productive work force. Further, if we reduce our reliance on many synthetic chemicals, we will preserve limited resources like natural gas and oil that are the starting materials for making synthetics.

One important disincentive to industry's acceptance of pollution prevention is the way profits and growth are calculated. We read in the paper about quarterly earnings and profit rates. Often the return on pollution prevention investments is seen as too far down the road to be worth the trouble. Long-term economic planning involving pollution prevention too often takes a back seat to the short-term quest for profits that is the driving force for America's corporations. Shortsightedness keeps prevention approaches from being implemented. Meanwhile, American industry continues practices that poison workers and consumers and damage the land, air, and water. Safe and economic toxic waste prevention is erroneously regarded as an extra cost, instead of an opportunity for industry to protect the environment while improving its strategic and competitive position. Pollution prevention can be profitable as well.

Pollution prevention can work for most industries with the possible exception of the synthetic chemical industry. A central part of the solution to the toxics problem is to reduce the most dangerous products and waste output. It may be that the petrochemical industry will lose revenues as the demand for toxics is reduced. But we don't have to worry about the DuPonts, Monsantos, and Exxons of the world. They seem to do well in any economic climate. As the idea of toxic reduction spreads, they will probably be the ones selling the organic gardening sets as replacements for some of the worst pesticides.

Transforming the chemical industry so that it generates less toxic waste may mean the loss of thousands of jobs. But if we need more solvents and they can be made from citrus, then it seems likely that the same number of workers, or more, will be needed to make the new safe chemicals. In any case, a real solution to the toxic threat must guarantee jobs or income at pay comparable to what workers were getting in traditional chemical industry jobs. A "Superfund" for chemical workers could be established that taxes the worst toxics producers to set up a pool of money aiding workers as certain product lines are restricted or eliminated. Meanwhile, the business of finding, developing, producing, and selling safe substitutes may actually create many new jobs.

WHY HASN'T GOVERNMENT STEPPED IN?

If there are solutions to the toxics crisis, why hasn't government stepped in to protect the public from industrial toxic pollution? The answer can be found in the laws and regulations that govern industrial pollution and in the government's will to solve the problem. Generally, our government's response to toxic hazards has been lax at best and scandalous at worst.

WEAK LAWS AND REGULATIONS

There are as many as 70,000 toxic chemicals in our air and water today. Yet only twenty-two of these chemicals are regulated under the Occupational Safety and Health Act (OSHA). Of thousands of air toxics in the environment, only seven are regulated under the Clean Air Act. Another law, the Toxic Substances Control Act, is supposed to ensure that only safe chemical products are on the market. But this law does not even require testing for long-term health effects such as cancer, reproductive problems, and birth defects. According to the Government Accounting Office and the congressional Office of Technology Assessment, between 80 and 90 percent of all chemical products have not been tested for their long-term health effects.

Moreover, current laws do not offer industry an incentive to clean up its toxic waste. Fines for workplace exposure to chemicals amount to little more than a slap on the wrist. The letter of the law and the enforcement simply do not encourage industry to invest in pollution prevention. Simply put, it pays to pollute. It is cheaper for industry to continue polluting in the short run than it is to invest in prevention strategies that pay off in the long run.

TREATING THE SYMPTOM

The regulatory approach currently aims to control the toxics problem by filtering out or treating the waste at the end of the pipe, stack, or vent instead of preventing the generation of waste in the first place. Prevention strategies, where toxic waste reduction and use reduction practices are in operation, constitute a much better way to stop toxic exposure. Technology is now available to reduce the use of toxic materials by means of shop floor changes and modifications of the production process. Moreover, acutely dangerous products can be taken off the market. But prevention has not yet been a major part of the U.S. regulatory system primarily because it would require retooling, capital changes, and investment in different industrial products and processes.

INADEQUATE FUNDING, LAX ENFORCEMENT

The EPA, OSHA, and other federal agencies with responsibility for controlling toxics are underfunded and understaffed. The federal budget allocates only enough money to inspect each of the 30,000 confirmed toxic waste sites less than once every fifty years. In real terms, the EPA's 1988 budget was equivalent to its 1978 budget—during a period when the agency's workload for toxics roughly doubled.

Enforcement of toxic legislation is clearly inadequate. In 1984, the Government Accounting Office released a study showing that 80 percent of all firms were not in compliance with the nation's toxic pollution laws. Imagine if 80 percent of us didn't pay our taxes! Currently OSHA, which is supposed to protect workers from toxic hazards, employs about 1,200 inspectors to cover 4 million workplaces. Since each inspector visits four sites per month, it will take seventy years to visit all of the workplaces in the nation at least once.

PIECEMEAL APPROACH

The government's response to the toxics crisis has been segmented. Government responsibility for toxics has been divided among a number of different agencies and divisions at the local, state, and federal levels. The resulting lack of coordination between agencies and divisions often has meant that a "solution" only created other problems elsewhere. In the 1970s, for example, the federal government told industry to stop polluting surface waters. Instead, industry dumped its toxics into landfills that have poisoned our drinking water. Now the federal government is saying no to landfills. So toxics are released out of incinerators or dumped into new deep-well injection units underground. Thus in many cases the strategy for controlling toxic waste has merely shifted toxic materials from one route of exposure to another.

BIAS TOWARD INDUSTRY

As inadequate as our federal regulatory programs are, government often seems determined to weaken them further. The EPA has been particularly lax in its approach to polluters. In the early 1980s, EPA officials indicated their intention to abolish much of the agency's enforcement and reduced its staff from 15,000 to 11,000 in 1986. The scandal that forced the resignation of EPA director Anne Gorsuch Burford and Superfund chief Rita LaValle revealed a disturbing relationship between industry and the EPA. Worse still, it revealed an administration willing to use cleanup funds for partisan political purposes. Meanwhile, at all levels of government the Political Action Committees of the chemical polluters donate millions of dollars to politicians and candidates. The challenge before us is clear.

THE TOXICS BILL OF RIGHTS

The problem of toxics and the environment requires renewing democracy as we make specific changes in chemical use and production. It requires moving America's economic machinery from a toxic to a nontoxic, or at least a less toxic, approach. It requires fundamental changes in the way we do our business—industry, agriculture, and energy use. Each year, the nation must measurably reduce the use and manufacture of the dangerous synthetic and toxic chemicals currently on the market.

We must enact laws that shift the balance of power in government—a shift that will give citizens and public officials more influence over what is produced and how it is produced. We call it environmental democracy. This approach is rooted in the highest ideals of American democracy. If industry currently has the right to chemically trespass into our air, water, soil, food, and bodies, then citizens must have the right to protect themselves, their neighborhood, and their workplace. Specifically we must have the right to know what these chemicals are, how they affect our health, and what volume of waste is produced in relation to the volume of product. It does the world no good if the replacement for CFCs is a chemical whose by-products create equal units of ozone-destroying chemicals as well as others that cause birth defects and cancer.

Citizens must have the right, moreover, to inspect the facilities, operations, and processes that put poisons into the public air and waterways. Citizens inspecting facilities with their own experts is a model of local participation that should be mandated by law. Citizens could then sit at the bargaining table with companies and negotiate for changes at the site of the problem. Under President Reagan, the Russians were given the right to inspect our most sensitive military facilities. Certainly citizens living next to chemical polluters must enjoy these same rights.

The right to negotiate for essential changes could produce "good-neighbor agreements" in which industry could agree to timetables for reducing environmental health and safety hazards. At the same time the common law must be preserved and strengthened to give a solid right to sue polluters and collect damages—not only for loss of health and property but also to ensure that it won't happen again.

Today citizens have little influence over decisions that affect their community's health and safety. The new national right-to-know provision of Superfund gives citizens information about toxics from industrial facilities in their communities, but it doesn't go far enough. Community residents and workers still cannot legally inspect hazardous waste landfills or facilities. Nor can they negotiate for cleanups with responsible parties. Empowering citizens with a "toxics bill of rights" would go a long way toward defining what is necessary to protect the public health. We must have:

1. The Right to Know
2. The Right to Cleanup
3. The Right to Compensation
4. The Right to Law Enforcement
5. The Right to Participate, Inspect, and Negotiate

6. The Right to Pollution Prevention
7. The Right to Be Free from Toxic Chemical Exposure

We must fight for these rights in many forums: in factories, at city hall, in the nation's courthouses, in the statehouses, and in the halls of Congress. Local citizen groups must take action to eliminate toxic hazards in their community. Workers must organize to demand occupational health and safety protections from management. Enactment—and enforcement—of toxics laws must be demanded at the local, state, and federal levels of government. New laws and campaigns against polluters must focus on:

- Expanded Superfunds to clean up toxic dumpsites.
- Pollution prevention programs that pretest chemicals for health effects, get the worst toxics off the market, reduce toxic waste, and prevent chemical spills and accidents.
- Full compensation through citizen suits for all victims of toxic poisoning. It's the right and just thing to do, and it also gives industry a powerful incentive to clean up and prevent toxic pollution.
- Increased enforcement and penalties for chemical polluters.
- Economic and technical assistance to small businesses to help them finance reductions in the use of toxics. Assistance must also be provided for chemical workers if jobs are lost during the transition to less toxics-oriented production.
- Full citizen rights to participate in all decisions governing toxics.

The toxic poisoning of our bodies and the environment is the biggest hidden health threat facing America today. We cannot, however, just leave it to the experts to solve the problem. If we do, we may reach a point not too long in the future when the toxic saturation of the environment and our bodies reaches epidemic proportions. We cannot afford to wait. Citizens must exercise their right to know about chemical hazards and their right to participate in industrial decisions that affect community health and safety.

Society has the know-how to solve the toxics crisis. The piece that is missing is citizen activism to pressure industry to get the solutions off the shelf and put into practice. The goal is simple: to make pollution prevention the highest environmental ethic—in each community, at each industrial facility, on the farm, within each state regulatory agency, and within the nation as a whole.

2

Organizing to Win

JOHN O'CONNOR

This chapter describes successful organizing approaches that citizen groups can use to press for—and win—solutions to their toxics problems. It explains the nuts and bolts of how to build and maintain powerful citizen groups and describes campaign strategies and actions that can result in toxic cleanup and prevention.

What is organizing? How do we build organizations from scratch? How do we define our issues? How do we strategize, take action, and maintain and strengthen our organizations? How do we win concrete victories? These and other questions will be explored. The approaches to organizing around toxics issues described here are certainly not the only workable approaches, but they are proven strategies that citizen groups have used successfully in many parts of the country and in other nations.

WHAT IS ORGANIZING?

Organizing in its simplified form is people working together to get things accomplished. Organizing is about people taking a role in determining their own future and improving the quality of life not only for themselves but for everyone. Those who organize communities to clean up or prevent toxic hazards share a belief that large numbers of people working together can gain greater control over their daily circumstances. Through their collective power, citizens can demand and win legitimate toxic cleanup and preventive actions. If you want to protect your community against toxic hazards, then you need to organize.

Examples abound of successfully organized citizens in all walks of life. Religious groups are good examples of the components necessary to build healthy organizations. Organized religions have weekly events where members participate and contribute money to sustain the organization. Unions with monthly dues have during the last century organized for improved wages and working conditions. Even large chemical producers are organized into big-spending lobbies that fight in the halls of Congress for regulations that permit dumping toxic products and waste into our neighborhood air, water, and land.

CONFLICT AND POWER: TOUGH CONCEPTS BUT NECESSARY

Organizing always entails conflict. This is not because people who demand toxic cleanups are hungry for battle. Rather, change through conflict is historically the way substantial improvements have been made in society. When citizens put forth legitimate demands for toxic dump cleanups, they are making demands that require a corporation to spend large sums of money. The community's self-interest is to get the dump returned to its natural clean state—the way it was before toxic waste was dumped. The industry's immediate self-interest, more often than not, is to protect its profits. This is their bottom line and their primary motivating force. The conflict lies in these competing interests.

We see continuous conflicts between organized religions, between unions and management, between banks and family farmers, between rich and poor. Life is forces in conflict: in nature, in society, among nations, classes, races, cultures, and sexes. Our entire legal system is based on an adversarial model that pits plaintiff against defendant in often nasty courtroom battles. Don't be afraid of conflict. It is an integral part of our open and democratic society.

Organizing in the case of toxics is about numbers of citizens taking action to solve toxic chemical and waste problems. It means using all the nonviolent, political, and economic tools available in order to win tactical victories and improvements. The history of organizing to solve toxics problems shows that while cooperating with polluters is certainly a desirable goal, hard-hitting and (sometimes) confrontational steps must often be taken to get them to respond.

What sort of conflict will you be engaged in? In your local toxics campaign, you will be trying to convince both government and industry to respect your right to live and work in a safe environment. You will want them to understand your concern for your families. In a very basic way, you will be pushing them to recognize your *humanity*—to recognize that no human being should have to live under the constant threat of toxic exposure, which can lead to cancer, birth defects, even death.

In this basic strategy, therefore, you must appeal to the humanity in your adversary—whether it be an EPA chief or a bank president. This does not mean you appeal to their pity. Instead, you move them to see the justness of your concerns. This may be a difficult task when you are confronting a company executive who's concerned primarily with short-term profits, but it's always a worthwhile pursuit. Once you get past the bureaucratic facade and confront people face to face, you'll find you get better results.

In many cases, of course, this appeal to humanity will be futile. It is also wise, therefore, to appeal to your adversary's self-interest. If it is in the company's interest to make money, and your constant protests and demonstrations are tarnishing the company's name and costing it contracts, then you negotiate with the corporate executives to stop your protests if they agree to your demands for pollution prevention. In general, corporate officials will understand the politics of self-interest a lot better than the moral basis of your demands for a safe environment.

Since your campaign is ultimately concerned with rights and humanity, even in the heat of conflict you should never use tactics that deny your adversary's humanity. This means that you should never use violence to achieve your objectives. There may be times when you need to use civil disobedience to illustrate the injustice of your plight, but you should never use violence to further your toxic cleanup campaign. Not only will you lose the respect of the community and receive negative press, but you will lose the moral bargaining position that citizens usually have in toxics campaigns.

Remember: To move people and take the actions necessary to protect the public health, you need to present information in a lively but accurate way. Battles, wars, lawsuits, and toxic cleanup campaigns are waged and won by promoting your position and downplaying your opponent's position. Although it is important to understand your opponent's view, don't get lost in the gray areas. Industry too often tells us that there is no problem. The history of industrial disease and toxic waste sites, however, shows that problems are discovered and solved *after* people are injured and die from toxic hazards, not because citizens were informed beforehand by chemical polluters. Your bottom line is the safety of the community and the workplace. Campaigns require the careful use of words, honestly stated, but in a way that mobilizes fellow citizens into action.

Just as *conflict* is one of those dirty words that must be reexamined, so is *power*. All organizations are associations of people seeking to increase their power in a given field. Whether it's organized utilities seeking higher rates, big oil companies seeking higher profits, or citizens seeking toxic cleanups, it's all a struggle over power. This could mean financial power, military power, or power to live in a world free from toxic hazards. Where toxics are concerned, real power means people's ability to force the cleanup or prevention of dangerous chemical exposure. For the chemical industry, it often means more toxic waste and higher profits. For the chemical producers, less pollution may mean less profit. But for most chemical *users,* which accounts for 80 percent of all industries, pollution prevention can in fact be profitable.

Part of the solution to the toxics crisis is changing the power relationships between people, the polluters, and the government. Too many toxics decisions in the past were made exclusively by the companies responsible for the pollution. Then, starting in the early 1970s, government began to regulate certain aspects of toxic pollution. Only rarely have the *victims* of toxic contamination been involved in decisions affecting their health and safety. In order to win protection against toxic hazards, citizens must gain power— through direct organizing as well as legislative change—to ensure that they are at the bargaining table when cleanup decisions are being made. Given corporate self-interest, combined with the limited budgets and staffing of government, an organized citizenry is needed to protect against threats to the public health. Only organized citizens can gain the power necessary to monitor these crucial health and safety issues.

SCIENCE AND ART

The ability to organize citizens to win environmental improvements is both an art and a science. It is a science because a systematic approach involving face-to-face conversation about the group's concerns will get you some new and active members. It is an art because it involves certain leadership abilities that are hard to quantify. Organizing is the power to enlist and lead people in ways that are bold and dramatic. It is the ability to challenge people's limitations and help them overcome those limitations. It is an understanding of human nature and an ability to engage people in action with precise timing. It is good judgment and organizational skills, but it is also having a vision of a better tomorrow and projecting it effectively. It is also the ability to have fun as you get there. As grassroots leader Esla Byroe-Andreola from the PJP Landfill campaign in Jersey City said:

"There has to be fun in our fight if we are to keep people involved. In fact, the fun is in the fight!"

The democratic and nonviolent forms of organizing advocated here are based on the following premise: To bring about a world free from toxic hazards, we need permanent self-funded toxics organizations that work primarily on a local level but also connect to state, regional, and national coalitions that promote policies to empower citizens and prevent toxic hazards. We believe that the growth and livelihood of all organizations require the direct participation of people on many levels—negotiating with polluters, lobbying legislators, holding accountability sessions with politicians, circulating petitions, writing letters, and even holding demonstrations.

It's not good enough simply to have the facts on your side (as toxics victims usually do). Action is called for. The bottom line for all toxics organizations is simply this: You must establish a relationship with polluters in which potential victims have more influence over health and safety decisions than they have today. The central objective of all toxics organizing is to pressure the polluter (or appropriate government agency) to recognize the legitimate role citizens have in protecting their communities. Citizens must have the right to know about the chemicals, the right to inspect the dumps and facilities, and the right to negotiate for solutions. Citizens should become the protectors of the environment and the watchful eyes on the chemical producers and users. In short, they should become guardians of the public health. But before we explore winning approaches, we've got to get organized.

HOW TO MAKE ORGANIZING WORK FOR YOU

GOALS, ISSUES, AND ORGANIZATIONAL FORM

A typical problem in the infancy of every organization is clearly defining your goals. You want to pinpoint your goals and find the best organizational means to get there. If the organization's leaders don't have a clear sense of purpose, and if they don't feel powerful enough to effect change, then it's very hard to get the rank and file motivated. The organization's vision must be compelling and exciting. It must give rise to a sense of urgency and hope. And it must move people to act.

Goals should be divided into short-term and long-term. A citizen group may define its long-term goal as a world free from the manufacture, use, and disposal of the worst toxic hazards. Its short-term goal may be getting action on the toxic dump down the street. But since even the short-term goal may take many years of organizing to reach, you should focus on a number of short-term subgoals—for example, getting the dump adequately tested, winning a neighborhood health study, and getting alternative water supplies.

The distinction between short-term and long-term goals is important. Unless you can accomplish your short-term objectives, you'll never be able to sustain the level of commitment necessary to reach your long-term objectives. After hours, weeks, and months of hard work, members need to feel that their work is paying off. They need to celebrate little victories. Little victories are the fuel that runs powerful citizen groups. Your long-term goal is a world free from toxic hazards. On the path toward that goal, you will push to get the local dump cleaned up. Then you will push to get local industry to reduce emissions, use safer chemicals, and a number of other realizable goals. If your goals on different levels are not defined—and then achieved—there will be frustration, stagnation, and decline from the lack of clear direction and winnable victories.

To choose and define your issues is a different matter. Defining an issue involves taking a goal, clarifying the power relationships involved, and choosing the path of action to achieve that objective. You must answer these questions: What is our self-interest? Who are the opponents? Who is the decision maker we will pressure to win the desired change? What is the exact power lever we will use to pressure the decision maker? Before you can map out your campaign plan, you've got to define the issues.

Generally, organizations decide to work on issues that are supported by the majority of fellow citizens, that offer realizable solutions, and that, when finally resolved, improve the conditions of the community at large. Saul Alinsky, a pioneer in community and labor organizing in the 1930s and 1940s, said that issues must affect large numbers of people and be "immediate, concrete, and realizable."

While the details of your issue presentation will vary from place to place depending on the needs of your audience, there are still a couple of rules. First, you should always address people's self-interest. If you are going door to door and you know that lead exposure from the local dumpsite can cause learning disabilities and mental retardation in children, you should discuss these dangers with mothers of small children. Second, you should always mention solutions when talking about toxic problems. Hearing the problems without hearing what you can do about them can lead to frustrated and apathetic citizens.

TYPES OF ORGANIZATION

As you figure out your goals, the issues to be worked on, and how to talk about them, you must also build a large local organization (if you are not already part of one). The most common ones are:

- A neighborhood organization made up of dues-paying members who live near a toxic pollution source
- A coalition of groups that might include senior citizens, unions, environmental organizations, and dumpsite groups
- A combination of a neighborhood membership base and coalition partners such as the local churches or senior groups

The most common organization fighting toxics on a local level is the neighborhood membership organization. This formation is generally made up of neighbors within a multiblock area closest to the dump or source of chemical pollution. An organization like this generally has a dues-paying membership, an elected leadership, committees to do research, membership drives, fundraising, and campaign planning and execution. Strong local organizations with lots of active members are a prerequisite to the significant state and federal policy changes that must be made to solve the nation's toxic chemical problems.

A coalition-style organization is made up of community institutions concerned about a toxics issue that are willing to lend their resources to a coalition effort. If it is a local coalition, perhaps not all the coalition members live next to the pollution source. Nonetheless, the local organization joins the coalition out of self-interest. A church, for example, may get involved not just because it is a "Christian thing to do" but because some of the parish is directly threatened. Failure to solve the problem may mean loss of property, threats to health, and loss of parish membership. A union without many members in the affected neighborhood may get involved because it needs help on a piece of legislation or because supporting the toxics fight gives the union a good image for its own organizing activities.

There are many good examples of coalition work on the state and national levels. The National Toxics Campaign (NTC), founded in 1984, is the largest coalition of unions, environmental groups, state citizens' groups, and grassroots toxics organizations working to improve the nation's toxic waste laws. In its first three years it brought together groups in over forty states to pressure Congress to expand the Superfund cleanup law—and succeeded.

An organization that combines a local or regional membership with institutional members is another option. Basically this option combines the two approaches discussed above. While this form is probably ideal, it generally takes longer to build than either of the other two. It also takes more energy and resources to put into place. Your organizational form generally depends on what you have to work with and varies from place to place, region to region.

RECRUITMENT

Cesar Chavez, the community and labor organizer who is now president of the United Farm Workers, was once asked by an aspiring young organizer, "How do you organize?" He said, "First, you talk to one person, face to face, then you talk to another . . ." "But, Cesar," the impatient youth interrupted, "how do you really get them involved?" Chavez replied, "First, you talk to one person, face to face, and then you talk to the next and then the next . . ."

The point is that there is no substitute, whether it's neighborhood or coalition organizing, for clear, concise, person-to-person talk. Whether it's doorknocking in the neighborhood or meeting with the parish priest or rabbi, the only way to begin is with personal conversations. There are three common approaches to recruiting members, volunteers, or coalition partners: doorknocking, house meetings, and institutional visits.

Doorknocking

Step One: Select your target area. Get a map of the general area and drive or walk through the neighborhood to figure out which homes are closest to the toxic site. Common sense tells you that those most concerned about cleaning up or preventing toxic emissions are the ones living closest to the problem.

Step Two: Prepare your clipboard. Its basic ingredients will include: petitions or contact sheets with spaces for name, address, and (especially) phone number; membership cards; a letter of reference signed by community leaders that introduces the organization and adds legitimacy; a fact sheet about the problem and organization; and a few newsclips about your organization's work.

Step Three: Prepare yourself mentally. Doorknocking is like climbing a big hill. When you're at the bottom looking up you ask yourself, "Do I really want to climb it today? Maybe I'll put it off until tomorrow." But when you start to climb you feel invigorated, and by the time you reach the top you realize it wasn't that hard. In fact, it was good for your health. Similarly, knocking on that first door can be a scary experience. What if they slam the door in my face? What if they're not interested? But as you get going you realize what a pleasure it is to meet new, concerned people. Not only will most people be interested, but most will sign your toxics petition and a good percentage will join your organization. As you progress, you realize that the hard work is rewarding. You develop new skills and learn from the people you meet. Remember: If you don't get out there and recruit you'll never have enough fellow citizens organized to win the dumpsite cleanup and protect children from the horrors of uncontrolled toxic substances.

Step Four: You've got your map, the clipboard is ready, you're ready, you approach that first door—but what do you say? First introduce yourself and the name of your organization. Then you must establish credibility by legitimizing your group. Next you have to engage the neighbor in conversation to ask what he knows or feels about the issue. If he is not talkative, describe the problem and get his opinions and concerns. Then point out the solution and give him the opportunity to take the path of action necessary to put the solution into practice. You must be able to overcome negative thinking and pessimism. You must know when to be low key and when to be fiery. There is no set formula on what to say or how to say it. Each doorknocker has to develop his or her own style, delivery, and membership appeal.

Having said this I will nevertheless suggest one approach I developed with community organizer Mike Bishop, an approach that has been used successfully in many communities across the country. This approach, called the "five-point rap," contains the key elements that need to be covered when you're trying to recruit members, enlist volunteers, or persuade people to turn out for an upcoming event. The five points are:

1. Identification (name and organization).
2. Legitimize your organization.
3. Engage and educate.
4. Membership.
5. Next event or meeting.

Obviously, the first two points are crucial when the neighbor's initial thought is "who is this person and why is she here?" Very quickly you cover these points, as explained in the following paragraphs.

Point 1: Identification. "Hi, my name is Lisa Hopkins, and I'm with FIST—Families Involved in Stopping Toxics."

Point 2: Legitimize Your Organization. "You've probably heard of us. We're the organization of residents who are fighting that toxic dump that's poisoning our air and water." At this point, it's a good idea to show the neighbor the newsclip of your organization's work. Don't hand the newsclip to the person since it will distract him or her from talking with you. If you hand them the clip, some people's response is to read it (or pretend to do so while they figure out a way to throw you off their doorstep).

Point 3: Engage and Educate. "We are going through the neighborhood today to see what people think we should do to get the toxic dump down the street cleaned up. Do you have any ideas about the situation, or do you think we should be working on other issues that are of concern to you?" Resident: "No, I just know what I read in the paper, and it wasn't much!"

Don't lose them. Use careful questioning to get your neighbor talking. If people are lectured, rather than being engaged in conversation, they are less likely to get involved. When people give their opinions they feel a sense of participation in the discussion and will be more open to joining the fight than if you just talk at them. Real conversation requires two parties. Ask them what they know about past dumping. Have they smelled the toxics or tasted them in the water? Such questions engage their participation. If you ask people questions and listen to their ideas, they feel that what they say matters. Your goal as an organizer is to leave each resident with the thought that he or she is important to the organization and the neighborhood's future.

Often the people will not have a lot to say—for many reasons—so it's important to give them more facts about the problem and the ways to solve it. That's the educational side to Point 3.

Doorknocker: "Well, the main reason you don't know what is in the water is because the polluter and the government have refused to give us information about what is in the water. FIST believes that we have the right to know what toxics are in our water and how the stuff affects our health.

"We know from some of our research committee's work that at the very least benzene and lead are at the site. We know that benzene causes leukemia—a form of cancer. Lead can cause learning disabilities in young children. We also know that the waste is less than a mile from the town's drinking water source. We have a petition we plan to present to the government and the polluters to test our water and get us an alternative supply if it proves to be toxic. Would you look it over and sign if you think it's appropriate?"

Resident: "Well, let's see it. But tell me what you really want."

Doorknocker: "Well, first we want your signature to win the proper testing and cleanup. As you probably know, the more signatures we get the better our chances of getting these things checked out."

Resident: "Well, okay, I'll sign, but I don't give out my phone number, you know."

Doorknocker: "Your phone number will not be given out, and will only be used to get back to you about important organizational business—like a meeting to get the water tested or something important regarding the neighborhood's health and safety."

Resident: "All right, then . . . here."

Point 4: Membership. Membership is the most important part of the entire conversation. Every person approached must be given an opportunity to improve his or her life. All must be given a straightforward membership appeal—an opportunity through collective action to protect their health and safety against toxic hazards. If you don't inform people of the importance of membership at the first interview, they usually say "I knew there was a catch to this" when the question is brought up later.

Membership is an important way to guarantee participation and turnout. Experienced neighborhood leaders and organizers will tell you that neighborhood meetings are more fully attended right after an intensive membership drive. People who join often say to themselves, "Of course I'm going to the meeting—I'm a member! I own a piece of the rock and I'm going to find out more about the toxic dump and what we can do." The greater the number of members that sign up and pay dues, the greater your organizational results will be.

Why is it important to pay dues as a member? First, it costs money to wage campaigns. You need money for leaflets, literature, travel, phones, postage, copying, and, if your organization gets big enough, for paid staff and office space. Corporations generally don't give to community organizing projects, especially if the company in question dumped chemicals at the site. Even if they were available, corporate funds usually come with such strings attached that the group would not be able to take the hard-hitting actions that are necessary to prevent toxic hazards.

The membership appeal must be done with ease and comfort. You must look the potential member in the eye, smile, and ask him to join. If you seem uneasy about asking people won't join. Back to the sample appeal:

Doorknocker: "As you probably know (nodding your head), our organization, like every other organization, needs money to accomplish our toxic cleanup campaign. Not much, but some. That's why we are on a membership drive. Membership is only $25 a year; that's less than $3 per month— less than the cost of a six-pack these days. The big issue is not the money, but rather the power that we have to improve the situation. The more dues-paying members we have, the better our chances of getting the toxic dump cleaned up. Would you like to become a member?"

Resident: "Sure, I'll join." (Hand him the card or the membership form to fill out.)

Point 5: Next Event or Meeting. What if your neighbor says, "No, I don't know enough about it yet"?

Doorknocker: "Well, then come to the next meeting this month and see what good work we're doing. Once you see us in action, I'm sure you'll want to join. Here's a flyer about the meeting that will be held at St. James Church, two weeks from tonight, June 1st, at 7:30 P.M. Thanks for your time. Nice talking with you."

Too often people make the mistake of telling the resident about the next big meeting or event *before* the membership appeal. The familiar response is, "Oh, I'll come to the meeting and then decide if I'll join." Membership, however, is the best guarantee of getting someone to attend the meeting, action, or event. People follow their money!

House Meetings

House meetings are another way to build your local toxics organization. Before you hold a big organizational event, organize several smaller meetings in members' apartments or homes. The host family can invite friends, neighbors, and relatives who might become active in the organization. Apart from recruiting, house meetings are a good way of developing the skills of new members. Often when new members enter an organization, there is not enough opportunity for them to take on the roles that challenge, develop, and test new leaders. Taking a leadership role in house meetings is the first step to developing the skills necessary to run meetings, plan actions, and build the organization.

The house meeting format is straightforward. The host welcomes everyone and introduces people to each other. Then someone (not necessarily the host) explains what the organization is, its goals and objectives, and how the group works. This explanation can be given by a new member who wants to take on a leadership role. House meetings give people practice in understanding and projecting the organization's mission. On the other hand, you may want an experienced leader to explain the organization's goals. They can project the necessary experience and confidence to recruit new members and volunteers.

Institutional Visits and Coalition Building

One of the most difficult jobs in organizing is building a coalition around a common purpose. If you want to fight toxic pollution in your backyard, the first step is to build a membership organization of people living closest to the site, since they are the ones who have the greatest self-interest. Once you have built your own organization, only then should you think about working in coalition with other groups. There are only rare exceptions to this rule.

Whenever you approach an organization to join in your efforts, you must appeal to that organization's self-interest. What benefits will other groups gain by joining your toxics coalition? If the neighborhood dump is not detoxified, for example, is there a danger that toxic chemicals could permeate the neighborhood to such a degree that it would have to be evacuated, as in the case of Love Canal? If you're trying to get a synagogue to join your coalition and the problem is as bad as Love Canal or Times Beach, you could suggest to the rabbi that there might not be a synagogue anymore if this toxic problem is not remedied. Always appeal to people's self-interest.

Here are some key questions to ask before approaching other organizations:

- What power would other groups bring to the coalition?
- What problems would other groups bring to the coalition?
- What does your group stand to lose by working in a coalition?
- What is the price of the support of other organizations?
- What are the issues to avoid?
- Under what sort of structure will the coalition function?
- What groups are potential coalition members?
- How will the coalition function? Who makes decisions?

Once you've figured out the answers to these questions, it's time to start talking to people. When you approach a potential coalition member, you can use a version of the five-point rap. First introduce yourself and tell them about your organization and the coalition that's being formed. Ask them about the issues they think the coalition should be working on. Describe your goals for the coalition. Then solicit their support (as in the membership appeal in the doorknocking format).

At each visit ask your potential coalition partner to help out in some way. Always ask for the big things first. If you ask them to send a representative to sit on the coalition board or for assigned staff time and they say no, they might just let you use the hall. If they say no to using the hall, they probably won't join the coalition. People basically like to help others in need. If institutional representatives are even slightly interested, put them on a mailing list and keep them informed.

In building coalitions, think what *you* can offer the groups you want to solicit. Bring your members to their fundraiser. Show up for their picket line. Coalition building requires good human relations. As West Coast organizer Tim Sampson says, "The flowers of organizational relations grow from personal interest, kindness, and cultivation."

Coalitions must be built locally, statewide, regionally, and then nationally to solve the country's toxic chemical crisis. But remember this central caution: Coalition attempts can be a dangerous distraction from building a powerful local membership organization. Build your neighborhood organization first.

One final note on all forms of recruitment: There is a saying that "organizations are either growing or dying." Growth depends on a permanent recruitment campaign. The lifeblood of all organizations is a constant influx of new members. All organizational power flows from the strength of its members. The more people you have, the more you can do to clean up and prevent toxic hazards.

BUILDING YOUR ORGANIZATION

Now that you have learned outreach skills, you need to spend eight to twelve weeks building your organization. Here we cover the four stages of a community organizing drive: groundwork, recruitment drive, organizing committee, and formation meeting. Your main job is to find new citizen leaders or new activists for your group. Basically you are trying to develop "new leaders" who have had little organizational experience. Your main job here is to find new citizens to develop into leaders through direct experience in three basic steps: (1) planning strategies and specific tactics; (2) executing the plan; and (3) evaluating your progress during and after campaigns.

Groundwork

Gather some basic information about the neighborhood. What is it called? Get precinct, ward, state representative, city council, state senate, and congressional maps so that people are organized in a way to exercise maximum political pressure. Get the basics on race, age, sex, religion, and income levels if you can. Find out what the key institutions are—religious institutions, employers, hospitals, schools (especially next to pollution sources), senior citizen organizations, and so forth. Who are the people of influence—clergy, union leaders, politicians, and the like? The groundwork phase should last two weeks. (We assume here that you have information on your pollution problem; if not, see Chapter 4.)

General Recruitment Drive

The recruitment drive generally lasts eight weeks—and the organizer or community leaders may be working more hours in this period than in any other phase of the drive. Get ready to spend *full* work weeks on recruitment. In addition to working five to six hours a day knocking on doors, the remainder of your time should be slotted for institutional visits, careful record keeping of all interested contacts on 3-by-5 index cards, research, new fact sheets, and planning for the organizing committee and house meetings.

Doorknocking should lead to seven or eight good conversations per hour. Whenever possible you should try to actually get in the door, but talking on the porch will do. Use the five-point rap described earlier. Make sure everybody signs a petition; names and phone numbers are the key pieces of information.

During the recruitment drive, ask everybody to join and get people talking. Remember, you're looking for potential leaders who are not only articulate but have a base of supporters through their affiliations—and also have some time and willingness to work. In the first four weeks, recruitment should consist of "cold" doorknocking in the late afternoon until evening. Generally, 3:00 to 9:00 are acceptable hours. Retirement communities can be canvassed earlier in the day. Saturdays and Sundays are also available— lots of people are home then. Keep careful records of homes that don't answer and go back at other times—some of the best leaders may not be home when you first show up. By the tail end of the fourth week and beginning of the fifth week, you can do home visits to set up house meetings and the first organizing committee meeting.

By the fifth week, home visits begin to replace a couple of hours of the cold doorknocking each day. Your purpose is to see if these people will agree either to sit on the organizing committee (if you think they're leadership material) or to hold a house meeting. Take time to find out what makes people tick. Are they part of a church or other organization? Who else do they know that might be interested in joining the local campaign?

House meetings serve two purposes: to recruit new people to the organizing process and to test leaders who might have potential—can they turn out their friends and neighbors and help orchestrate the meeting? There should be at least four house meetings as part of the drive from weeks five through eight. A typical agenda includes introductions, discussion of issues, explanation of the organization, collection of dues, and recruitment strategies.

The Organizing Committee

As you do the cold doorknocking and visits with church clergy and other institutions, you should be looking for people to lead the organization through the organizing committee. We're not necessarily looking for the leaders of the institutions themselves to lead the group. Rather, the minister or rabbi may have rank-and-file members who may be interested. Again, what we are doing is developing new leaders.

There should be at least four organizing committee (OC) meetings in weeks five, seven, and eight. At the OC meeting your new leaders come together to build an organization around the pollution problem that sparked their interest. Ideally, the meeting should be held in a member's house or a neighborhood center or church. The meeting should focus on the pollution issue with a subsequent discussion of the need to organize. If the organizer has done his or her home visits properly, everyone at the OC meeting will already be predisposed in favor of organizing. A typical agenda at the first OC meeting might include:

1. Introduction
2. Discussion of issues (ideally the polluter or another target)
3. Decision to organize
4. Dues collection
5. Recruitment plan and timetable
6. Time, place, and chair for the next OC meeting

As part of the recruitment plan we recommend that you designate the last three Saturdays of the organizing drive as "doorknocker days" when you train the leaders in the five-point rap and you all go door to door for a few hours. The date, time, and place of the formation meeting should be selected at the first OC meeting so that flyers can be made the next day for general distribution. The second OC meeting should be a general repeat of the first.

At the third OC meeting you should plan the campaigns. Use the strategy chart and discussion on planning in this chapter as a starting point. You must make a decision at these meetings to invite the targets (corporate, political, or regulatory figures who have decision-making power) to the formation meeting. Recruitment planning must be a part of all meetings. At the final OC meeting a day or two before the big formation meeting, it is important to do some role playing. Go over each person's part in the meeting. Who will mark "yes," "no," or "maybe" on the scorecard at the front of the meeting hall? Prepare for all the "what-if's." If the targets say no to your legitimate demands, what are the steps in the campaign? Who will do the membership appeal? How will officers be elected? Who will ensure that those present sign up for the working committees of the group?

The Formation Meeting

The first phase of a successful formation meeting is getting the largest number of people to attend. If you follow the Overkill Method described below, you should have one hundred or more people at your first formation meeting. The key to turnout is to have at least two thousand names and phone numbers from the petitions that you call *twice* before the big meeting. If the meeting is on Thursday, for example, everybody should be called once on Monday and all callers should keep a list of yes's, no's, and maybe's, as well as who needs a ride to the meeting. The second call should come the night before with only the yes's and maybe's called back. ("We just wanted to know how many chairs to set up. Are you still planning on attending tomorrow?")

The phoning should be done by organization volunteers. This is a test to see if people will really do work for the new organization. You can find out by giving each caller a sheet with twenty names or so along with columns for yes, no, maybe, and transportation (for people who need rides). This sheet can be picked up the day before the meeting by the phone tree captain or the organizer.

You can mail to people as well. Get a bulk rate permit and review the reverse street guide from the library. Get the organizing committee to sign the letter and instruct volunteers to help with the mailing. Residents should receive the mailing two weeks before the meeting. The mailing should have the letter about your new organization and a flyer about the big meeting.

What about the Overkill Method? It simply means that you want people to hear about the formation meeting six or seven times. Get the time, date, and place in religious bulletins several weeks before the meeting. If you're really persuasive, you'll get the minister or rabbi to announce the meeting at the weekly sermon. Try getting flyers to the bingo halls, the senior citizens' events, and other gatherings with large numbers of people. Get it listed in the newspaper and announced on the radio. Try to make news several days before the event that feeds into the big community meeting. The morning before the meeting, send out the "Tonight" flyer. In 2- or 3-inch bold print this flyer should say "TONIGHT" and then in smaller print "Come to the meeting to reduce toxic pollution . . ." and then the time, date, place, and a phone number for more information.

The formation meeting itself should serve several purposes: to educate people about the nature of the problem and the power of the organization; to put your demands to targeted officials; to design the steps that will move people into some form of mass action; to establish committees to get people to work; and to recruit new members. Here's a typical agenda for that crucial meeting:

1. Introduction and welcome by the chair
2. Testimony regarding the problem
3. Decision to wage a campaign
4. Demand to the targets
5. Dues collection
6. Open discussion
7. Announcement of the next steps

Now that you're past your first big formation meeting, it's time to do more planning with your key leadership.

PLANNING THE CAMPAIGN

Every organization, whether it's a basketball team, business, church, or toxic waste cleanup campaign, must make a detailed plan of activities to meet its objectives. When you formulate an organizational plan, you figure out the specific steps to take within a set time in order to achieve your short-term or long-term goals. K. C. Jones, former coach of the Boston Celtics, was asked why his basketball team had been so successful. "Besides the talent," he replied, "it's been careful planning that has gotten us where we are today. If plan A doesn't work, we switch to plan B, and if that doesn't work we switch to C, and so on down the line." Good planning is often the difference between winners and losers. In some ways, proper organizational planning is like planning a trip. You must figure out the strategy of how far to go, for how long, and at what cost. How much of the trip will be work? How much will be leisure time and celebration? Once your long-range strategy is in place, you must decide daily what tactic to use to advance your group.

Lee Staples, a leading community organizer and author of *Roots to Power,* writes that "any plan should first recognize the basic principle that power flows from numbers." The best plans take lots of hard work and the contribution of lots of organizational members. Moreover, strategizing requires "a systematic analysis of the positive, negative and undetermined factors which will give a good indication of the campaign's chances for success. There are two ways to help tip the balance in favor of victory—increasing the helping forces and decreasing the hindering ones." When fighting to stop pollution, your organizational strategy must recognize that "organizations draw their power from their ability to affect the factors of your opposition's needs, i.e., money, legitimacy, resources or what they hope to accomplish."

Organizational planning means deciding "what to do with what you got." Resources—both people power and financial power—are key considerations. If it takes a thousand people to carry out a particular action and you have only a hundred volunteers, you'd better go back to the drawing board. Similarly, if you are about to organize committees around four newly discovered dumpsites while fighting for cleanup legislation at the state capitol, and you've got $10 in the organizational kitty, you'd better do some fundraising fast or make sure that fundraising is carefully built into every campaign step.

Strategy and tactics are the two parts of planning. Strategy is figuring out how to win the one-mile race; tactics are the individual steps you take over the course of the mile. General strategizing happens when people imagine the contest, figure out the consequences of different steps, and then select the actions, the timetable, and the organizational process for winning. When you select your tactics, you should consider the following points:

- Will the proposed action establish the moral legitimacy of your group?
- Is the action true to your members' experiences and concerns? (See the section on Taking Action.)
- Will the action be carried out in a way that fulfills your organization's general concerns?
- Will the action attract new members and give others an opportunity to build their leadership skills?
- Will the action provide your group with positive visibility (such as media coverage)?

When you have figured out your strategy and tactics, get your ideas down on paper. First write out a sentence or two that clearly state your organization's plan. (Example: FIST will put direct pressure on the companies that dumped at the site to win a commitment for a speedy and thorough cleanup.) Once you select the date for accomplishing your goal, work backwards and decide what needs to get done by what deadline and schedule that into your timetable.

Always consider the next steps and options before the close of each action or phase. Let's say you meet with the head of your state EPA. If it becomes clear that the official is not responsive to the community's concerns, be ready to suggest the *next* step to your membership in order to give them a sense of urgency and continued involvement. (Example: "We've got to go to the official's boss—the governor—if we're going to get the help we need.") One way to figure out this strategy and the timetable is to use the accompanying strategy chart and look at all the pieces at once. (See Table 2-1.)

TAKING ACTION

Now that you've built your base of citizen support and developed a plan, it's time to take action. Actions are the steps taken to advance your organization's agenda—petitioning, lobbying, educational events, and so on. There is a specialized form of action called *direct action* that has been used by dozens of antitoxics organizations across the country. You take direct action when your organization dramatically, forcefully, and nonviolently confronts a designated power with a set of specific demands. Direct action often provides the necessary leverage to move the designated target to meet your organization's demands.

Both polluters and their official regulators often consider the use of direct action "improper," "counterproductive," "establishing blame when we're

TABLE 2–1

Campaign Strategy Chart

Goals

1. What are your long-range goals? (Example: cleanup of all dumps.)
2. What are your short-term goals? (Example: get air and water tested at the local dump.)
3. What is your definition of victory? What is the specific change you are seeking?
4. What demands will you make to appropriate targets?

Organizational Considerations

1. Will your organization be stronger after the campaign?
2. What specific areas is your organization trying to strengthen?
3. Will your campaign get new members and allies?
4. Will your campaign develop current leaders and new ones?
5. How will money be raised throughout the campaign?
6. What potential problems exist? What do you stand to lose through your campaign?
7. What resources does your organization bring to the campaign?

Building Membership and Allies

1. Why would new members and allies join your organization?
2. Who else could new members or allies bring into your organization?
3. Who might be alienated by new members and allies?
4. What power do new allies and members have to persuade targets to make needed changes?

Targets

1. Who has the power to meet demands or solve problems?
2. Who must you reach before you reach targets?
3. What are the strengths and weaknesses of each target?
4. Who is the target's boss? How does this person hold power—by voters, by appointment, or by ownership?
5. What are the self-interests of all targets?
6. What conflicts of interest might each target have?
7. What are the new targets if you get into a new jurisdiction? (Example: get polluters investigated under the price-setting law.)

Research Needs

1. What facts are missing on the problem?
2. Where do targets live, work, and play?

TABLE 2–1 (*Continued*)

Campaign Strategy Chart

3. Who are the regulators at the local, state, and federal levels, and what are their powers?
4. Can research be done in ways that build neighborhood or membership involvement? (Example: health studies.)

Actions

1. What are the options for action? Remember: Actions should be fun, dramatic, and hard-hitting but within people's standards of acceptability. See the List of Direct Actions in the next section.
2. What action is most threatening to the target?

Timetable

1. Dates of actions
2. Dates for meetings to evaluate and adjust your plans
3. Dates to end the campaign
4. Dates for celebration

all to blame," "un-Christian," "petty harassment," and even "illegal." While direct actions may be confrontational, they are an effective and long-standing tradition in America, a legitimate and time-tested way of fighting for justice and equality. Direct action is rooted in the colonial history of America. Samuel Adams, Paul Revere, and others dumped tea off ships in Boston Harbor in direct defiance of the British Empire. They gave a strong message to the British: "No taxation without representation!" Dr. Martin Luther King, Jr., one of the nation's greatest social change activists, organized many direct actions, such as the bus boycott in Montgomery, Alabama, as a way to end segregation laws. When Dr. King saw injustice, he would "walk his talk," as one of his top assistants once said. Citizens sometimes need to take strong measures when they discover their neighborhoods are being poisoned. When direct action is done well, it gets positive results.

While the kind of direct actions you undertake are limited only by your imagination, there are two points to keep in mind. First, the best actions include the largest numbers of people. Second, while the event itself is important, don't forget these four fundamental stages:

- Careful planning, including reconnaissance and mapping of the location

- Practice by means of role playing
- The direct action itself, where your designated leaders make demands, rouse the crowd, and guide the event
- The post-event review to determine what was gained, what was lost, and what needs to be done next

During the event, don't get distracted by the media. Direct actions are too often spoiled when the leaders of a group get pulled away to do a TV interview instead of following the polluter who's slipping out the door. To avoid this you'll need an excellent press kit that includes a press release, a background summary of the issues, past press clips, a list of demands, and a copy of good quotes from your leaders. (See Chapter 6 on media relations.)

Most direct actions try to bring about an instant response to your legitimate demands. At other times you'll try to force the target into negotiations where you can systematically present your program for a toxics solution. Sometimes you can get a commitment from a polluter at a direct action, but you'll need to follow up with negotiations to nail down the concessions he made.

Before you roll into action, though, it's important to define victory. "A win can result from an opponent's agreement to do something, stop doing something, report back, give information, give recognition, or recommend something to a higher authority," says organizer Lee Staples. Your members must understand what a victory is—that is, under what conditions will you allow the company to continue doing business as usual? Is the polluter's agreement to two out of four demands enough? Before you undertake the action, you must answer such questions as "how do we score a win?" and "what are the next steps?"

Listed below are various actions that have been used by toxics organizations around the globe. You only have to read the newsletter put out by the Citizens Clearinghouse for Hazardous Waste to learn of new approaches evolving daily. The list of direct action ideas is nearly endless. But if you select the direct action approach, you need to give careful consideration to local conditions, the experience of your membership, and the timing of your action. Penny Newman, leader of the Concerned Neighbors in Action fighting to clean up California's Stringfellow acid pits, sums up "action thinking" in the following words: "You must take action to improve your community. As a leader and an organizer, you must decide what is dramatic and effective at the moment, but at the same time, what people will feel comfortable with. You can push people a little bit, but you can't push too far beyond people's experience." In proposing actions—especially direct actions—you must not go too far outside your membership's experience.

List of Direct Actions

1. Voting: At an event where you want the opponent to agree to a good cleanup, take a vote on how the official did. Add up the yes's and no's and maybe's, then give him a grade on his performance (such as D+ or C or B). Tell him his performance isn't good enough and the group has no alternative but to approach his boss.

2. Petitioning: Do some quick doorknocking or set up shopping mall tables to gather signatures. Present them to your senator as you arrive unannounced at his Ritz-Carlton Hotel fundraiser.

3. Issue the Challenge: Visit the homes or offices of state representatives that won't meet with your group over important waste reduction legislation. Along with fifty of your neighbors, present them with a pledge and a deadline for answering. Talk to their neighbors if they don't answer.

4. Picketing: Picket in front of a senator's exclusive fundraising dinner.

5. The "Tough Tour": Take an obstinate official with you on a tour of the local toxic waste dump. Hold him accountable to your specific demands.

6. Rally in Action: Schedule a large event with speakers, music, and food. Turn the rally into a debate with an invited official. Later, present him with your community's toxic prevention demands.

7. Militant Letter-Writing: Collect a letter from your allied canvassers and hand-deliver it along with your cleanup demands to your target's office. Let the target know that if he doesn't respond to the letter, your group will escalate its activities.

8. Parade or March: March with 100,000 toxic activists from the Washington Monument to Capitol Hill and demand toxics reduction. A marching band and the American flag would indicate the truly patriotic tenor of your campaign.

9. Teach-Ins with Demand Sessions: Hold a teach-in, where a designated opponent hears from toxics victims. Put specific demands to the target and argue for your position.

10. Call-Ins: With 100 volunteers, tie up the corporation's switchboard at the headquarters building. Everybody should be asking to speak with the targeted executive about the toxics issue.

11. Exposé: Bring press crews on a discovery tour of toxic barrels

dumped in the woods. Then take them along to an action or the owner to demand the right to know what's in the barrels.

12. Public Hearings: Go to city hall, take over a hearing (grab the microphone), and filibuster with your community concerns. Make the officials play by your rules. "Is that a yes or a no, Mr. Executive? What do you think, neighbors? Well, it looks like your company's proposal for this new incinerator is unacceptable to the neighborhood."

13. Militant Ads: These are probably not worth it to struggling people's organizations. This is where you attack your opponent with all the ammunition you can muster—a messy tactic (not to mention the money you'll need to defend yourself in the courts from the target's libel suits).

14. Award: Take an award directly to the polluter—for example, the "Number One Toxic Dumper of the Year" award.

15. Balloon Release: Release balloons in front of the senator's office with a card attached that says, "Tell your senator to vote for a strong Superfund toxic cleanup bill—(401) 353-2045." Get the story (and the senator's phone number) printed in the newspaper.

16. Homage to the Dead: Funerals of toxics victims can turn into powerful street demonstrations, as we see today with blacks in South Africa.

17. Sit-In: This means sitting down and occupying your opponent's floor space. Organizations must be careful, though, for these actions can lead to arrests. Massachusetts Fair Share occupied the regional EPA headquarters in Boston in 1982 and demanded that they get Ann Burford on the phone to negotiate over a cleanup proposal. After talking with her, the organization got a commitment for stronger cleanups at two sites.

18. Legal Suits: A lawsuit is not direct action, but you could organize a citizens' court regarding the site or do mass filings in federal court—a tactic that would mix legal strategy and direct action. (See Chapter 9 for more information on using legal strategies in toxics campaigns.)

19. Caravan: Lead a procession of cars from the dump to the polluter's backyard to deliver the cleanup challenge.

20. Vigil with Demands: Hold a candlelight vigil at a landfill and count the numbers of trucks rolling in. Don't leave from the front gate until officials agree to your demands. Wear space suits if possible to protect yourself from the toxic hazards.

21. Toxic Labeling Action: Make up a label that reads "Danger: Toxic

Pollution" and put it on products stacked on the store shelves that you want to see banned because of their toxicity. With this tactic, it's also useful to give customers leaflets to educate them about the products they should avoid buying.

22. Honk-In: In this version of the caravan, you surround the target office with 100 cars and honk horns until you get the meeting.

23. Blocking Traffic: With bodies or in cars, stop or stall traffic. Sit-ins on streets or busy intersections during rush hour are ideal.

24. Mock Funerals: Bury your "symbolic dead" on the polluter's front lawn.

25. Walk-Out: Organize the members of the town meeting or the health board to walk out when the company seeks permission to site a landfill. Get them to boycott meetings until the dump company dramatically changes the scope of its proposal.

26. Membership or Account Withdrawal: Have several hundred people at the same time withdraw their savings and checking accounts from a bank that is financing a company poisoning your neighborhood.

27. Staying Home: Love Canal mothers refused to send their children to a school that was built on top of a toxic dump.

28. Consumer Boycott: Your group and its allies agree not to buy the polluter's products or services. At the same time, you try to persuade *all* consumers to participate in order to protect the public health. It's very hard to win these campaigns when one neighborhood takes on a multinational chemical corporation. It's a different story, though, if you enlist large institutions such as unions, senior groups, churches, and environmental organizations on your side. You must have a good media plan that enables you to talk directly to millions of Americans. The successful Nestle's boycott took ten years and millions of dollars.

29. Alternative Market: If the supermarket isn't willing to sign an agreement to stop selling produce with pesticide residues, tell consumers where they can buy safer fruits and vegetables.

30. Strike: Organize workers to leave the worksite until health and safety demands are met. In 1973, the Oil, Chemical, and Atomic Workers, under the leadership of Tony Mazzocchi, organized a nationally coordinated strike against Shell Oil over workers' health and safety demands. In the late 1960s and early 1970s, students struck schools over Dow Chemical's recruitment on college campuses.

31. Dual Government: If the government won't respond, elect neighbor-
    hood health and safety officials to inspect problem areas and negoti-
    ate for cleanup and prevention. Usually this is part of an overall
    strategy for much broader social change—as blacks are now doing
    in South Africa.
32. Selective Buying: Let's say the polluter manufactures sporting
    goods. Your organization and its allies should buy only the basket-
    balls from the polluter's competitor. If you stop buying basketballs
    from *all* the producers, you don't have the economic leverage of
    helping the competitors and hurting the target.
33. Citizen Enforcement: Citizens can force government and corpora-
    tions to recognize the citizen's right to know, to inspect, and to
    negotiate over health and safety issues. (See the next section.)
34. Civil Disobedience: You've tried everything, but they are still dump-
    ing poisons. Now it is time to cite the Declaration of Independence
    and higher moral laws as you practice civil disobedience with large
    numbers of people. In 1979, Lois Gibbs took EPA officials hostage
    and won stronger public health protection at Love Canal. In 1983,
    blacks and whites in North Carolina got arrested trying to stop PCB
    dumping in a mixed neighborhood in Warren County.

THE THREE RIGHTS MODEL

The Three Rights Model is an approach that groups have been using successfully all across the nation. As a precondition, though, you must have
an organization with lots of people, established goals, a plan, and a willingness to do hard work. In neighborhood health and safety campaigns,
citizens should try to establish a relationship between the neighborhood organization and the owners or management of the polluting facility.
The relationship can be cooperative. Often, however, it is confrontational
because of industry's unwillingness to allow citizens to participate in its
decisions. In this relationship, citizens must *win* the right to participate
in the toxic hazards decisions made by the company. Our premise is
that citizens must be party to health and safety decisions in order to
protect themselves from corporate negligence and government inaction.
Government often lacks the resources and the political will to get
the job done while many industries are shortsighted and driven strictly by
profit.

The Three Rights Model includes:

1. The right to know about all actual or potential chemical exposure and the health effects from these chemicals
2. The right to inspect dumps and polluting facilities
3. The right to negotiate directly with responsible parties over the solutions to public health threats

Where do these rights originate? Rights are principles of human behavior that, strictly speaking, cannot be given to people or taken away. They exist inherently in the relationship between citizens, government, and even corporations. Where toxics are concerned, citizens must have the right to protect themselves through knowledge, inspections, and negotiations, as long as the polluter still has the legal right to chemically trespass into the community's air, water, and land. By now it is common knowledge that toxic chemicals know no boundaries. Thus decisions regarding chemical pollution are no longer a private matter but must be open to full democratic participation. Remember: Health and safety are everyone's business. Exercising these rights, however, takes strong, well-organized citizen groups.

While these rights are beginning to be recognized by local, state, and federal legislatures, one has to wonder what would have happened if toxic waste had been an issue during the American Revolution. If King George III had owned poisonous and polluting petrochemical plants, certainly citizen participation rights would have been written into the Constitution and Bill of Rights.

Eventually these three rights will have to be written into law in order to guarantee true toxic waste protection and prevention. We cannot wait, however, for city councils, state legislatures, or Congress to act. We must exercise these rights, case by case, to create a groundswell of citizen support and action that will be the basis for improved laws. Ultimately these new laws will lead to specific environmental improvements and will empower citizens with the rights to know, to inspect, and to negotiate—thus giving citizens the right to act to protect the public health.

Given the lack of an adequate response by all levels of government and business, citizens must take up the fight to enforce proper protection against toxic hazards. Citizens must be the watchful eyes on the changing technologies, on the shop floor, and on the environment. Citizens must, in a sense, be regulators. Critics might ask, "Aren't you taking the place of the government?" The answer is clearly no. Instead, we are acting as a backup to government and fulfilling a coordinating function that government doesn't provide. As we have seen, the regulatory laws are so segmented that an agency's response to a specific hazard can actually create problems in other environmental media (the toxics shell game). Citizens pushing for toxic protection rights must act to ensure that the EPA's air division does not simply shift the toxics from the smokestack to the river or landfill. (See Chapter 9 for specific guidelines in dealing with regulatory agencies and companies on toxics issues.)

Direct neighborhood campaigns against corporate polluters are the best approach to toxics problems because:

- Citizens are forced to learn a lot more about dumps or factory pollution than if they simply left the problem to government.
- Citizens can pinpoint the real source of many of their health problems—that is, the company and its executives who make decisions that result in toxic exposure for residents and workers.
- Citizens armed with the proper technical tools (which we will learn about in the following chapters) have a much better chance to guarantee protection than the understaffed, underfunded, and uncoordinated local, state, and federal agencies. Government's power to solve toxics problems is multiplied many times over when coupled with an active citizenry.

THE RIGHT TO KNOW

If you can get a company executive to a meeting, the first step in the Three Rights Model is to claim the right to know about the types of chemicals that have been dumped or are being used, manufactured, stored, transported, or discharged by the industry in question. Under the new Superfund legislation, citizens now have the right to know what chemicals are invading their neighborhoods or are being used in the workplace. Under the new law, companies must report their discharges into the community's air, water, and land. In 1987, the first year that companies reported their discharges, U.S. industry reported dumping 22 billion pounds of toxic chemicals into the environment. The right-to-know law also allows citizens to review "material safety data sheets," which describe the short-term and long-term health effects of the chemicals used in a plant. While this information is an important new tool for citizens, it doesn't include all the toxic chemicals that industry uses and it excludes companies that use less than 10,000 pounds of toxic chemicals each year. The list of chemicals needs to be expanded—and more companies need to be brought into compliance with the law.

The new Superfund also authorizes the creation of local and state planning committees to plan in advance for serious chemical accidents. These committees should have citizen representation and can become a powerful source of information about a company's chemical management and safety practices. Because they were given broad information-gathering powers, citizens can use these committees to exercise their right to know.

Citizens and workers must know about all the health effects of toxic chemicals. Workers must be trained how to handle hazardous materials safely. In addition, citizens must demand that industry provide a chemical audit or survey of the plant. By audit we mean that citizens must know how much of the chemical comes into the plant and how much leaves in the form of both products and waste.

Here are some typical right-to-know demands that citizens can make to dumpsite owners or industrial operators:

- A list of all the companies who have dumped at the site
- A list of all wastes dumped at the site—types, amounts, and health effects
- A list of wastes being generated or stored at the factory
- A list of all chemicals being used at the firm and information about their long-term and short-term health effects
- A chemical audit of each substance used
- A description of the pollutants coming out of the stacks
- A description of the pollutants being dumped into the community's water or sewers
- A description of the chemicals being produced or manufactured by the firm
- Information about transportation routes for shipping wastes or chemical products
- Information about the firm's emergency plans in case of a spill or accidental release
- A description of the company's insurance plan covering potential damages
- Results of all tests or monitoring done by the firm on any of their environmental or occupational problems

Companies may argue that releasing this type of information will reveal trade secrets that will allow competitors to put them out of business. The issue of trade secrets does have some legitimacy, since competitors could replicate a product from information about its chemical constituents. But trade secrecy arguments are often an industry smokescreen to obscure the health and safety issues. Citizens fighting toxic pollution have no interest in promoting a company's competitors. Whatever argument industry uses, toxics activists believe that the right to know about hazardous chemicals far outweighs any trade secrecy claims by industry. (See the trade secrecy discussion in Chapter 7.)

The right to know about a company's chemical use and disposal does not go far enough, however. Neighborhood inspections must be done to verify this information, investigate the specific problem areas, and find the solutions to the public health threat.

THE RIGHT TO INSPECT

The right to inspect the local dump or factory is most often claimed at the same meeting where the right to know is asserted. If a company dumps enough toxic waste into the environment, the site can become a Superfund priority dumpsite under EPA's supervision. Once the site is covered by Superfund, the polluting company can inspect the dump, take its own samples, and then negotiate with EPA over the cost, timing, and extent of the cleanup. Thus corporations have the power to protect their financial interest through participation rights, yet the citizens who are threatened by hazardous waste don't enjoy the same rights. They do not have the right to inspect, take their own samples, and sit at the bargaining table to ensure that the public health is protected.

If you can get the dumpsite owner or polluter to agree to a neighborhood inspection, find a friendly expert who can help your neighborhood committee with the inspection. The experts generally used by citizen groups include industrial hygienists, environmental engineers, and other public health scientists. Industrial hygienists are experts on workplace hazards—doctors of the shop floor who can tell you what's right, what's wrong, and what needs to be done to reduce toxic hazards. Environmental engineers have different specialties, but generally they are knowledgeable on technologies to reduce air and water pollution. Hydrogeologists are experts who understand soil, rock, and water formations and know where the chemicals go once they enter the ground. National organizations like the Citizens Clearinghouse for Hazardous Waste and NTC have compiled lists of experts who can aid your organization's efforts at affordable costs. (See Chapter 5 for a complete description of how to conduct a neighborhood inspection.)

All experts should organize training sessions for the local group so that average citizens can learn how the process works. Once the inspection is done, the experts and the committee should write up a description of the hazardous problems and several solution options. The neighborhood committee must then decide what to demand of the company in order to deal with the hazards.

Inspection should take place periodically to ensure that workers and the neighborhood are protected against dangerous conditions. The effort to establish a permanent relationship between residents and corporations—so that residents exercise growing influence over health and safety conditions—must include inspections that end in corporations taking action to correct and prevent toxic hazards.

THE RIGHT TO NEGOTIATE

Once the neighborhood inspection has provided citizens with information about a company's health hazards, you need to sit down with the dump or factory operators and list the changes that will make the factory and neighborhood healthier and safer places. But first a caution or two about negotiations. Negotiations alone are never enough to win. It is in large events and actions that citizens can win the incremental shifts in power needed to convince polluters they must clean up and prevent toxic threats. Negotiations serve best to solidify what has been won in direct action. Remember, then, that actions drive negotiations.

Don't negotiate when you can be outmaneuvered or when it is too costly to your organization (if it means an end to action, for example, or if the negotiated benefits go to the leaders and not to the general membership). An accountability mechanism must be established to ensure that negotiations work for the benefit of the neighborhood, not just the members at the bargaining table. (See Chapter 9 for tips on negotiating strategies.)

With these cautions in mind, we return to the Three Rights Model. Let's say your neighborhood has found that the local polluting factory makes asbestos brake linings. Asbestos causes cancer. Your group wins the inspection and finds high dust levels on a shop floor as well as dangerous air emissions. The inspection report by your group's industrial hygienist lists seven options to reduce the hazards: an electrostatic precipitator; a baghouse filter; a scrubber; a mechanical separator; a taller smokestack; a closed-loop system that isolates and recovers the hazardous material; or a safer substitute for asbestos. The first four options are cleaning devices for shop floor ventilation systems. With these options air emissions would be reduced, but with little relief for the workers. In this case, the best option might be the closed-loop system, which would require a company investment to reduce both workplace and environmental emissions. In conjunction with these efforts your group could get its representative in Congress to push for a ban on asbestos products and at the same time get a research grant for the company to develop safer alternatives.

For each situation, there are many possible negotiated solutions with a company. These may range from simple maintenance changes to the use of safer chemicals, total detoxification of the dumpsite, getting the company to use less populated areas for its chemical transportation, or more complex pollution prevention systems. Local groups will be faced with tough decisions on which approach to pursue, but these challenges must be faced if citizens are to control the ever-increasing toxic threats to their children, their homes, and their neighborhoods.

CAMPAIGN STRATEGIES

What if the company refuses to recognize your neighborhood health and safety rights? More often than not, the dumpsite operator or chemical firm will not simply open its gates and allow the inspection. Even if they do allow the inspection, they may refuse to negotiate over the solution. What then?

Citizen groups across the country have been using a number of approaches to get companies to recognize their rights and take protective action. Direct action, covered extensively in the previous section, is always recommended. But there are three other strategies that we will discuss here: using the "arsenal of agencies," putting your issues into the electoral arena, and organizing a corporate campaign.

ARSENAL OF AGENCIES

If the company won't give you information, allow an inspection, or negotiate for solutions to their pollution, then your organization must pressure government agencies to enforce these rights. If the company refuses to tell you, send a large neighborhood group to visit the EPA and demand that *they* find out what the company is dumping. We need to impress upon government that the problems of toxic exposure are all interrelated. We are looking for solutions that do not simply shift toxics from one route of exposure to the next but, rather, prevent or reduce exposure to local residents at the same time. Typically, government agencies regulate just one aspect of the total toxics problem. This is why, when using the government to get the problem solved, you must go to several agencies to address a firm's air, water, solid waste, and occupational hazards. You'll need to become familiar with EPA, OSHA, and state and local regulatory agencies.

Between local, state, and federal authorities there are some fifteen agencies or boards with regulatory power over a firm's operation. There are local fire departments that regulate flammables, there are local zoning boards and local health boards, there is a group that enforces electrical codes, there are state air, water, and hazardous waste divisions as well as similar divisions at the federal level. Enforcement of the laws is often less than adequate to protect the public health, but at least they are a step in the right direction.

Once you call in inspectors from several local, state, and federal agencies, the company in question may decide to come back to the bargaining table and deal directly with your neighborhood group. Using the "arsenal of agencies," citizens may, beyond securing the minimal improvements stipulated by law, actually pressure the company to recognize their right to participate.

When using the agencies, remember these points:

- Demand the inspection with large numbers—a letter doesn't get effective action.
- Once the inspection is done, meet with agency officials (again in large numbers) to demand that the company reduce the toxic hazards found in the inspection.
- Make sure the solution is effective and does not simply move barrels into someone else's backyard.

THE ELECTORAL ARENA

If you can't get the agencies to do enough, remember that the *bosses* of local, state, and federal agencies are mayors, governors, and the president, respectively. If you can't get enough cleanup funds, government enforcement, or support for new laws, you can bring the message home to politicians that if they don't deliver on your issue, your organization will vote them out of office. An organization can undertake voter education or direct actions to make it clear that citizens shouldn't vote for a politician who supports polluters. Election years are an especially good time to get politicians to deliver on your particular health and safety problem.

In Massachusetts, in 1982, seventeen local groups came together under the coordination of Massachusetts Fair Share, a statewide citizens' action group. As a united front, they brought their demands to the head of the state environmental agency. When the commissioner refused to deal with them, they demanded a meeting with the governor. When he too refused, the group picketed several of the governor's fundraisers with hundreds of people in the state's biggest cities. The governor was forced to negotiate and meet half of the group's demands. When he wouldn't budge on the other issues, the group declared electoral war. The following month Massachusetts had a new governor.

CORPORATE CAMPAIGNS

Corporate campaigns are citizen efforts that use economic and political power to get companies to make changes. As in most campaigns, there are three basic steps: intelligence gathering, planning, and execution. In researching corporations, you examine the web of power relations and interlocking interests that make up a company. You then use this information to design a strategy that will make it extremely awkward for the company to continue resisting your group's demands.

Citizens have the power to conduct these campaigns in many arenas: as consumers, as bank depositors, as investors, as members of churches, as union members, as insurance policyholders, as shareholders, and in many other ways. Through an assortment of creative economic, political, and media-related actions, citizens can pressure corporations to clean up and prevent toxic hazards.

3

Corporate Campaigns

PETER OBSTLER AND RICHARD KAZIS

Sooner or later, and usually sooner, citizens trying to improve the quality of their lives by reducing exposure to toxic hazards have to confront the companies that produce, use, transport, and dispose of hazardous materials. Whether the company is a Fortune 500 multinational or a local hauler, whether the problem is an abandoned dumpsite or a working petrochemical plant, significant improvements require private firms to alter their ways of doing business. This is something that private firms generally resist.

The challenge for citizen activists is always this: How do we get the companies responsible for the problem to take us seriously, to take responsibility, and to make the necessary changes? What makes firms sit up and pay attention?

WHAT IS A CORPORATE STRATEGY?

One traditional way citizens have organized to protect themselves has been to push federal, state, and local governments to enforce existing laws, issue better regulations, and pass new laws. Most environmental laws of the past two decades were enacted because of intense public pressure. Over the past ten years, however, the government has become less and less responsive to citizen pressure for pollution prevention. In general, government has become more interested in protecting the polluters rather than the affected citizens. The long struggles for the reauthorization of Superfund and for

Superfund site cleanups are typical of the battles citizens must wage to get the government to respond to their needs.

Increasingly, activists are realizing that new tactics are needed if polluters are to be made more accountable. Consequently, people involved in the toxics movement are developing new strategies to challenge offending companies directly and to force them to deal with citizen concerns. At the local, state, and national levels, the toxics movement is broadening its tactics to include campaigns targeted at particular firms and specific problems. As a result, citizen organizations are developing more sophisticated research and thinking about corporations and their behavior.

Highly visible and ambitious campaigns targeted at irresponsible firms are certainly not new. In the early 1960s, Ralph Nader took on General Motors in a public campaign to improve automobile safety. Through the 1970s, the INFACT campaign challenged the Nestle Company and organized an international consumer boycott that won changes in Nestle's marketing of infant formula to Third World mothers. Labor unions fighting for fair contracts have, at times, developed broad-based public campaigns designed to increase their leverage with employers. In 1974, the Oil, Chemical, and Atomic Workers (OCAW) enlisted the support of major environmental groups to put more pressure on Shell Oil to resolve a contractual and health and safety dispute. Perhaps the best-known union-led campaign that used public pressure to force a firm to change its practices was the long campaign of the Amalgamated Clothing and Textile Workers Union (ACTWU) to win contracts at the notoriously anti-union J. P. Stevens Company.

In recent years, as American corporations have become politically and economically more powerful and citizens have found their recourse to government agencies more restricted, community and labor groups have found advantages in developing strategies that focus labor and community pressure directly on private firms. OCAW is currently fighting BASF, the world's largest chemical company, in Geismar, Louisiana, and is trying to build broad public support around safety concerns at that facility. The United Mine Workers and the anti-apartheid movement have joined together in an ambitious consumer boycott of Royal Dutch Shell.

These efforts are often labeled "corporate campaigns" (though they might be more accurately called "anticorporate campaigns"). The efforts described here were organized at the national or international level to challenge dominant firms in their industries. Such campaigns are not easy to conduct or to win. They require detailed research, capable organizers, lots of money, and a motivated organization able to locate and apply pressure to the corporation's weak links—whether they are financial, legal, organizational, or related to public image. But as the Nestle boycott and other efforts indicate, while the obstacles to these campaigns are formidable, they can be overcome. Corporate campaigns can yield significant, even precedent-setting, citizen victories.

Large-scale, highly visible, national campaigns are only one type of corporate campaign led by citizen and labor groups. There are other, less ambitious, but equally important corporate campaigns in progress in communities around the country, including many targeted at relatively small local polluters. If your organization is trying to force a firm to stop dumping effluent into the local stream, for example, or is demanding that a company improve its chemical accident emergency planning procedures, these are important corporate campaigns.

In reality, citizen groups conduct corporate campaigns all the time—though often they don't know that what they're doing is called a "corporate campaign." Sometimes they lack the skills, the research capability, and the resources to develop a campaign that pinpoints and then attacks the firm's vulnerabilities and brings it to the bargaining table. But increasingly the focus of grassroots activism is expanding beyond the regulatory arena to include direct pressure on firms responsible for creating and perpetuating serious toxic hazards.

This chapter will help you plan creative and effective campaigns against corporate polluters. The goal is to help citizen activists think more clearly and coherently about this emerging strategy—and to offer guidelines for doing the requisite research and campaign development. In the following sections, we examine the essential steps of a successful corporate campaign: research, campaign development, and execution. We then present a case study of a successful local cleanup campaign and an outline of ongoing efforts to develop national corporate campaigns targeted at the chemical industry. (Chapter 9 outlines numerous strategies for pressuring industry to clean up its act.)

RESEARCH AS INTELLIGENCE GATHERING

To figure out how to tackle a private firm, you have to study the company—its finances, product lines, litigation record, and so on. There is a lot to learn. And this can be a problem. It is easy to lose the forest for the trees, to start collecting more and more information while forgetting the purpose of the research. Remember: The ultimate goal is to get the company to change its polluting ways. The research is designed to provide an understanding of how the company works, where its power lies, how decisions get made—and, most important, how you can make it worth the firm's while to listen to you.

Because of this danger, it's often helpful to think about corporate research not simply as data collection but as intelligence gathering. The goal is not "knowledge for knowledge's sake" but knowledge that helps press the campaign forward and win the objective. You don't need to know everything about a company, but you do need to have a clear sense of what kinds of information are important. You also need to know where to obtain specific information that will help increase your leverage in bargaining with the company.

WHAT INFORMATION IS IMPORTANT?

Corporations in the same line of business can differ dramatically along many dimensions—financial health, corporate structure, labor/ management relations, environmental record, corporate culture, reputation in the community, political activity of owners and managers, and more. You cannot develop a strategy targeted at a corporation without having a clear picture of the company's nature and character. The more you know about your target and its specific vulnerabilities, the more appropriate your strategy and tactics are likely to be.

Here are some of the questions that corporate research can help you answer:

- What kind of company is this? What products does it make? What are its consumer product lines? Where are its facilities located?
- Who owns the facility in question? Does the corporation operate at several sites? Is it a subsidiary of a larger firm or is it the owner of smaller subsidiaries?
- How many employees are there in the facility? Are they represented by a union? What is the history of labor/management relations at the facility and in the company?
- Has the company had any legal problems in recent years on toxics or worker health and safety issues? Is there litigation pending that might be relevant to your demands on the company?
- Would pressuring the board of directors help your campaign? Who are the board members? What do they do? What are their connections to other businesses, banks, universities? Where do they live?

- Is this company in sound financial shape? Is it well regarded in the financial community? How much debt does the company have? Who are its key creditors?
- Has the company recently shifted its corporate strategy, its product mix, and so forth? Has it recently acquired other companies in order to diversify or strengthen its position?
- What role does the company play in local, state, and national politics? Is it a leader in political action or a follower of others in the industry or the community? Does the firm contribute heavily to political candidates? Which ones?
- The firm you are researching has been identified as a major dumper in the abandoned landfill in your neighborhood. Has that firm been named as a potential responsible party at any Superfund sites?
- You think you might be able to pressure the firm with threats of disinvestment by union and other pension funds if management does not deal with you. How do you find out if the company is publicly traded? How do you find out which pension funds hold how much of the firm's stock? And how are you going to figure out whether such a strategy is viable?

Of course, these are only a few of the questions you might want to answer. As you begin to think about strategy and tactics, other questions will inevitably emerge. But if you know where to look—and, often, who to ask—you can find very detailed answers to key research questions. First you need to know what you are looking for. Then you have to figure out how to get the information. Finally, you have to be patient and ready to dig long and hard for nuggets of information buried deep in publicly available sources.

STRUCTURING THE RESEARCH

The following checklist provides a helpful way to think about the research you may need to do. It is taken from a superb guide to doing corporate research called *Manual of Corporate Investigation,* prepared by the Food and Allied Service Trades Department of the AFL-CIO (see Resources). The checklist can help you organize your research and strategic thinking about corporate targets by providing ways to break the tasks into small pieces:

1. Administrative Information
   - Company history
   - Management structure and history
   - Plant location and activity
   - Divisional breakdown
   - Boardroom personality

2. Financial Information
   - Sales
   - Profits
   - Cash flow/liquidity
   - New stock issues
   - Indebtedness
   - Assets/liabilities

3. Products/Services
   - Rank
   - Product diversity
   - Competition
   - Plans and prospects

4. Corporate Environment
   - Interlocks
   - Principal investors
   - Pollution record
   - Litigation/law firm
   - Bankers
   - Insurance company
   - Acquisitions/mergers
   - Influence of government regulations and contracts
   - Public relations
   - Political connections

5. Labor Relations
   - Contract analysis
   - Attitude and tactics
   - Level of organization
   - Labor organizations involved
   - Personnel profile
   - Company's NLRB record
   - Overseas labor record
   - Pension and insurance programs

RESOURCES

Luckily for citizens, there are many places to get information about a company. Often the company itself can provide you with lots of good information about its holdings, current liabilities, products, and board of directors. Libraries and state and local government offices can also be treasure troves for gathering intelligence about a company.

COMPANY DOCUMENTS AND SEC REPORTS

The place to begin doing corporate research on publicly traded companies (that is, companies whose stock can be purchased through brokerage houses) is with the information public firms provide their stockholders and the Securities and Exchange Commission (SEC). The most important of these sources are:

- Annual Report: The company's yearly profile of itself presents, usually in glossy form, information on the company's history, management, financial condition, plant locations, and future plans.
- Form 10-K: This annual report to the SEC provides a wealth of information about the firm's products and services, its markets, its employees, pending legal proceedings, properties, large securities owners, financial statements, and directors (including remuneration and background).
- Proxy Statement: This document is distributed to shareholders before the annual shareholders' meeting. The proxy statement is especially useful for information about mergers and acquisitions and about the wealth and holdings of the company's directors and executive officers.
- Form 8-K: This form is available from the SEC reports on major corporate changes—such as changes in control of the company, acquisitions or disposition of assets, resignation of corporate directors, and bankruptcy/receivership.
- Form 13-F and 13-F Tabulation: The 13-F Tabulation is useful in finding out about the major institutional owners of a company's stock (such as union and church pension funds). The 13-F reveals where investment and voting discretion of stock and convertible bonds lies and which banks and investment companies have a large interest in the firm.

The Annual Report, Form 10-K, and the Proxy Statement are available from the company. All the other forms are available at the SEC's public reference rooms in Washington, New York, Chicago, and Los Angeles.

STATE AND LOCAL INFORMATION SOURCES

Important information sources can be located in the offices of state and local government—particularly for privately held companies that do not have to report to the Securities and Exchange Commission. One key resource for any group doing corporate research is the telephone directory for appropriate state, city, and county governments. The following records can be quite helpful:

- Corporation Records: Filed with the secretary of state.
- Partnership Records: Useful in tracing real estate deals and partnerships and determining an employer's personal wealth and business allies.
- Financing Statements: Filed with the state whenever a firm borrows money and uses real property as collateral.
- Court Records: An incredible amount of very useful—sometimes even damning—information about a company, its managers, lawyers, allies, and enemies can be gathered from civil case records of circuit, district, superior, and other courts.
- Recorder of Deeds: Deed and mortgage information on the company's real property holdings are available at the recorder (or registry) of deeds, usually located in the county courthouse.
- Tax Assessment Records: The local tax assessor's office can provide information about the assessed value of a firm's or individual's property (which is usually lower than market value).
- Pollution Information: The new federal right-to-know law (called Title III) mandates public access to information about a company's chemical storage and toxic emissions. This information is housed both at the EPA and with each state's Emergency Planning Commission. For information about Title III filings, call the EPA's Community Right to Know line (800-535-0202) or the EPA's Title III Reporting Center (202-488-1501).

Don't forget your local library, particularly if your city has a business library. Also check the resources of the Chamber of Commerce, trade associations, and the Better Business Bureau.

INFORMATION ON CORPORATE EXECUTIVES

Any large public or university library's business reference collection will include the following sources of information:

- *Dun & Bradstreet Reference Book of Corporate Managements*
- Standard and Poor Register of Corporations, Executives, and Directors
- Dun & Bradstreet Million Dollar Directory
- A variety of *Who's Who* volumes, including the *Chemical Industry Directory and Who's Who* (published by Benn Publications in London)
- Local *Social Registers*

Important information about individuals can be gleaned from these reference volumes.

INFORMATION ABOUT BANKS

Banks can be a good target for corporate campaign strategies. Banks that provide financing for the target firm or have a special business relationship with the company through interlocking board members and other connections can sometimes be pressured by visible community action.

What bank are paychecks written on? Does the bank providing corporate finance hold management's home mortgages? At what date? There are a lot of ways in which banks play direct and indirect roles. Information on banks is available from the various federal and state agencies that regulate bank practices. The agency that keeps track of the bank you're targeting depends on the type of bank—commercial, savings and loan, and so on—and whether it is state or federally chartered. Here are some key information sources on banks:

- Comptroller of the Currency: Banks file with the office of the Comptroller of the Currency annual reports, proxy statements, and other reports similar to those filed with the SEC by publicly traded nonbank firms. This office is in Washington, D.C.
- Federal Deposit Insurance Corporation (FDIC): Member banks file complete reports twice a year with the FDIC in Washington.
- Federal Home Loan Bank Board (FHLBB): Savings and loan associations that issue stock must file proxy statements with the FHLBB in Washington. And any savings and loan insured by the Federal Savings

and Loan Insurance Corporation (FSLIC) must file financial reports twice a year with the board.

- Securities and Exchange Commission: Bank holding companies that are public companies must file the full range of SEC reports.
- Federal Reserve Board (FRB): Bank holding companies that are members of the Federal Reserve system file with the FRB.
- State Banking Commissions: For information on state-chartered banks, go to your state's regulatory agency.
- Community Reinvestment Act: One result of grassroots activism in the 1970s was the passage of the Community Reinvestment Act, a federal law that opens bank loan practices to public scrutiny. Every bank must provide a public statement about how it is serving the community, including a summary of loans to low-income residents. These statements, available from the bank, can provide the basis for objections to the bank's application for new branches, relocations, mergers, and acquisitions. They are potentially important sources of information and strategic levers.

FEDERAL GOVERNMENT SOURCES

In addition to the SEC and banking agencies, other federal offices can be a treasure trove of information. The trick is finding the right office and actually getting the information (often with the help of Freedom of Information Act requests). Regulatory agencies with the most detailed and easily accessible information include the Environmental Protection Agency, Occupational Health and Safety Administration, Equal Employment Opportunity Commission (EEOC), Office of Federal Contract Compliance (OFCC), Federal Election Commission, Federal Communications Commission, Federal Trade Commission, and Interstate Commerce Commission. For an investigation of toxic hazard producers, of course, EPA and OSHA records are critical. EEOC and OFCC records can reveal race or sex discrimination in the company. Here are some shortcuts to help you locate relevant information:

- *Federal Regulation Directory:* a handbook on information sources; available from *Congressional Quarterly* in Washington
- *Federal Information Sources and Systems:* issued by the Comptroller General of the United States; available from the Government Printing Office

- *Federal Fact Finder:* a handy alphabetical guide to over a thousand federal offices; available from Washington Researchers, a private firm in Washington, D.C.

For an excellent treatment of federal sources on environmental and toxic information about specific firms, see Chapter 4.

LABOR RELATIONS SOURCES

It is often essential to understand the labor relations histories and trends of target firms. Key sources include:

- NLRB election and unfair labor practice data
- Interviews with relevant union representatives at the national, regional, and local levels
- *Daily Labor Report,* published by the Bureau of National Affairs in Washington
- Department of Labor forms LM-10, LM-20, and LM-21, which provide information on employers' use of union-busters

The best way to proceed here is to get in touch with experts within the labor movement at the AFL-CIO and its departments (the Industrial Union Department, for example, or the Food and Allied Service Trades Department) or the international union that represents workers in your target firm or industry.

CASE STUDY: A LOCAL CORPORATE CAMPAIGN

Citizen groups, as we have seen, are often involved in corporate campaigns at the local level—campaigns where they have to force a company to be a more responsible member of the community and to respond to concerns of local citizens. These campaigns take a variety of forms, depending upon the character of the adversary and the organizational strength and sophistication of the citizen group. In this section we'll take a detailed look at one such local corporate campaign—one that was waged successfully by Lowell Fair Share in Massachusetts. The goal of the campaign was the cleanup of the Silresim Chemical Corporation's hazardous waste site in Lowell. After careful research, the group focused its campaign on a large local bank with direct ties to the company and the site. As you can see from the following description, the combination of basic research with a creative campaign strategy can yield significant results in the resolution of toxic hazard problems.

While corporate campaigns have grown in complexity and sophistication over the last decade, not all corporate campaigns require a lot of complicated research and vast financial resources. No doubt the most visible national corporate campaigns—such as the J. P. Stevens campaign waged by clothing and textile workers (or the recent campaign by FAST)—call for research, tactics, and resources generally beyond the scope of local grassroots organizations. Even so, local groups have waged very successful corporate campaigns with only the most basic corporate research and minimal resources.

BACKGROUND

The Silresim Chemical Corporation is an abandoned and bankrupt hazardous waste recycling facility. The site is located directly adjacent to a moderate-income residential neighborhood in Lowell, Massachusetts, known as Ayers City. For several years, citizens from Ayers City, who were organized as part of Lowell Fair Share, battled city, state, and federal regulatory agencies for timely, effective, and safe cleanup of the facility. Moreover, the residents requested actions from the appropriate government agencies to address their concerns about health problems and deteriorating property values caused by the site.

Initially the campaign strategy focused exclusively on the public-sector agencies. This "arsenal of agencies" approach yielded significant victories, but the basic issue of "who pays for cleanup and how much" was not resolved. Agency representatives had begun to stall campaign activities by arguing that although threats to the residents' health and safety did exist, there was absolutely no more funding available for future remedial actions at the facility. Further, state health officials reasoned that since the facility went bankrupt, only responsible industrial parties could be held financially accountable for cleanup activities. Such accountability could only be secured through lengthy, complex, and costly court litigation.

To overcome this roadblock, the neighborhood residents of Lowell Fair Share had to implement a direct strategy to pressure private parties to provide funds so that cleanup could continue. They believed that a campaign against a private-sector target with sufficient funds could yield the money necessary to proceed with the cleanup. Moreover, they felt that such activities might pressure the government agencies to search for other public-sector funding sources because of further negative publicity surrounding their effort to get private industry to pay for cleanup costs.

RESEARCH

The campaign did some basic research to identify a target. The first step was to search Silresim's title and deed records. The group obtained the title and deed information by going to the City of Lowell's tax assessor's office. The title and deed revealed facts about the facility, as well as the source of financing for the construction and operation costs. The funding source listed on the deed was the Union National Bank, a large local institution.

According to the deed, Union National had granted several major loans or mortgages totaling in excess of $500,000. Former employees, moreover, interviewed by residents, said that the bank was also involved in the actual management of Silresim in an effort to recoup the bank's mortgage investments in the financially failing corporation. This information provided Lowell Fair Share with a legitimate private-sector target that had the financial ability to assist in the cleanup efforts. Moreover, the bank was a local target whose headquarters were situated in Lowell. Strategically, the bank provided residents with a readily accessible target (unlike the other potentially responsible companies at the site, which were located in other parts of the country).

Residents followed up this valuable lead by doing some research on the Union National Bank. They obtained a Form 10-K and an annual company report from the bank headquarters. The Form 10-K and annual report provided the organization with the following key information:

1. A list of the board of directors and key financial officers at the bank included the bank president and chief executive officer, who would become the central target of the campaign; key board members of the bank, including the publisher of the local daily newspaper; several key local business people; and a top executive in an environmental consulting firm that was bidding with the regulatory agencies for work contracts at the Silresim cleanup.
2. The Form 10-K and annual report revealed that the bank was not a local bank but a wholly owned subsidiary of State Street Bank, a huge multinational Boston-based financial institution.

3. The annual report revealed some interesting financial situations in which the bank was directly involved—including a recently filed suit against the bank by the Massachusetts attorney general claiming monetary damages for the Silresim cleanup to date.
4. The documents revealed several large financial projects the bank was currently involved in, including a $20 million financing project for the Hilton Hotel Corporation in Lowell.

Residents supplemented this research with several other easily accessible items:

- By petitioning the secretary of state, they obtained information about the bank's financial election contributions to local, state, and federal officials.
- By writing the bank, residents obtained a Community Reinvestment Act (CRA) statement listing the activities and investments that directly affected the neighborhoods in Lowell. This information revealed a financial and board relationship with the YWCA of Lowell, a nonprofit organization on which several local Fair Share members had board member seats. Eventually one YWCA became another focus for the campaign.
- By checking the Lowell phone book, residents found home address information on the bank's president and other key bank officials.

These basic and accessible pieces of research gave the Ayers City residents all the information they needed to design and wage a simple but direct corporate campaign to win cleanup concessions at Silresim. To recount briefly these five pieces of information and where they were obtained:

1. A title and deed search obtained from the city tax assessor's office
2. A bank corporate Form 10-K and annual report obtained from bank headquarters
3. Bank election campaign contributions obtained from the secretary of state of Massachusetts
4. A bank Community Reinvestment Act (CRA) statement obtained from bank headquarters
5. A list of the telephone numbers and home addresses of key bank officers

WAGING THE CAMPAIGN

Once residents had pinpointed an appropriate and legitimate corporate target and obtained the relevant research, they designed a coherent and calculated campaign plan. The plan began with a campaign platform that listed specific demands on the bank and a basic statement about the bank's moral and legal responsibility to meet these demands. The platform demands were:

1. Union National Bank should place in escrow the entire amount of money ($1.5 billion) for which the Massachusetts attorney general was suing them to recoup public cleanup costs already spent at the site. Such funds could constitute a quick out-of-court settlement with the state rather than expensive and lengthy litigation. The funds, furthermore, should be set aside and immediately allocated for future cleanup activities so that progress at the site could continue.
2. Union National Bank should provide all residents within a quarter-mile radius with a buyout option on their present homes at "fair market value." (Many residents had trouble selling their homes; others needed to move away due to serious health effects.) In addition, the bank should provide these residents with low-interest mortgages to purchase new homes.
3. Union National Bank should use its corporate standing to pull together a cleanup conference regarding Silresim. It should also solicit funds from all other privately owned responsible cleanup parties at the site.
4. Union National Bank should use its corporate standing with state and federal agencies and elected officials to secure additional public-sector funds for cleanup. This meant using its political clout to place Silresim on the federal Superfund program's National Priority List (NPL), thereby making it immediately eligible for federal emergency money.
5. State and federal agencies should ban Arthur D. Little, a Boston-based environmental consulting firm, from bidding on health and cleanup contracts in the future because of "conflict of interest" status concerning the firm's management connections with the bank's board.
6. Subsequent to the preceding demands, Governor Edward King of Massachusetts should appoint a Special State Police Task Force to

investigate any criminal allegations of the bank's involvement with actual site management.

7. State and federal election candidates should not take any PAC or direct election contributions from the bank or parties or officials associated with the bank.

8. Union National Bank should work with local residents to establish a trust fund to cover medical damages, both immediate and long-term, believed associated with the Silresim site.

Note that residents did not expect to win everything listed in these demands. They wanted the program to provide them with a strong bargaining position for eventual hard-core negotiations with the bank.

Fair Share publicized the program and kicked off the campaign by holding a press conference outside the bank's headquarters. They delivered a formal letter to the bank president and demanded that he negotiate on the bank's behalf regarding the residents' demands. The press conference produced its desired goal of giving their campaign high visibility through TV and press reports. The press conference not only succeeded in focusing attention on the bank's role in the Silresim disaster but reshaped the way the media perceived the responsibility issue for the Silresim cleanup.

The bank president promptly responded to the group's demands by issuing a media press release dismissing their claim of the bank's moral and legal responsibility as "childish and immature." Under no circumstances, he said, would he or any other bank official negotiate or meet with local residents on the issue.

The following week, using information from the telephone book about the bank president's home address, the group executed a series of "direct action" events to press their program and escalate the campaign. Seizing upon the bank's new advertising slogan—"Better banking, closer to home" —more than 100 Ayers City residents picketed branch offices while Fair Share members with local Union National checking accounts closed their accounts at bank offices. When bank officials tried to stop the group from doing this, local residents climbed aboard buses to take their cause to the bank president directly at his home in the wealthy suburb of North Andover.

Carrying signs that read "Better Banking Closer to Home: Silresim Chemical Corporation—Thanks a Lot!" they piled out of the buses and picketed outside the bank president's lush estate. Citizens unveiled a huge draft check with the bank's logo, which read "Pay to the order of the taxpayer of Massachusetts . . . $1.5 billion." They posed for press and TV photographers holding signs that read "Hey Dick, you made us sick" and

"UNB sign on the line." When the bank president refused to appear, bank security personnel in black cars were surrounded by chanting residents demanding a meeting with him.

The action escalated the publicity around the campaign effort. A huge front-page photograph appeared in the local newspaper of residents carrying signs and props on the banker's front lawn. Besides the photo, several lengthy articles described the campaign and there was a pro-campaign column on the op-ed page. The paper also carried a damaging photo of a bank security agent covering his face with his hands. The caption read: "Shy—Residents Picket Bank President's Home."

The high-visibility campaign began to pay off. First, the advertising agency that designed the bank's "Better banking, closer to home" slogan called the bank to ask if they would call off the ad campaign or begin negotiations with the citizen group. Several minutes later, the bank president's office called to say that he would agree to "discuss" the issue with a few leaders from Fair Share before the week was out.

At the end of the week, Fair Share had its first negotiating session with the banker. He and the bank refused to admit any responsibility or to negotiate on the demands. Residents, however, were ready with their next tactic. Lowell Fair Share members who had relations with the Lowell YMCA succeeded in organizing the YWCA board to pull its portfolio, valued at $750,000, out of Union National Bank. Moreover, they requested meetings with Hilton Corporation and the federal banking regulators, charged with Community Reinvestment Act (CRA) implementation, in an effort to tie up proposed bank projects.

Later that month they succeeded in getting state officials to deny Arthur D. Little the health study contract at the Silresim site because of the group's claim of "conflict of interest" between the bank and the consulting firm. They also persuaded Governor King, then running for reelection, to look into allegations concerning the bank's involvement in the management of Silresim.

The results of this campaign surprised even the most skeptical members of the organization. While further negotiating sessions yielded minimal progress on the group's demands, other agencies, which prior to the campaign had been silent, began to surface in the cleanup effort.

First, the attorney general's office announced that it was close to an out-of-court settlement with the bank. A settlement was concluded later that year for $250,000.

Second, a week after the YWCA divested its investment portfolio with the bank, Senator Paul Tsongas, a Lowell resident, announced that Silresim had been "fast tracked" to the top of the Superfund's NPL and would receive emergency federal money so that the cleanup could continue.

Third, a week later the state announced that a $100,000 health study would be provided and that local residents would participate in the selection of a contractor.

Fourth, Governor King announced a commitment later that summer for additional long-term funding from both state and federal authorities.

Fifth, EPA established a "trust" of the 200-plus potentially responsible parties who came together to provide private-sector assistance to the Silresim cleanup. To date, more than $800,000 has been earmarked for cleanup efforts at Silresim.

Finally, the issue of a bank's liability in a hazardous waste site was successfully established for the first time. The *Wall Street Journal* covered Fair Share's corporate campaign on the front page. The *Journal* referred to the campaign as groundbreaking and suggested that the handwriting was on the wall for bank liability in future hazardous waste cases.

CONCLUSION

The Lowell Fair Share campaign was far from a total victory. The corporate strategy did, however, achieve the principal goals that local citizens had originally set—to force the government and the responsible parties to continue the cleanup of the Silresim site.

The bank gave in on several demands. But the real lesson in this corporate, or anticorporate, campaign was the profound effect it had on the public sector—it produced millions of dollars for additional cleanup efforts and won other key concessions from government officials. "I never realized how much power these guys [the bank] really have with government agencies at all levels," remarked Phyllis Robey, an Ayers City resident. "Crack down on a bank and they can really work miracles if it's in their self-interest."

The moral of the story is that a citizens' organization with limited resources and a little basic research was able to mount a successful campaign against a multi-billion-dollar financial institution. No matter what your local group's resources may be, a well-designed corporate campaign can be extremely effective in winning victories on toxic hazard issues.

4

Getting Information

KEN SILVER

Gathering information is a key step in your toxics campaign. In many cases, knowledge is power. The more you know about the source of toxic pollution affecting your community, the stronger your case will be when you publicize your demands to the press and enlist the support of the community. Besides, your opponents will take you seriously when they see that you have the sources to back up your facts.

Information and research are never ends in themselves. In the complex world of toxic chemicals, you must always guard against the threat of endless information gathering. Information is only useful if it leads to action. Research is only useful if it leads to organizational decisions about strategy and tactics. Remember: No matter how many facts you assemble, you'll still need to organize your community to deal with your pollution problem. Facts don't move industry and government—people do.

The unifying concept of this chapter is the *toxics cycle*—the process by which chemicals are extracted, synthesized, formulated, transported, used, and ultimately disposed of in the environment. At least eight federal agencies have authority to regulate different stages of the toxics cycle. This chapter gives you the tools you need to collect information from a diversity of sources (federal agencies in particular) about each stage in the toxics cycle. The kind of research described here will also help your community target the opposition and make a strong case to meet the community's needs.

If you're concerned about a polluting company, then you'll probably want to gather information about the chemicals it emits from its plant, who's on the board of directors, and whether the company has ever been fined before for illegal dumping. In your research strategy, you'll be concerned with exposing and documenting problems, but you may also find out some things along the way that will be crucial to solving the company's toxics problems.

In researching *Cutting Chemical Waste*, a report that examines what twenty-nine chemical plants are doing to reduce toxics, scientists for the group INFORM found that information in government files was "fragmented and incomplete." To get complete information, INFORM went directly to the companies and asked for their files. A well-organized community group can do the same thing.

Your local toxics group should first try to get information from the company that concerns them. Many company spokespersons, however, will politely tell you they can't release "confidential" information about the company. Other times, they may respond that they are putting the information together and you won't hear from them for six months. Even if they gave you all the information you asked for, how would you know it was true? Only by going to independent sources—government files, libraries, workers in the plant—can citizens check the accuracy of information provided by the company. If you suspect a local company is part of the toxic pollution problem, here are the questions to ask:

1. Potential Hazards
   - What does the company produce?
   - What materials or chemicals are used in the company's production processes? Ask for their Title III filings that outline their chemical use and emissions.
2. Corporate Information
   - Who are the company officers?
   - What corporate information is available?
3. Worker Health
   - Has the company been cited for worker safety violations?
   - Has the company violated worker discrimination laws?
4. Air
   - If the company is suspected of polluting the air, what chemicals are involved?
   - Has the company violated air quality standards?
5. Water
   - If the company is suspected of polluting water, what chemicals are involved?
   - Has the company violated water quality standards?

6. Hazardous Waste
   - Does the company generate, treat, store, or dispose of hazardous waste?
   - Has the company been cited for any violations of its hazardous waste permit?

FINDING OUT WHAT A COMPANY PRODUCES

To find out what a suspected polluting company produces, first check the Industrial Directory for your state. Published by the Chamber of Commerce or a private publisher, the directory (sometimes called the "manufacturing directory") classifies firms according to the Standard Industrial Classification (SIC) code. SIC codes categorize businesses according to the goods and services they provide. The federal government's *Standard Industrial Classification Manual*, a fixture in most library reference sections, defines industry-by-industry classification codes. Two-digit industrial codes are general; four-digit codes are more specific.

RIGHT TO KNOW

Under the Community Right-to-Know law (SARA Title III), companies must submit information about the chemicals they use, store, and emit at their facilities (Title III, Sections 311, 312, 313). Much of this information is available through your local Emergency Planning Committee, the local fire department, and the state's Emergency Planning Commission. You can also get it from the company directly, if they will give it to you. The national right-to-know legislation enables a citizen interested in a certain factory to obtain a concise list of the chemicals used for that plant, while the Section 313 data for the first time provide citizens with information about the firm's toxic emissions. Together the Section 311–313 filings will include these essential pieces of information:

- Trade name of the product
- Identity of the chemical ingredients
- Chemical Abstracts Service (CAS) number
- Concentration of each chemical in the mixture
- Amount of material on-site

- Location of material on-site
- Emissions of specific chemicals and their amounts

Citizens are just beginning to use the Community Right-to-Know law. Many local toxics groups are beginning to understand that this law is a powerful tool in their campaigns. (See Chapter 7 on toxics and the law.) Because companies fought so hard against passage of this right-to-know legislation, you can expect some firms to try to take advantage of loopholes in the law to impede your access to essential information. Obstructive firms may use the following tactics:

- Information Overload: By submitting a lot of useless information, companies can bury you in paper. Precious hours can be wasted sifting through stacks of documents for a few essential facts. If you find yourself in this situation, focus your search on the essential pieces of information listed above.
- Vague MSDSs: The material safety data sheet (MSDS) is the common currency of chemical health and safety in the workplace. MSDSs are the information filed under Section 311 of Title III. They are usually two- to four-page summaries of how to protect yourself when working with a particular chemical. But even a complete collection of MSDSs that are 100 percent accurate will be of limited value to you since they never disclose the amounts and locations of chemicals on site. For that information, you'll need to obtain the Section 312 inventory form. Far from being highly detailed, the MSDS often fails to disclose the precise identities and CAS numbers of chemicals named in trade-name products and mixtures. Generic terms such as "an aromatic hydrocarbon" might be used to conceal the presence of toluene, for example, or "a chlorinated alkene" might be used to mask the presence of trichloroethylene in a solvent. Remember the "Four B's" when trying to get information out of the government about a polluting company: Bureaucracy's bark is bigger than its bite.

Under the law, EPA was mandated to set up a publicly accessible database of emissions data (Section 313 information) for all U.S. companies emitting large amounts of toxic chemicals into the environment. The database, called TOXNET, is being managed by the National Science and Medicine Library. Anyone with a computer and a modem can get access to this network. To find out how to get hooked up into this database, call (800) 638-8480.

THOMAS' REGISTER

To supplement the Industrial Directory and Title III filings, *Thomas' Register* is a good source to learn more about the details of a specific product. Comprised of several oversized green volumes (easy to spot on the library shelves), *Thomas' Register* is essentially an advertising mart for companies to sell their products. Companies pay to be listed here. In the company index you'll find an "asset rating" that tells you how much the company is worth. Under "Products and Services" you'll find the company listed alongside many of its competitors. In the same section (or in the "Catalog File") you may find a picture of the product.

A picture of a product can be very helpful, especially when it's something you've never seen or heard of before. If you discover the company you're researching makes "rheostats," for example, you can find a picture in the Products and Services section of *Thomas' Register*. From the photo it is clear that metal, plastics, and perhaps some wire go into the production of rheostats. This picture doesn't tell the whole story. But with it you'll be able to gather bits of information about how materials, machinery, and labor come together to make the product—and what you might expect to find in the factory's waste stream. There are a great many other library sources for gathering information. Consult the Resources section at the back of the book.

A note of caution: American industry is incredibly diverse and constantly changing. Not every industrial process will be adequately described in library sources, but additional information can be found in government files. Moreover, workers at the plant itself know what is involved in the production processes. Through conversations with workers, you may gain clues to determine what chemicals may be present in a factory's waste stream.

TIPS FOR ANALYZING THE INFORMATION

You needn't consult *every* information source. Set a cutoff point for gathering information, then begin to sort out what you've assembled. Here are some important questions to consider.

Are there several industrial methods to make the same product? Which ones are used by the factory in your community? Let's say you're researching a chloralkali plant that produces chlorine and sodium from brine. According to some of the library sources, two processes may be used. The difference is crucial: The mercury electrolytic cell process causes mercury emissions, whereas the diaphragm electrolytic cell process leads to asbestos waste problems. Some processes may use safe chemicals that don't lead to toxic emissions. If a firm is using a toxic chemical process even though safe substitutes exist, the community can demand that the company change processes.

Can hazardous by-products be generated by the production process? For example, highly toxic dioxins and dibenzofurans may be associated with the manufacture and use of chlorophenols, commonly used as wood preservatives and chemical intermediates in the synthesis of drugs.

D> the library sources recommend safer chemicals that may be substituted for highly toxic materials? The following book, conveniently arranged by SIC codes, describes in detail the steps some companies have taken to substitute safer materials and reduce their toxic waste: *Proven Profit from Pollution Prevention: Case Studies in Resource Conservation and Waste Reduction* by Donald Huisingh, Larry Martin, Helene Hilger, and Neil Seldman.

GETTING INFORMATION FROM GOVERNMENT AGENCIES

After Love Canal, Three Mile Island, and Union Carbide's chemical disaster in Bhopal, India, few people are comforted by the thought that the "government is protecting us." Particularly in the 1980s, federal regulatory officials eased up on enforcement of health, safety, and environmental laws. Moreover, the government has been quietly instituting policies that reduce the amount of information gathered by federal agencies. The president's Office of Management and Budget (OMB) tightly controls the information-gathering activities of federal agencies. A government-wide policy adopted in 1981 limits the circumstances under which agencies may grant "fee waivers" to organizations and citizens who request information under the Freedom of Information Act (FOIA). In sum, fewer people now pay more money to get less useful information.

Fortunately, huge veins of information about workplace and environmental health hazards still run deep through government agencies' files and computer systems. Bringing it to the surface, though, requires the patience of a prospector and the skill and luck of an underground miner. There's gold in those files—if you can find it.

HOW TO DEAL WITH GOVERNMENT WORKERS

In the best of all possible worlds, government employees would have the time and inclination to help any citizen who sought information about toxic hazards in his community. A mere telephone call to the agency would be answered by a knowledgeable, sympathetic, and patient person willing to listen and completely research the problem at hand. In fact, bureaucracies do have "Public Affairs" offices for that very purpose. But the people who staff them tend to have limited experience and lack the specialized knowledge to be sufficiently helpful. Their standard answer is "I'll get back to you." Rarely do they provide you with more than a few morsels of information. Often they are more concerned with presenting a positive image of the agency than serving the public. And, as information dispensers, they can also keep tabs on the information your organization possesses and thereby anticipate any controversies that may arise.

Getting past the Public Affairs staff is essential. Several hurdles may stand in your way. First, how do you know which office within an agency to call? Particularly in the federal government, a citizen can get an endless series of referrals from office to office without ever finding anyone who will say, "Yes, I'm responsible for that." By the fifth or sixth phone call, you may wind up at the first office again. If you're calling long distance to your state capital or Washington, this could lead to excruciating headaches and an expensive phone bill.

TIPS ON TARGETING FEDERAL OFFICES

More than twenty laws contain fragments of regulatory authority over toxic substances and are enforced by eight different agencies. The toxics terrain is mapped out on a large scale in the book *Federal Activities in Toxic Substances*, part of the EPA's Toxic Integration Information Series. Although it costs $30 and was written in 1983, it is the only comprehensive, accessible guide to "who does what" to control toxics in the federal government. It lists the specific government offices that collect and analyze information when new regulations are proposed and current ones enforced.

You can get the most out of *Federal Activities in Toxic Substances* by using it in conjunction with another highly detailed book: the Washington Monitor's *Federal Yellow Book*. This is essentially a phone book to federal departments and agencies. The Yellow Book allows you to find the "information specialists" who manage information for the regulators. Using the

Yellow Book, for example, NTC located the employee who oversees EPA's computerized database on pesticide plant locations. When we spoke to him, he acted as if he hadn't received a telephone inquiry in years. Although a Freedom of Information Act request was necessary as a formality, he proved to be extremely helpful, talkative, and an invaluable resource.

The *Federal Yellow Book* also allows you to see how the various offices, branches, and bureaus are organized. People change jobs frequently within the federal government; but barring large-scale reorganization, the functions of the various branches and their phone numbers remain the same. (Since both *Federal Activities in Toxic Substances* and the *Federal Yellow Book* are pretty expensive, try to persuade your local library to purchase them.)

With some luck and persistence you may eventually find an agency employee who knows where to find the information you seek. At this point, diplomacy is the key. Developing a trusting relationship with this person could be a tremendously useful long-term asset. Moreover, long-time agency employees who've moved around from program to program can be treasure troves of knowledge and offer wide-ranging contacts.

More likely, you'll meet up with government employees who are wary of activist organizations. They may be under pressure not to give you the information you seek. They may, for example, be pressed by lack of time. The scientists and specialists who know where information is located have assignments, projects, and deadlines just like anybody else. The time it takes to help you may upset their schedule.

Moreover, agency policy may require FOIA letters. Although the agency employee may have the time and inclination to help you, some agencies require you to file Freedom of Information Act requests for even the simplest kinds of data. These policies serve a twofold purpose: They ensure that supervisors know exactly what information their employees release, and they control the release of "confidential business information" (CBI), or trade secrets, that may be contained in information submitted by regulated companies. For example, the Toxic Substances Control Act requires stiff penalties, even jail terms, for government workers who leak CBI. New employees of EPA's Office of Toxic Substances receive a rigorous indoctrination course in the personal, career, and criminal consequences of releasing CBI. When you're told to file an FOIA letter, the agency employee is simply protecting his or her career.

Finally, there's sometimes a general reluctance to share information with the public. You may run across agency employees who immediately try to discourage you from finding the information you seek. Sometimes they're new employees who don't want to seem ignorant. With an air of great authority they may tell you that the information "doesn't exist." Be sure to ask how long they've been with that particular office. Worse, they may be deeply entrenched bureaucrats who derive their self-esteem from a sense of power—and derive their power from the simple possession of information. Arrogance and self-importance usually go hand-in-hand with such an attitude. Another type of naysayer is the one who's afraid that the information you're after will simply mean more work for them—more field inspections, more press calls, more evenings at the office. Finally, you may find some future stars of "60 Minutes" standing in your path: bureaucrats who know that the information you seek will make their agency—or themselves as individuals—look bad. They may be terrified by the thought that a serious problem documented in their files has received no agency attention—and you've just reminded them of it. For all of these reasons it may be necessary to work around certain individuals.

HOW TO USE THE FREEDOM OF INFORMATION ACT

The Freedom of Information Act (FOIA) is the law that governs your access to information in the federal government's files. FOIA may be the single greatest tool ever created for health, safety, and environmental protection. First enacted in 1966, later strengthened by amendments in 1974, FOIA has been used to unearth information that has ultimately saved thousands of lives, prevented untold health and environmental damage, and saved consumers millions of dollars. For example:

- Forty-six factories along the Ohio River were ordered to cease sewage violations after EPA documents obtained by the *Louisville Courier Post* in 1981 showed that they were dumping hazardous chemicals into the river. The Ohio River serves as a source of drinking water for communities downstream.
- Public Citizens' Health Research Group obtained Food and Drug Administration documents linking the drug Darvon to 11,000 deaths and 80,000 emergency room visits between 1968 and 1978. Subsequent government actions led to a 33 percent reduction in Darvon prescriptions and decreases in deaths and emergency room visits.
- The Union of Concerned Scientists used FOIA to obtain caches of government files that revealed safety and management deficiencies at scores of nuclear power plants around the country.

Here's a short description of UCS's search for nuclear plant safety documents and how their good relationship with one Nuclear Regulatory Commission FOIA officer won them access to the "Nugget File":

> While reviewing a set of documents written by a senior Nuclear Regulatory Commission (NRC) official, Dr. Stephen H. Hanauer, which were reluctantly turned over to us, we happened across a "buckslip" initialled to Hanauer. A buckslip is a standard transmittal form used by the bureaucracy to route memoranda and documents from one office in the federal labyrinth to the other. This particular buckslip transmitted a document from "S.H.H." to "E.P.E." The document being transmitted was not attached to the copy of the buckslip we received, but the buckslip itself contained a handwritten message: "This one is too good to pass up." And, in the corner of the form, there was the notation "Nugget File dtd. 8/15/72."
>
> We immediately telephoned Dr. Hanauer and questioned him about this file, which had never been mentioned in public by the Atomic Energy Commission (AEC) or the NRC. Hanauer confirmed our guess: the Nugget File was a special, internal file, maintained personally by Dr. Hanauer for the last ten years, on serious accidents and deficiencies at U.S. nuclear power plants.
>
> The Union of Concerned Scientists (UCS) asked the NRC, under the provision of the Freedom of Information Act, to make public the entire contents of the Nugget File. NRC responded by making public a listing of just the titles and dates of the documents in the file, but not the documents themselves. This would have necessitated an enormous search of ten years of files to get the actual documents in the file. We were able to prevail upon Mr. Joseph Felton of the NRC staff, who has always processed the UCS Freedom of Information Act requests with impeccable courtesy, to have the Nugget File itself copied and placed in the NRC Public Document room. Finally, the 12-inch-thick stack of nuclear safety documents squirreled away by Dr. Hanauer became available for public perusal. (UCS, *The Nugget File,* p. 2.)

Even though it's a federal law, effective use of FOIA still depends in large part on serendipity, skill, and personalities. Fortunately for the Union of Concerned Scientists, the first batch of documents they received contained the telltale buckslip. It was only useful because UCS had the skill to spot important information.

With a little patience and practice, neighborhood citizens' organizations can make effective use of FOIA. The first step is to learn to write iron-clad FOIA letters that leave the agency no option but to give you the information you need. You needn't be a lawyer to learn this art. Get a copy of *Using the Freedom of Information Act: A Step-by-Step Guide*. Perhaps the best bargain in all of official Washington, this pamphlet is a concise roadmap through the bureaucratic labyrinth for lay people.

Like many other tools, the Freedom of Information Act is bifunctional. You can use it in a general way as a "divining rod" or you can use it in combination with other tools in a more precise manner. Your choice of technique depends on how much time you have to target the precise office in the federal government that's likely to have the information you need.

Divining consists of writing a broadly worded letter to whichever federal office you think may have the information that concerns you. Often this method yields satisfactory results. But, as in any big organization, the government's right hand may not know what the left hand is doing. A report developed by one branch of EPA may never come to the attention of the branch you are dealing with; or it may never find its way into the regional EPA library. A well-meaning agency employee who tries to respond conscientiously to a broadly worded FOIA request may not know all the places to look for the most pertinent information.

By way of contrast, *targeting* your FOIA letter to specific offices and databases (information systems) within the federal bureaucracy has two obvious advantages: First, you're more likely to get exactly the kind of information you need; second, you can be certain that a thorough search will be conducted.

HOW TO DEVELOP A SEARCH STRATEGY

Three levels of government may have information on the company you are researching: federal agencies' headquarters offices in Washington, federal agencies' regional offices, and state agencies. For each step of the toxics cycle (workplace, air, water, waste, and so on), you'll have to request information on the company from these three levels of government. By understanding the relationships between the three—and your organization's probable relationship to each of them—you can decide where to concentrate your efforts.

The job of the headquarters office in Washington, D.C., is to set standards and guidelines. The job of the regional office is to carry them out. Headquarters plays a supervisory role, collecting and analyzing information about the day-to-day activities of the regions. Although regions tend to have more up-to-date and detailed information on specific companies, headquarters employees may be more willing to share the information they've got. Far removed from the community, headquarters employees are less concerned about the political consequences of citizens' organizations using official data to fight local companies. Regional employees tend to be more cautious, since they're in the direct line of fire when industrialists and their political allies fight back.

Taking these generalities into account, a good strategy to use with FOIA is to move from the general to the specific. First, write an FOIA letter to agency headquarters requesting information on the company or geographical area you're interested in. Use the information you get from headquarters to compose your FOIA letter to the region. Ask the region for details on agency actions "including but not limited to" the activities described in the information from headquarters. Finally, use your state's open-records law to gather information on the role (if any) that state agencies have played.

Almost every environmental law contains provisions for the federal government to "delegate" enforcement authority to state government. It is not uncommon to have enforcement authority pass back and forth over the years, or for the federal government to delegate enforcement authority for only a narrow slice of the law to a state agency. Clarify which level of government was responsible for what and when, particularly if you are trying to document a long history of violations.

The willingness of state agencies to provide information to the public will vary from state to state. Traditionally it has been the pro-industry bias of state government that has compelled Congress to create federal regulatory agencies. In recent years, however, many state health and environmental agencies have made valiant efforts to take up the slack created by recent cuts in federal programs. But few states have adopted laws and regulations that are stronger than federal standards.

In many cases, the factory in question will have been granted a permit by the state regulatory agency. By first arming yourself with information from federal government files, your group can deal with state regulators from a position of knowledge and confidence. The state bureaucrats will know you're serious. Moreover, there's nothing a state agency fears more than being stripped of its delegated enforcement authority by the federal government—and losing its federal grant money.

Here are some do's and don'ts for researching toxics:

- DON'T get caught shouldering the burden for devising technical solutions to a company's toxics problems. That's what engineers and consultants are paid to do.
- DO use the information you acquire about chemicals and industrial processes to gain a general idea about the changes needed to safeguard the community. Potential problems uncovered by research can support

basic demands, such as the right of a citizens' group to bring in its own experts to inspect the factory. These experts can then make detailed recommendations that the group can present as demands to the company.

- DON'T get stuck on the research treadmill where action is repeatedly postponed "until we have more information."
- DO use the telephone to gather information. Business executives often volunteer important information on the phone to college students doing research for term papers.
- DON'T let staff people monopolize the research.
- DO involve members of the organization in doing research.
- DO talk to workers at the plant.
- DO find a government depository library at a nearby university or main library in a large town or city. Depository libraries receive the most useful NIOSH, EPA, and congressional documents.

HOW TO USE COMPUTER DATABASES

The computer revolution is alive and well in Washington, D.C. Among the leading users of information technology, federal agencies have massively retooled their headquarters and regional operations to improve efficiency in the collection, analysis, and dissemination of information. To target your FOIA letter for information on a specific company in your community, you need to know which computerized databases to check.

One of the greatest victories to emerge from the 1986 Superfund reauthorization was the passage of the Community Right to Know provision (SARA Title III). For the first time citizens can find out about a company's chemical releases into the environment. The database of SARA Title III is called TOXNET and may be the first database you should access to find out what your local company is dumping into your community's air, water, and soil.

In the back of the book, in the Resources section, you'll find numerous computerized databases containing information on toxic contamination problems in communities across America. They range from the bird's-eye view, "Facilities Index System" (FINDS)—a complete listing of facilities regulated by the various programs and branches of EPA—to narrow inventories of specific sources such as underground injection wells. From the descriptions in the Resources section, you can figure out which computer systems may contain the information you need. A phone call to the agency will help you verify whether a search of that system is likely to bear fruit. (But don't let this person simply shunt you to a state agency.)

The following tips can reduce delays in getting a response to your request:

- Write one FOIA letter for each computer system you want searched. Standard procedure at EPA and other agencies is to wait until all the searches have been completed before mailing any part of the package. One malfunctioning system, or a key employee "out on leave," can bog down the entire process. Spread your separate FOIA letters over several days; don't send them all on the same date. If you're a member of an organization, enlist other members to send FOIA letters in their own names for particular databases.
- Always include a daytime phone number on your letter.
- Don't be discouraged by the specter of monetary fees for the information. If you're a representative of an organization working in the public interest, the Freedom of Information Act entitles you to a fee waiver. Many agencies may deny your initial request for a fee waiver and send you a bill along with the computer printouts. You have thirty days to appeal. Most legitimate citizens' organizations are eventually granted a reduction or fee waiver.
- Follow up with weekly phone calls to the FOIA officer or person handling your request until your package is "in the mail."

Despite their many benefits, you should be aware of the limitations built into computerized databases maintained by federal agencies. Upkeep of these national systems depends on cooperation from regional offices. At EPA, for example, the degree of cooperation depends on the program branch and region involved. (Regional employees rarely have anything good to say about "headquarters employees.") Still fewer state agencies cooperate with the EPA office in their region to provide the necessary computer data unless they are required to do so. Many state agencies maintain their own internal computer systems. Routine reports to EPA, some say, take too much time. Others claim that routine reporting deprives them of an effective negotiating tactic with polluting companies: They threaten to report them to the federal government if they don't abide by state regulations.

Here is a list of the computer systems that state agencies are likely to maintain for internal use. Use your state records law to obtain information from these sources.

1. Hazardous waste
   - Waste disposal, treatment, and storage enforcement system
   - List of active landfills
   - List of abandoned dumpsites (a state "ERRIS list")
   - List of sites covered by the state Superfund law
2. Air pollution
   - List of stationary sources covered by criteria pollutant regulations
   - List of stationary sources covered by air toxics regulations
   - Air enforcement tracking system
   - Emission inventories
3. Water pollution
   - Reports submitted by public and private drinking water suppliers
   - Water quality monitoring data for rivers, lakes, and streams
   - List of NPDES (or SPDES, "S" for state) permit holders and specific effluent limitations
4. Transportation
   - List of road accidents involving hazardous materials

FINDING INFORMATION ON WORKER HEALTH RECORDS

OSHA INSPECTIONS

Companies that use toxic substances in amounts large enough to catch the community's attention may well have had serious chemical health and safety problems affecting workers in the plant. Documenting past inspections by the U.S. Occupational Safety and Health Administration (OSHA) is a good way to learn about chemical "hot spots" inside the plant. Since OSHA's follow-up to inspections is often lax or nonexistent, the findings from your research may eventually help to revitalize safety and health concerns among workers at the plant.

Write an FOIA letter to request copies of all inspection reports, correspondence, citations, and documents that relate to the plant. Address it to the nearest OSHA field office. (OSHA field offices are beneath the regional offices.) To find the address, check the phone book under "United States Government—Labor Department." It would not hurt to send the same letter to the nearest regional OSHA office.

OSHA REVIEW COMMISSION

Companies may appeal OSHA citations and penalties to the OSHA Review Commission, an independent three-member panel. The commission's decisions are published annually by the Bureau of National Affairs in *Occupational Safety and Health Cases*. (Try a law library to find this publication.) You can find an index to employers in the back of each volume.

The OSHA Review Commission's Executive Secretary's Office maintains a "case tracking system." It contains the most recent information on active and recently decided cases, as well as cases taken to the U.S. Court of Appeals. To get information on the company you're dealing with, submit an FOIA request to: Freedom of Information Officer, Executive Secretary's Office, OSHA Review Commission, 1825 K Street NW, Washington, DC 20006.

NIOSH HEALTH HAZARD EVALUATIONS

The National Institute for Occupational Safety and Health (NIOSH) performs occasional workplace inspections called Health Hazard Evaluations (HHEs). HHEs are published as technical reports and are listed in the NIOSH publications catalog. Searching in the sixth edition (most recent) by the type of product made at the plant is unreliable. To find out whether an HHE has been published since 1981 on the plant you are interested in, contact the NIOSH Division of Technical Services at (513) 841-4287.

STATE WORKPLACE INSPECTIONS

In about twenty-five states, federal OSHA regulations are enforced by a state agency. For businesses located in these "state-plan" states, federal OSHA is not likely to have records. Instead, the state agency, usually located in the state labor or health department, will have the inspection records.

Where federal OSHA is the enforcer (in "non-state-plan" states), it may still be worthwhile to check the state agency's records. Some state industrial hygiene bureaus were established before enactment of the federal OSHA Act of 1970 and have maintained their workplace inspections. Though often ineffectual as enforcers, these agencies may have valuable information in their files.

WORKER COMPENSATION CLAIMS

Every state government administers a workers' compensation program. Records of claims filed against a company for work-related illnesses, deaths, and injuries are sometimes in the public domain. Evidence of workers' compensation claims dating back many years can demonstrate a company's long familiarity with—and possibly its apathy toward—chemical hazards.

Discretion here is advisable: Before approaching the state agency, check around with the Coalition of Occupational Safety and Health (COSH) group or trusted compensation attorney who represents only victims. COSH groups are progressive groups within the labor movement concerned with occupational health issues for workers in industrial facilities. Your request may be the first of its kind filed with the workers' compensation board. Many state boards may deny your request for access to these files because of their concern for privacy. Because your motive is community-oriented, not work-related, they may also use this as an excuse to deny you access. You'll be in a stronger position to see the files if you are armed with legal precedents in which the board has granted access to unions, attorneys, news reporters, or, ideally, community residents.

WORKER DISCRIMINATION

Worker discrimination records can disclose instances of corporate denial of basic rights. Minority workers have traditionally labored in the jobs with the greatest health risks. Women have been denied employment in industrial processes that may affect their reproductive organs.

The federal Equal Employment Opportunity Commission covers the entire country. File FOIA requests with the nearest district and regional offices. You can get the address by calling 1-800-USA-EEOC. In your letter, ask for information on the company, not mentioning claimants' or parties' names. Many states have established independent antidiscrimination commissions. Use your state's open-records law to obtain information from them.

OBTAINING INFORMATION ABOUT AIR POLLUTION

In searching for information on a company's air emissions, you need to be aware of a major cleavage in federal air pollution regulation: criteria air pollutants versus toxic air pollutants. Under the Clean Air Act amendments of 1977, EPA was given a strong mandate to control six so-called criteria pollutants—sulfur dioxide, particulates, carbon monoxide, ozone, nitrogen oxides, and lead. Generally, criteria pollutants are a public health concern when emitted in large quantities (usually on the order of several tons per year) from industrial facilities. By contrast, toxic air pollutants are a public health threat at levels as low as one part per million. (Lead actually fits into both categories: Tons are emitted from the tailpipes of vehicles that use leaded gas, while levels as minuscule as a few parts per million can cause irreversible health problems.) Overall, though, two fundamentally different regulatory approaches—and therefore two different sources of information—come into play.

Another important law to be aware of is Title III of the new Superfund reauthorization. Under this national right-to-know law, companies using or producing toxic chemicals must report their toxic releases into the air, water, and land. Each company must complete a "Form R" (also known as "Section 313 data" for the provision in the law that mandates emissions reporting) that identifies which chemicals in what amounts are being released into the environment. For information about using Title III information, see the Resources section at the end of the book. (See also Chapter 7 on the law.)

CRITERIA AIR POLLUTANTS

Under a provision of the Clean Air Act, EPA was authorized to set emission standards for chemicals that are hazardous because they are emitted in large quantities into our air each year. These are known as *criteria* pollutants.

State Implementation Plans

State agencies play a pivotal role in enforcement of the Clean Air Act. They are required to draw up State Implementation Plans (SIPs) to meet and maintain federal air quality standards. These plans include specific emissions limits and cleanup timetables applicable to major industrial facilities and other "stationary sources." SIPs are available for public inspection. If the company you're dealing with is a major industrial polluter, that fact may be revealed in the SIP—in which case a sizable cache of engineering studies, correspondence, and other information is almost certainly on file with the state agency that authored the SIP.

State Agency Files on Nonattainment Areas

Major urban areas were given until 1982 to reduce pollutant levels to below ambient standards. Areas that failed to meet this deadline were designated "nonattainment" areas. Existing industries in nonattainment areas are required to install "reasonably available control technology"; new plants and major emitters must be built with more effective pollution controls ("lowest achievable emission rate"). If you live in a nonattainment area and you're dealing with a big company, the responsible state agency has probably collected a lot of information about plant emissions. If the plant was built in a nonattainment area after 1982, agency files probably contain a long trail of paper related to the permit process.

Computerized Databases

The Resources section identifies several computerized databases maintained by the EPA that contain information on emissions, ambient concentrations, violations, and enforcement actions involving thousands of stationary sources across the United States.

TOXIC AIR POLLUTANTS

In contrast to the elaborate regulatory apparatus in place to control criteria air pollutants, EPA has barely scratched the surface to control toxic air pollutants. Under the National Emission Standards for Hazardous Air Pollutants (NESHAP) program, standards have been established for only six hazardous air pollutants (asbestos, benzene, vinyl chloride, beryllium, arsenic, and mercury). Two additional toxic air pollutants (radionucleides and coke oven emissions) have been officially recognized by the agency, though no standards have been set. The six standards that have been set require "no visible emissions" and prescribe certain control technologies to achieve this requirement.

Compliance Data System

Stationary sources of toxic air pollutants are described in the EPA's Compliance Data System. (See the Resources section.)

Research Triangle Park

Since the late 1970s, a great deal of EPA's air toxics work has been done through the agency's Office of Air Quality Planning and Standards at Research Triangle Park, North Carolina. To assess the severity of the air toxics problem and the feasibility of certain control technologies, EPA scientists have conducted field studies at dozens of chemical plants and other major industrial facilities. Frequently these studies have been conducted for EPA by private contractors. When they are published, such studies are generally abstracted in *Government Reports Abstracts*. But an FOIA letter to EPA at Research Triangle Park might turn up studies not yet in the public domain.

OBTAINING INFORMATION ABOUT WATER POLLUTION

COMPUTERIZED DATABASES

The Resources section summarizes the major EPA computerized databases that deal with drinking water and sources of water pollution. EPA's main repository of ambient water quality monitoring data is the computer database STORET. It contains monitoring results collected by local, state, and federal agencies at more than 600,000 sites across the country. The sites include sewage treatment plants, effluent pipes from industrial facilities, and drinking water wells. Data can be retrieved two ways:

- Latitude and Longitude Search: All water monitoring data for facilities in that area, or some subset of that information, can be retrieved. If a certain chemical shows up in the water, for example, STORET can be searched for local companies that discharge that chemical.
- Entire Body of Water Search: Data are stored according to "hydrologic accounting units," a coding system devised by the U.S. Geological Service for rivers, lakes, and streams in the United States. EPA employees can usually find the code for the water body you are researching; codes can also be obtained from the National Water Data Exchange. Information on point sources of water pollution is contained in EPA's Permit Compliance System.

DRINKING WATER SYSTEMS

Mere detection of chemical contaminants in drinking water supplies does not prove how the chemical got there. But combined with other sources of information, drinking water analyses are an important link in the chain of evidence connecting industries to discharges of toxic substances.

Under the federal Safe Drinking Water Act (SDWA), anyone who owns or manages a public drinking water supply must monitor for chemical contamination. State and federal agencies may also conduct their own water analyses. The results of these analyses are available from three principal sources:

1. Water supplier's annual and triannual SDWA monitoring reports: The water supplier may provide copies upon a customer's request.
2. EPA's Federal Reporting Data System (also known as the Public Drinking Water Database—see the Resources section): This database catalogs monitoring violations and other SDWA requirements in drinking water supply systems.
3. State agencies: EPA's Federal Reporting Data System only lists violations of the Safe Drinking Water Act reported by state and local government agencies. More comprehensive monitoring data for particular water supplies may be collected separately by the state agency delegated authority for enforcement of the act.

OBTAINING INFORMATION ABOUT THE TRANSPORT OF TOXICS

Transportation of hazardous materials is gaining increasing recognition as a threat to the health and safety of American neighborhoods. Over 1.5 billion tons of hazardous materials are transported in the United States each year. More than half of this (927 million tons) moves in the nation's fleet of 467,000 trucks. Another 549 million tons is transported by ships and barges. Railroad cars haul the remaining 73 million tons. Hazardous materials include flammable gases, petroleum products, radioactive materials, and toxic commodities. The term also includes hazardous wastes, though wastes constitute only 3 percent of all hazardous materials.

A complex patchwork of federal, state, and local regulations attempt to address the problem of transporting hazardous materials. At the federal level alone, six agencies have some jurisdiction; within the Department of Transportation (DOT), five separate offices are involved. Within this patchwork, the Office of Technology Assessment recently noted several gaping loopholes in the public's protection from hazardous materials in transit: insufficient training of local public safety officials; serious underreporting of accidents and shipments; and the fact that DOT does not regulate intrastate shipment, only interstate shipments.

Sources of information on hazardous material shipments through communities are, not surprisingly, somewhat primitive. In the early 1980s seven jurisdictions received grants from the Department of Transportation to develop comprehensive hazardous material management plans (Central Puget Sound Region; San Francisco Bay Area; Indianapolis; Memphis; New Orleans; Niagara County, N.Y.; and Massachusetts). A report summarizing the DOT's program, which was then called the State Hazardous Materials Enforcement Development (SHMED) program, is available by calling (202) 366-4439. Some states and cities have initiated their own studies of hazardous material management.

Government systems are unable to track the flow of hazardous materials. The greatest progress made to date in tracking these shipments has been to start with inventories of fixed facilities. Right-to-know laws are uniquely suited to developing such inventories. Once the stationary locations of chemicals are known, it is relatively straightforward for government agencies to ask local companies where the hazardous materials are coming from.

Right-to-know laws do not, however, cover transportation per se. Early in the development of the right-to-know movement, activists decided to steer clear of the thorny issue of federal preemption created by the Hazardous Materials Transportation Act, the main federal law concerned with this issue. Nevertheless, citizens can use the national right-to-know law (Title III) to develop inventories of fixed facilities in their communities. Well-organized citizen groups may then be able to leverage information directly from companies—although no law explicitly requires it—on how hazardous raw materials are transported to their plant and where end-products go when they leave a facility. The Environmental Policy Institute has developed model legislation for local governments attempting to regulate the transport of hazardous materials. It strongly emphasizes information gathering. (Contact Fred Millar at 218 D Street SE, Washington, DC 20003; 202-547-5330.)

The most efficient way to gather information on hazardous material transport through your community may be simply to go out and look for it. Under DOT regulations, trucks and railroad cars containing hazardous materials must be identified with a four-digit code number called the "DOT" or "UN" number. On trucks, the number usually appears on a diamond-shaped placard on the side of the truck or as large black numbers on a bright orange sticker. On railroad cars, it is a little tougher to spot—the UN/DOT number is usually stenciled along with lots of other numbers on the side of the car.

The book for deciphering what chemicals these codes represent is DOT's *Emergency Response Handbook*. Armed with this book you can directly survey the trucks and railroad cars carrying hazardous materials through your community. A Saturday afternoon spent with the DOT book and a pair of binoculars down by the railroad tracks or alongside the highway might yield powerful ammunition for passage of a local disclosure ordinance covering the transport of hazardous materials.

Of course, nothing gets attention like an accident. Several government databases keep track of hazardous material "accidents" and "incidents." The DOT's Hazardous Materials Information System is the main system and is described, along with the others, in the Resources section. Data can be retrieved by date and geographic area from all of the systems. From some systems you can even obtain listings of all accidents involving a particular chemical. Although no accident involving that chemical may yet have occurred in your community, examples of accidents from other communities can spur efforts to tighten local laws and regulations.

5

The Neighborhood Inspection

RICHARD YOUNGSTROM

Hazardous waste dumps continue to receive significant media attention and regulatory action. Less attention, however, is paid to the actual source of hazardous waste, air pollution, water pollution, and catastrophic accidents: the workplace. A neighborhood inspection is one approach that citizens can use to address their concerns about toxic chemicals and safety hazards—an approach that does not depend solely on regulatory authority or voluntary efforts by industry. It is a do-it-yourself strategy that encourages a "good neighbor" approach by management and alternative solutions to environmental problems. It tries to incorporate management's economic concerns and labor's health and safety concerns.

WHY A NEIGHBORHOOD INSPECTION?

A neighborhood inspection can be a valuable strategy for several reasons:

- It's an action-oriented strategy to protect yourself and your family and to organize your neighborhood.
- It can teach you what prevention really means: taking action before something tragic happens.
- Unlike legal and regulatory activities, the neighborhood inspection is a direct challenge to corporations to change the way they do business.

101

When these bedrock issues of the workplace are addressed, management responds.

- The struggle for the right to know, the right to inspect, and particularly the right to negotiate has evolved from the struggles of workers and unions to establish essential rights. Workers can be important allies and their tactics and strategies can be helpful models for action.

THE LIMITS OF REGULATION

The regulatory process has its limitations. The real issue in every neighborhood campaign for hazardous waste cleanup, toxics use reduction, or accident prevention is the community's concern about adverse health effects. Various outside authorities can be helpful. Since all public servants are susceptible to pressure from the community, it certainly helps to find a sympathetic official or researcher who's willing to push, bend, or use the law to the best possible interest of the community. Nevertheless, there are serious limitations to seeking help from these sources:

- Regulators must operate in their specific area of jurisdiction and follow the rules of their organization. Health and safety officials are not concerned with the environment; environmental officials cannot enforce toxic reduction in the workplace.
- Research and public health investigators must "prove" there is a problem by showing an excess number of disease victims in order to support the community. Not only does this process take a long time, but waiting for victims has obvious limitations as a prevention strategy.
- Elected officials at all levels must weigh their involvement and support against political and economic realities. At best, they deal with their constituencies, which include business interests, in an evenhanded way.
- Fire officials, zoning boards, and other licensing agencies and inspectors can all be used effectively if there's a specific violation of their regulations. But even in the most favorable political climate, none of these bureaucrats can institutionally represent your concerns.

THE ACTION-ORIENTED STRATEGY

Since it is the community that has the most to lose from environmental threats, the community must in a real sense become the regulators. A neighborhood inspection with technical support is a manifestation of this kind of action. The neighborhood inspection can also help you organize your community. You may first organize your neighbors around a specific issue that needs to be resolved. But this step may lead to longer campaigns and other issues of health and safety. In situations where your organization should be continued, the neighborhood inspection is a way to approach other problem areas, look for trouble, and practice prevention.

PREVENTION

It's essential that the community promote the concept of pollution prevention. This simple approach is designed to anticipate problems based on all available information and then intervene to make changes before there are victims—like putting the traffic signal at the busy intersection *before* a child is hit by a car. Many people claim to practice prevention, but the concept has been distorted by such ideas as cost or risk/benefit analysis, blame-the-victim notions, and a widespread "compliance mentality" on the part of business.

Cost/benefit analysts base their decisions on bottom-line cost and presume that some risks to health, even preventable risks, cannot be avoided. A blame-the-victim mentality presumes that most injuries and disease cannot be prevented because people are accident-prone or inherently susceptible to certain diseases. Even well-meaning health promotion activities or wellness programs assume that most illness is caused by a person's "unhealthy behaviors," not occupational or environmental exposure. Finally, business interests regard prevention as minimal compliance with the law. This view disregards the fact that all laws and regulations represent, to a greater or lesser extent, a compromise between economic and health considerations—that is, the profit-oriented interest of business and the health prevention interest of workers and the community.

In contrast to the after-the-fact regulatory and political approach, a neighborhood inspection deals specifically with the community's concern and confronts the source of the problem in a prevention-oriented way. The inspection and written report can provide key technical assistance by focusing demands and channeling efforts toward the real problems—those that are the most serious or require the most investigation.

CHALLENGING MANAGEMENT RIGHTS

By incorporating a broad view of the issues, the inspection strategy challenges management's inherent position that the risks associated with its operation must be borne by workers and the community while the corporation enjoys the profitable benefits. Management would prefer to deal with these issues through government officials or legal channels. They are not accustomed to dealing with angry and informed neighbors inside their plants. From this position, pressure for change can be very effective—particularly when the community understands the workers' concerns.

WORKERS AND UNIONS AS ALLIES

When the fight for a clean environment moves to the workplace, the workers in the plant, like it or not, become involved. The preventive approach to toxic substances is bound to affect them, and whether they're organized into unions or not, they may see the campaign as a direct threat to their jobs and livelihood. This is, of course, a valid concern that management may try to exploit. But it can also be your opportunity to broaden the fight, suggest different strategies, and make the demand for a clean environment include job protection and a safe workplace. The workers' fight for a safe workplace and the community's fight for a safe neighborhood have much in common:

- Management sometimes counters the union's attempts to have its health and safety experts inspect the workplace through claims of private property and trade secret disclosure. Community activists, by contrast, have had an easier time gaining entry to plants for neighborhood inspections. This situation is likely to change, however, and the unions' hard-won experience in this struggle will be useful to the community.
- The unions' emphasis on collective action can be useful to the community. The rallying theme of worker organizations—"An injury to one is an injury to all"—is no less important to community organizing.
- The primary strategy for reducing occupational health problems is called *engineering control*. These concepts, such as substitution of less hazardous materials for dangerous ones, can work hand in hand with strategies for reducing the use of toxic substances.

Many of the ideas presented here may be new to community activists; this is particularly true for workplace and union issues. But the fight to protect your community will be more successful if it draws from the new strategies and collective action suggested here. In the following sections, we'll take a look at the issues and details of this new strategy. As with all new ideas, however, discussion, education, understanding, and adjustment to local conditions must be incorporated into the campaign.

THE KEY ISSUES

Once citizens take their local prevention campaign beyond the plant gates and begin to challenge the way a company does business, there are two issues that require careful consideration and strategic planning: worker attitudes and management resistance. Grassroots activists are only beginning to form a bridge to workers in dangerous factories. In too many local environmental struggles, the community and the workers have been at odds with each other. To be successful in a local fight, however, there are ways to incorporate the concerns of workers and enlist their support. In places where workers believe their jobs are on the line, they're not likely to support you. But even in these situations, there are ways to at least keep workers from opposing your fight. By addressing workers' attitudes head on, you'll have better leverage when you confront management resistance.

WORKERS' ATTITUDES

Incorporating workers and their unions into neighborhood campaigns is always a complex and difficult task—not only because of the issues raised around the workplace but also because of workers' attitudes and divisive management strategies. Health and safety (inside the workplace) and the environment (outside the workplace) are dealt with as separate issues by government, the media, the community, and workers.

American workers have been organizing themselves into collective groups to represent their interests for more than a hundred years, using tactics of strength in numbers, membership education, and collective bargaining. In the area of health and safety, however, workplace hazards are often accepted as part of the job, an attitude that has interfered with organizing efforts.

In contrast to the worker's acceptance of risk, community members expect their neighborhoods to be free from the risk of pollution of any kind. The refusal to accept even a low risk of disease (as compared to the attitude of workers inside the plant) is the driving force behind the campaign against plant emissions, hazardous waste, and other "risky" activities. Understanding *why* workers have accepted workplace risks of injury and illness may help you to change their attitude. The main issues are these:

- Management generally views health and safety as secondary to production and tends to get involved in the issue only because of regulatory or union pressure. Workers generally fear their jobs will disappear if they speak up. A sense of powerlessness leads to acceptance of the hazard: "It's part of the job" and "What can I do about it?" are phrases often heard on the factory floor. Plant closings and layoffs are often blamed, incorrectly, on health and safety regulations.

- Misinformation, propaganda, and human nature have also contributed to the problem. If a chemical is being used at work, there's often an assumption that "someone" must have checked it out. It's hard for people to believe that management often doesn't know the hazards of materials to which they expose their workers (and the community).
- Management often blames "unsafe workers" for accidents and "hyper-susceptible workers" or "lifestyle factors" for cases of occupational illness. Workers hearing a half-truth over and over may come to believe it themselves.
- The long-term nature of occupational disease makes health issues difficult to address when there are more pressing needs—a job to put food on the table.
- The issue of risk/benefit ("We don't live in a risk-free world, you know") is distorted. Workers, consumers, and the community are asked to accept the risks of disease and environmental damage while management takes the major share of benefits.
- Injured or ill workers drop out of the work force. Since only the survivors are seen, there's a belief that "it won't happen to me."
- The workers' compensation system—the sole remedy for injured or ill workers—does not deal with prevention. Benefits are paid to workers *after* their exposure and illness. Meanwhile, the corporation's insurance policies minimize the true financial impact of inadequate health and safety efforts.

Clearly workers should become more involved in workplace health and safety issues and in environmental issues. The following facts can help you get them involved:

- Since workers in plants often live in the community, they can find themselves in double jeopardy. They are exposed to toxics both at work and at home.
- Understanding the long-term hazard of cancer in the workplace can help workers to understand the long-term hazard of cancer in the environment. There is no level of "zero risk" for any cancer-causing chemical or material.

• Workers often know their jobs are hazardous but accept the risk because high wages allow them to provide a better life for their families. But understanding that there may be risks to their families as well may help to get them involved in an inspection campaign. These risks involve direct exposure (such as asbestos brought home on clothing), the risk of reproductive hazards to both sexes, and the risk of environmentally induced disease.

MANAGEMENT'S RESISTANCE

As the center of our economic system, the corporation is identified with jobs, prosperity, even patriotism. In this hallowed context, the workplace is seen as private property and all attempts to impose socially beneficial changes are seen as a threat to profits. The system first demands that the problem must be proved to exist. Have the carcinogens Company X released into the environment caused any cancers? When environmental disease is in fact discovered after the many years it takes to develop, costly changes are resisted on the basis of past practices. ("We have always done it this way.") Communities that want inappropriately located firms to move or to be shut down inevitably meet with strong corporate and government resistance. Even when the community's demands are less radical than closing the plant—such as reducing the use of toxics—resistance to change is nearly always encountered.

Since environmental cleanup—installing pollution control devices and managing hazardous waste, for example—costs time and money, corporations oppose, delay, and lobby against these requirements. In the workplace, the same tactics are practiced but the community's demand for changes is seen as a more direct threat to the corporate structure. Companies have always resented government regulators coming into the workplace and telling them "how to run their business."

Our response to corporate resistance should not be to back down or compromise the nonnegotiable demand for a safe workplace, a clean environment, and job protection. Indeed, we should see the growing corporate opposition to change as an encouraging response to our action. Our position is clear: Companies should pay for their use of our air and water and for the consequences that result from the materials they use or misuse. These consequences should not be, as management argues, the price we pay for progress. Instead, solving these problems should be part of their cost of doing business.

THE KEY PLAYERS

Using the neighborhood inspection is opening a new front in the fight to clean up the environment. It is not a substitute for the other tactics you may want to use. Moreover, the inspection is not a polite open-house invitation to tour the plant after hours. It is a walkaround inspection that generally takes as much time as the community can win and management will allow. Although it is not a detailed look at a firm's operations (that step could come later), it should be done with technical assistance and a clear understanding of issues, tactics, and goals. In thinking about a neighborhood inspection, different interests are involved: the community, plant owners or managers, workers, unions, government or regulatory officials, and the industrial hygienist or other expert you'll use. In the following sections we'll assess different approaches for dealing with these key players.

THE COMMUNITY

"You always keep your house cleaner when you're expecting company." This simple truth points to the fact that winning a plant inspection by the community can be a victory in itself, regardless of whether the plant is forced to implement the community's demands. Not only will the plant be cleaner, but the community's demonstrated concern can have a lasting effect, particularly if ongoing contact is negotiated.

Seeing the inside of a factory can be educational as well as important in understanding workers' concerns about occupational exposure. Because plants are considered private property by management, few people know how familiar household products are produced. The dirty, dangerous conditions in many factories contrast sharply with "the good life" and "gusto" presented in advertising. Moreover, the community inspection may point to violations of the Occupational Safety and Health Act. OSHA violations, although not the primary focus of the inspection, can be used to show noncompliance with the law and be incorporated in your demands for change. They can also indicate areas of concern in the plant and can be used to gain support among workers. An inspection may also point to areas where further investigation for medical problems (which are likely to appear first in workers) is warranted.

The community must decide whether the inspection will be used to confront management or to gather as much information as possible for future activities. This decision is significant, for it will determine how much the community should tell management about the inspection, the involvement of the media, and so on. Generally a cooperative strategy is most useful, but some situations may call for a more confrontational approach. (See Chapter 2 on organizing.)

MANAGEMENT

In general, management will view the community's involvement in health and safety issues as an unwarranted intrusion into its private affairs. When pressed, it will usually respond to the community as if the issue were one of public relations that will disappear with a few kind words and gestures. Nevertheless, management is beginning to understand that dealing with the community is necessary, and this trend is likely to continue.

The most effective argument to present to management is that what happens in the plant will have a direct effect on the community. Thus the effects of business decisions are also the "business" of the community. There are many examples of spills, fires, and explosions that have killed people and damaged property; the Union Carbide disaster in Bhopal, India, is the most vivid example. (See Appendix E, in this chapter, on how this unprecedented tragedy could have been prevented.)

Even routine safety hazards can cause accidents in the plant and lead to fires, explosions, or chemical spills that have serious consequences in the community. Even more important, all plants use materials that become more toxic (and widespread) when there is a fire. The 1981 Lynncorp Plastics fire in Lynn, Massachusetts, for example, produced toxic smoke from burning PVC (polyvinyl chloride) that spread through a heavily populated downtown area. Because pollution knows no boundaries, citizens have the right to participate in corporate decisions that ultimately affect their community's health.

Environmental audits and management of the toxics cycle should be encouraged as alternatives to mere compliance with workplace and environmental regulations. If management has prevention-oriented control of its processes and materials, it will have little trouble with legal compliance issues. Some industrial consultants are promoting this approach, and management should be pressed to follow up the inspection with this kind of assistance.

WORKERS

"We are the community," said a Chevron refinery worker. This statement illustrates some of the issues you'll confront in dealing with workers. It's essential for workers to understand the concerns of the community. But this is not going to happen unless *you* understand the situation and the use of unifying tactics. With an understanding of the worker's fear of job loss, management's control (especially in unorganized plants), and other issues, citizens can begin to contact workers and their unions and involve them in the campaign. In addition to simple strength in numbers, there are other reasons to involve workers:

- The advantages of a unified community/worker approach to toxics are obvious, but workers can also provide unique information to support the campaign. They may know when there are process upsets, routine discharges, or even illegal dumping that may affect the community. They may know what materials are being used in the plant. And if they don't, they have several ways to obtain this information not available to outside groups: the OSHA "Access" standard (1910.20), provisions of the National Labor Relations Act, and their own contract (if they are organized).
- When there's a union involved, it is even more important to make contact, for the union can become an ally. In one case, a group was concerned about polychlorinated biphenyl (PCB) contamination but didn't know there was a union in the workplace. When they contacted the union, they learned that the union was as concerned about PCBs as the community and reacted favorably to the group's activities.

Tactics for involving workers can include many approaches. In all cases, workers in the local plant should be invited to meetings and encouraged to participate. Workers may want to get involved simply because it's their neighborhood too. Fear of reprisal from employers may dampen this involvement, but they may be able to participate anonymously. Whether workers get involved or not, the campaign should take care not to lump workers in the plant together with management as part of the problem. Rather, you should continue to see the issues of the campaign as directly affecting workers too.

Unions that offer a basic level of job protection to their members are better able to get involved and can be approached in different ways. (See

Appendix D: A Primer on Unions.) For example, the union local is likely to have an office where the campaign can meet with union leaders away from the workplace. Goals and strategies can be discussed in this setting, including the question of how a neighborhood inspection could help workers in the plant.

Many national unions, through various programs, now have health and safety staff people who are technically knowledgeable about how their plant operates. They can be a valuable technical resource to the campaign directly or, if that isn't possible, they may be able to assist the campaign by providing educational materials or classes for workers in the plant. Through this contact, workers may better understand the concerns of the campaign and the true risks they may be facing. (A listing of national union programs is provided in the Resources section at the end of the book.) Unions may also be interested in organizing workers in unorganized plants that are the subject of antitoxic campaigns. Technical assistance, including consultation services for plant inspections, may be possible in these circumstances.

GOVERNMENT

Companies must comply with an assortment of laws and regulations (federal, state, and local) governing their use, handling, and disposal of hazardous substances. Since enforcement of these measures is often inadequate, you may discover in your campaign that the company in question is not in compliance with a number of regulations. Its violations will give you good leverage (with both the company and the regulators) in pushing for improved toxics use and waste management practices. But mere compliance with the law is probably not the main goal of your campaign, so you'll need to be cautious in exercising the various strategies:

- Don't depend on the government to do everything. The laws don't go far enough, and most agencies monitor only their own regulations. Keep a broad view of the issues, set your own goals, and think in terms of enlisting the aid of politicians and regulators to win your objectives.
- Regulatory agencies are accustomed to dealing with companies (which can be an advantage), but they do so in a friendly business climate. Forcing a company to clean up its act may lead to closed-door negotiations between the company and the regulators. Don't let this happen. Push hard for the right to participate in regulatory activities or negotiations.
- Politicians and government officials are accustomed to dealing with

the petitions of their constituents, a point in your favor. But they are also accustomed to appealing to the widest possible audience of potential support, of which the business community is a significant part. They can be pushed, but not too far.

- Avoid the trap of the negative result. When a situation is studied—such as a community health research project—and there is a negative result (that is, the study did not find excessive risk or a definite connection to a specific material or situation), there are two possible interpretations. You could conclude that since the study did not find anything, there is no problem—case closed. But you could also conclude that the study, given its scope and limitations, could not find a connection that may nevertheless exist. Overworked bureaucrats will be attracted to the first interpretation, but the second is closer to the truth in most environmental and community health issues. The Woburn, Massachusetts, leukemia cases are a good example: Until a second study investigating water consumption in affected homes was undertaken, no connection could be made between contaminated well water and the cases of childhood leukemia.

- In many cases, contact with lower-level officials in the various regulatory agencies who actually do the fieldwork can provide a more accurate picture, for politically sensitive department heads may influence their agency's public statements. It may be hard to find these people, but local resources like COSH groups may be able to help. COSH groups (Coalitions for Occupational Safety and Health) are nonprofit labor-based organizations concerned about workplace hazards. (See the Resources section.)

THE INDUSTRIAL HYGIENIST

As a society, we probably depend too much on the experts for advice and especially decision making. If an expert makes a statement, we are conditioned to believe him or her without finding out whose interest the expert may represent. Moreover, expert information is often presented in a mystifying manner in order to maintain control over knowledge that might lead to action. In fact, the community is made up of many people who are experts—experts in what is best for them and their families. Still, it can be useful to have the advice of concerned people who have initials after their names. Good expert advice can often point the campaign in the right direction, lead to useful alliances, and discredit the "you're not an expert" argument. Two cautions, however, should be kept in mind:

- Remember that your experts are not your leaders. They are part of your strategy to win demands decided on by the collective organization.
- If expert advice is useful to the campaign (and that is the bottom line), it must be understandable to community members. If your expert cannot demystify and communicate the information, find another one.

In contemplating a neighborhood inspection, a logical choice for expert advice is the industrial hygienist. This specialist is trained in plant health and safety issues and should have a good understanding of where to find the greatest toxic threats in a facility. In what may be the most successful citizen campaign involving a neighborhood inspection, the Quinsigamond Village Health Awareness Group, a local citizen group in Worcester, Massachusetts, approached the Lewcott Chemical and Plastics Corporation to do an inspection. Lewcott Chemical was the focus of community pressure because of odors and concern about potential health hazards. The community organizers contacted a local union industrial hygienist for technical help and arranged an inspection of the plant. The inspection found that Lewcott posed significant hazards to the community and was inappropriately located in a densely populated urban setting. (For the inspection report see Appendix B at the end of this chapter.)

Most of the industrial hygienists employed in the United States work for industry. These experts are not likely to be sympathetic to your community's issues; in fact, you may encounter them in their defense of the company's position. Other industrial hygienists work for state and federal agencies, and a growing number work for labor organizations or are associated with COSH groups (see Appendix C). These professionals are the obvious choice for allies. The following issues should be considered:

- Controlling occupational hazards is part of the industrial hygienist's job—and this specifically includes *engineering control*. Engineering control means eliminating the problem at the source; it means using safer and less polluting materials, changing the process to reduce exposure, and, in general, reducing the use, handling, and storage of hazardous materials.
- Industrial hygienists who work for labor organizations or are associated with COSH groups are also experienced with workers and worker issues. This experience is invaluable in making worker/community connections and addressing workers' concerns.
- Although many free services may be available through local universities, COSH groups, and regulatory groups, industrial hygienists and

other professionals normally charge for their services. Their fee will generally range from $25 to $125 per hour plus expenses. Financial arrangements should be discussed fully before the work begins.

- Generally you'll hire the consultant to do a walkaround inspection that will last a few hours and then complete a detailed report of what was found. The agreement should also cover training for the group before the inspection and availability for questions and technical assistance after the inspection.

- Management may oppose or try to limit the scope of the inspection. You should anticipate their resistance while pushing for as complete an inspection as possible, which should include at least five community representatives. If the scope or time allowed for the inspection is limited, don't abandon your strategy. You'll be surprised how much can be seen and analyzed by an industrial hygienist in a very short time. Even if the company has significant advance notice of the inspection, it won't be able to disguise what is really going on.

- There are significant differences between inspections of "user" industries and "producer" industries. Chemical producers may react quite differently to your recommendations than chemical users. These differences may not be significant when you're dealing with individual plants, but they should be understood and dealt with if necessary. The safety of the community and the work force are of primary importance.

Other experts may be useful to your campaign. In deciding whether to enlist their aid, the same issues listed above should be considered. *Chemists* study the structure and behavior of chemicals. Environmental chemists or biochemists will be especially knowledgeable about human health and environmental issues. *Biostatisticians* do mathematical comparisons of data to determine whether significant effects have occurred. They usually work on studies with epidemiologists. *Doctors* treat diseases. If they specialize in occupational or community medicine, they'll be helpful with the health effects of chemicals and with health surveys. *Engineers* are trained to design things. Environmental engineers, sanitary engineers, and chemical engineers might be especially useful in your campaign. *Environmental scientists* and *ecologists* have a broad background including biology, chemistry, engineering, and epidemiology. They can be useful in evaluating pollution problems. *Epidemiologists* study the patterns and causes of diseases in populations. They are useful if there are questions about health surveys. *Geologists, hydrogeologists,* and *hydrologists* study issues of rock, soil, surface water, and groundwater. They are useful for water pollution and hazardous waste questions. *Toxicologists* study the toxic effects of chemicals.

CONDUCTING THE INSPECTION

A neighborhood inspection is only one means of promoting a safe and healthy environment for your community. It does not preclude calling for other inspections or regulatory action, but it does allow the community to exert some control over local toxic problems. Unlike official regulators, community members can take the broadest possible perspective of the issues. It's useful to see the inspection in the context of your overall organizing strategy:

- Step 1: Recognize and document the problem. (Although the problem probably initiated the campaign, the inspection can fill in the details.)
- Step 2: Formulate demands that will solve the problem. (The inspection can suggest changes and help you formulate specific demands.)
- Step 3: Choose strategies to win the demands. (The inspection may suggest new strategies that have not been recognized.)

The following sections outline the essential elements of the neighborhood inspection.

PREPARATION

First, familiarize community members with the plant: what is manufactured or processed there and how it is done; the history of the plant in the community; regulatory activities; general observations about topography, climate, weather, water supplies, and population patterns; incidents of spills, fires, explosions. This information can be obtained from various sources including word of mouth, the local library, and general reference sources. (See Chapter 4 for tips on how to do research and obtain information.) The Preinspection Information Request (Figure 5-1) is a model for what information to request from management.

Second, consider finding an expert to assist with the inspection. In conducting a neighborhood inspection, there's a direct parallel to the practice of industrial hygiene, so the industrial hygienist is often an ideal expert.

1. What products or services are manufactured or provided at this facility? Is there a plant layout and map of the facility available, as well as a locale map showing the location of the nearest neighbors? What environmental or occupational control systems, such as local exhaust ventilation system, waste treatment, and air pollution controls, are in place at the facility?

2. How many employees work there? Is it more than a one-shift operation? Are employees represented by a union? Is there a health and safety committee at the facility? Is it a joint labor/management committee? Are contract workers used for handling hazardous waste or other jobs inside or outside the plant?

3. Is there a health and safety program at the facility? At the corporate level? (Is it written?) What health, safety, or environmental professionals are on staff? Are any available to you from the corporate level? Are they retained as consultants, or are they part of the organization?

4. Are any of the following activities done on a regular basis: environmental monitoring (inside and outside the facility), medical surveillance programs, employee training? Are respirators used on a regular or emergency basis in the plant? (Please provide details of these programs.)

5. Has the facility been cited for violations of any municipal, state, or federal regulations (DEP, OSHA, EPA, Right to Know, DOT)? What accidents, process upsets, spills, and the like have occurred at the facility in the last year? In the last five years?

6. What chemicals or raw ingredients are used, stored, processed, or discharged (into the air, water, soil) at the facility? (Please give quantities, locations, and methods of shipping and receiving.) Has a mass balance audit been performed?

7. Are there written programs for any of the following: emergency action plan, Hazard Communication (OSHA) Program, RCRA compliance, environmental contingency plan, spill reporting procedures, fire plan/fire brigade, hazard assessment (worst-case scenarios, plume maps), emergency preparedness plans (SARA Title III), or similar descriptions? (Please supply details and copies.)

Thank you very much for your cooperation in providing this important information about your facility.

Figure 5–1. *Preinspection Information Request*

Third, be sure to provide some training for those who will actually go into the plant. Remember that the major focus of the inspection is on prevention—finding situations that can be hazardous before there are any exposures or ill effects.

SAMPLING

The issue of sampling can be very complex and is often misunderstood. Although sampling is often seen as the definitive answer to questions about occupational and environmental exposure, it is subject to the same variables as other issues: How and when the samples are taken and who takes the samples can strongly influence the results. Sampling usually involves knowing what it is that you want to measure. There is no universal "hazard meter" to tell you there is a problem, and analyzing a sample for *everything* is prohibitively expensive. Moreover, evaluating sample results is open to wide interpretation. Sometimes there are standards to which the sample results can be compared, but often there are none. For these reasons, and because management will usually not permit samples to be taken during the inspection, comprehensive environmental sampling is neither technically nor economically feasible. There are some things that can be done, however.

It's always useful to look at sampling data that have been collected by regulatory agencies or by the company itself. (See Chapter 4 on obtaining information.) These data can then be evaluated by your group and by friendly experts. For example, most regulatory authorities require that samples be taken to document toxic exposure before violations are issued. Taking a preventive approach, however, one could look at these sample results and decide that *any* detectable level of contaminant constitutes overexposure. This approach is particularly useful when you are dealing with known or suspected carcinogens, teratogens, allergens, and mutagens for which the conservative view suggests there is no level above zero that does not involve some risk.

In general, sample results can be evaluated by asking three questions:

1. Is it *accurate*? Where, when, and how was the sample taken and analyzed?
2. Is it *legal*? How does it compare to known standards, guidelines, or recommendations?
3. Is it *hazardous*? According to published studies and other known information, should you be concerned regardless of the legality?

You may demand that the regulatory authorities do sampling based on the company's track record or on limited sampling done by your group or an outside consultant.

Useful information can also be collected through direct observation or simple measurements. These include:

- Bulk samples of water may show color, sediment, or odor and can be tested easily for pH (acidity), bacterial content, and other factors.
- Visible smoke, fumes, and dust may indicate faulty operation of ventilation systems.
- Smells (describe them) and irritation to the eyes, nose, and throat are important indicators.
- Some easy-to-use, direct-reading testers are designed for occupational exposure but can also be useful for environmental samples. The "universal tester" with its cheap, disposable tubes for various materials (vapors and gases) is the most practical for this purpose.
- Just knowing that a certain material is present may be enough information to act. Asbestos, for example, can often be tested by state regulatory agencies or screened using a simple and inexpensive test. Screening kits are also available for semiquantitative analysis for PCBs.

The National Toxics Campaign has the capability to conduct state-of-the-art sampling for toxic materials in the air, water, and soil. In fact, NTC operates the only citizens' environmental testing laboratory in the nation. The lab can be a valuable resource for collecting samples during an inspection. It can also be used to conduct preliminary sampling to identify toxics outside the plant gates. The data can then be used to call for an inspection and to pressure the company into making preventative changes. Contact the NTC office for information on how you can use the laboratory to do testing in your community. Questions about the feasibility and utility of various kinds of sampling and testing can be answered as well. (See the Resources section.)

THE INSPECTION

All factories have a flow of material: Raw material is received; it is moved, handled, processed, and stored; then the finished product and wastes are shipped or disposed of. It's most useful, therefore, to tour a plant in this logical sequence from start to finish:

- Receiving: What comes into the plant and from where? Is there an inventory? Are there procedures for handling different products? Are there written procedures? Are there special precautions for hazardous substances? What are they? Does management know what the hazards are?
- Handling, Processing, Storage: Remember that spills and fire hazards are greatest during transfer operations and movement. Look at the amounts stored, the arrangement of tanks and storage, exits, safety equipment, evidence of spills, sources of fire or heat, and housekeeping.
- Operations: Ask to see the operations performed. The inspection is not just to look around the plant; it is to see how equipment, systems, processes, and procedures are used. Have them explained in detail.
- Shipping: How is the product or waste shipped: drums, bulk, other means? How often? Are flammables marked? Are they segregated during storage? Are there any regulated areas? Have this all explained in detail.

The following list of questions can help you to focus on specific areas of concern. For many people this may be the first time they've been in a factory. So take your time, ask a lot of questions, and have the processes fully explained.

Before you go into the plant, these are the things to look for:

1. Is there any outside storage? Is there visible evidence of spills? Are there nearby water sources? Is there adequate security (fences, gates, lighting, watchmen) to keep children from playing in hazardous areas?
2. How close is the plant to nearby residences?
3. Are there ventilation systems, vents, or other equipment on the roof? Are cleaning devices installed? Is there evidence of discharges (stains on roof, building, ground)?
4. Are there vents, overflow pipes, or other potential discharge sites other than on the roof? Is there evidence of spills?
5. Have any wastes been stored or buried on the site (by current or previous occupants)? Are these wastes exposed? Could they be disturbed?
6. Will this company be accountable to the legitimate concerns of the community? How will community complaints be handled?

Once you are inside the plant, here's what to look for:

1. General housekeeping is a good indication of the overall program. Are work areas clean and orderly? Are equipment and materials kept out of aisles and in designated areas? Are spills cleaned up? Is there adequate lighting? Are periodic safety inspections done?
2. Are fire protection systems installed, inspected periodically, and tested at least annually? Are there adequate fire extinguishers fully charged, conspicuously located, and inspected regularly? Does the fire department know what chemicals are used here?
3. Are there any electrical problems (exposed wires, open electrical boxes, temporary wiring)? Is the employer familiar with the National Electrical Code? Are there areas where explosion-proof electrical equipment is used?
4. How and where are compressed gas cylinders stored? Are they chained? Are caps installed? Are oxygen and fuel gases separated?
5. How are flammable and combustible liquids (oil, paints, solvents, others) handled, stored, and transferred? Are safety cans, storage cabinets, and storage rooms used? Are there any sources of ignition such as open flames, hot metal, smoking areas, or welding?
6. Are other chemicals properly stored? Who checks? Incompatible chemicals like acids and cyanides, acids and bases, and many other substances must be segregated to prevent inadvertent contact. Is there a plan for bringing chemicals into the plant? Is it a written plan?
7. Are there strong odors, irritation of eyes or nose, visible smoke or fumes in any areas?
8. What do warning labels and signs warn against?
9. Are there any ventilation systems to protect employees? Do these systems have air cleaning devices before discharge?
10. What emergency and other arrangements have been made with the police, fire department, town and state officials, and federal authorities such as DOT and EPA?
11. What maintenance is done on storage tanks, processing facilities, transportation vehicles, ventilation systems, fire protection equipment, and the like? What is the schedule? Is it written?
12. Are any "unknown" materials (such as waste) handled? How?
13. Are any areas routinely monitored (inside or outside) for air, water, or surface contamination? Are there areas where workers are routinely monitored (for example, for lead exposure)? Areas where respirators (or other protective equipment) are used? Why?

14. Are there areas where carcinogens, teratogens, or allergens are used? What precautions are taken? What about asbestos, lead, vinyl chloride, arsenic, cadmium and other heavy metals, plastics, solvents, and sand (silica)? How are they used?

15. Are there emergency procedures for accidents, fires, spills, and the like? Are drills conducted periodically? What arrangements have been made with state, local, and federal officials? Firefighting equipment (extinguishers, sprinklers)? Where are emergency procedures kept?

16. Is there a list of *sources* of the materials processed? Will they change? Is information on the hazardous materials handled available at the facility? What about mixtures and potential chemical reactions? Are there any plans for waste reduction and hazardous material use reduction?

The "Safety and Health Guide for the Chemical Industry" published by OSHA in 1986 is a good question-format checklist for plant inspections. Although it was written for the chemical industry in the wake of the Bhopal disaster, it applies to toxics use in all industries.

AFTER THE INSPECTION

Where do you go after you've done the inspection? You may not have seen the whole plant in detail and you may not have seen it at its worst, but you've taken a major step that can be very useful in the overall campaign. After pausing to give yourself credit for this small victory, it's time to move on to the next objective. You have exercised your right to know about materials used in the plant; you have won and exercised the right to inspect; now it is time to sit down with management and demand the right to negotiate. What will the company do to solve the problems you have uncovered?

Just as management usually resists the exercise of your rights to information and an examination of the workplace, management will be reluctant to accede to your demands in negotiation. As you move toward the resolution of the issue, it's important not to let up on the campaign. The organizing (including workers), media attention, rallies, and other tactics should all continue and even be increased to keep up the pressure.

By definition, negotiation is a give-and-take process. Each side will try to get the most and give up the least, but both sides will give and get. Be prepared and be sure you understand the process. What is most important to your group (your bottom-line demand)? What would you be willing to give up or compromise on? These are crucial issues that should be discussed fully before sitting down with management.

A written report of the inspection plus detailed recommendations are an essential element of the inspection process. This should have been done by the consultant you hired. (See the sample report in Appendix B.) The consultant who did the inspection (and any other experts such as a lawyer) can also be helpful in the negotiating process. Now let's look at some examples of successful action after a community inspection.

When East Boston residents were concerned about vehicle emissions from a tunnel, they demanded an inspection. Their organizing effort and the attention the inspection brought to the issue eventually resulted in a change in the toll collection arrangement. Eliminating the exit toll and doubling the entrance toll resulted in fewer traffic problems and fewer emissions to the community.

After inspecting a hazardous waste disposal facility in a residential neighborhood, citizens of Dorchester, Massachusetts, used legal assistance to negotiate with the company. The company agreed to move the hazardous dumpsite to a more appropriate location, but to keep the rest of the business (paper recycling) in the same place. As a result of the community's efforts, a major fire after the move did not involve toxic waste.

With the help of local politicians, citizens of Worcester, Massachusetts, became involved in a relocation group after their community inspection of a chemical and plastics facility. The company agreed that their chemical processing plant was inappropriately located and agreed to look for alternative locations. The consultant who did the neighborhood inspection was hired by the relocation group to come up with site criteria for the move:

- Protection: The site must be selected to protect the community and maintain environmental integrity.
- Prevention: The plant must be designed and run to prevent harm to the community and damage to the environment. Plans must be made to minimize the effect of accidents.
- Public Confidence: Programs to address legitimate concerns of the community now and in the future must be developed.

In the end, the company agreed to these criteria and relocated elsewhere.

In Baytown, Texas, citizens working with the National Toxics Campaign began negotiations with Exxon Chemical Company to reduce the toxics threat posed by their chemical plant. As a result of months of discussion and review of Exxon chemical releases, the local group and NTC developed a model set of toxic prevention measures that Exxon could implement to reduce their use and emission of the worst chemicals. Appendix F is a copy of the toxic prevention report and requests for the Exxon plant. Although this report is specific to the Baytown plant, it gives you a sense of the overall goals for a local toxic prevention campaign. Remember: The inspection is only one step on the road to protecting your community. Negotiating with the polluting company is the next step. (For information on negotiating with firms on inspections and toxics reduction, see Chapters 9 and 10.)

APPENDIX A: EXAMPLES OF NEIGHBORHOOD INSPECTIONS

Target: Lewis Chemical Corp.
Inspected by: Massachusetts Fair Share (Hyde Park)
Date: March 27, 1981

Following concern about hazardous waste (solvent) reprocessing, this neighborhood inspection, the first in the nation, found serious fire and explosion hazards. The plant exploded and burned on May 25, 1983.

Target: Geochem Inc.
Inspected by: Massachusetts Fair Share (Lowell)
Dates: August 12, 1981; February 12, 1982; August 20, 1982

At this hazardous waste processor located near the abandoned Silresim Corp. site, the owner cooperated with the community and installed a sprinkler system and earthen berm and complied with other recommendations made by the inspection (with savings on fire insurance premiums). Additional inspections have been conducted by the community.

Target: Qualatron Electroplating Inc.
Inspected by: Massachusetts Fair Share (South Worcester)
Date: October 22, 1981

This small electroplater is located in a residential neighborhood. Incompatible chemical storage (acid and cyanide) and other safety hazards were noted during the inspection. Due to the inspection, a two-rinse system is now used to reduce discharged waste.

Target: Carr Leather Co.
Inspected by: Massachusetts Fair Share (Lynn)
Date: March 10, 1982

This tannery, located in a residential area, produced smells and drew other complaints from the neighborhood. A one-hour inspection yielded a description of the operation and areas for future investigation. Contact was made with the local union representing workers at the plant (UFCW) but was not followed up.

Target: Sumner & Callaghan Tunnel (MassPort Authority)
Inspected by: Massachusetts Fair Share (East Boston)
Date: May 21, 1982

Neighborhood concern over tunnel emissions (carbon monoxide, lead, diesel exhaust) led to this tour. Measurement of hazardous materials in ventilation exhaust air was recommended and other issues were discussed.

Target: Suffolk Services, Inc.
Inspected by: Massachusetts Fair Share (Dorchester)
Date: February 3, 1983

This paper recycling and disposal firm began a hazardous waste business in an inappropriate residential area. The inspection, accompanied by a television crew, received good publicity, noted several problems, and recommended a negotiated settlement between the company and the community to relocate the hazardous waste business. Owing to the community's timely action, a major fire at the site in 1986 did not involve toxic materials.

Target: Lea Manufacturing Co.
Inspected by: Massachusetts Fair Share (Metro-Everett)
Date: March 15, 1983

This chemical manufacturing firm was located in a residential area where blue deposits and other issues created concern. Some general health and safety issues were raised, but no major problems were noted during the inspection.

Target: Tillotson Corp.
Inspected by: Massachusetts Fair Share (Metro-Everett)
Date: May 2, 1983

This business and the Lea Manufacturing Company were located in an old DuPont plant where the neighborhood was concerned about waste disposal. A serious chemical storage problem was noted where hundreds of chemicals were stored alphabetically. Proper storage to avoid incompatibility prevented a potentially serious accident.

Target: Environmental Waste Removal
Inspected by: Waterbury Citizens' Action Group (Waterbury, Conn.)
Date: July 1983

Concerned about the presence and handling of hazardous waste, including chemicals, waste oils, and flammable solvents, this group conducted an inspection of the 24-acre site to learn about the operations. A four-hour inspection raised more questions than answers, but recommendations were made for increased worker training, better labeling, correction of safety problems, and consideration of relocation out of the city center. A follow-up was done in 1986.

Target: Fisher Scientific Co. (Allied Chemical)
Inspected by: Citizens' Organization for Pollution Prevention (COPP) (Bridgewater, N.J.)
Date: September 23, 1983

Shortly after this chemical packaging plant was opened in 1974, chemical odors and contaminated groundwater and wells began to be noticed. This inspection evaluated current and future remedial actions by management and recommended site improvements, better groundwater monitoring, more information and involvement for COPP, and development of a toxics reduction plan.

Target: Blue Hills & Northeast Neighborhoods
Inspected by: New England Community Environmental Elimination Project (Hartford, Conn.)
Date: October 15, 1985

Following concern about benzene-containing material oozing through a parking lot, a project was begun to create an "environmental profile" of several neighborhoods. Using land-use maps dating back to 1927 and neighborhood residents' testimony, areas were targeted and a walkaround inspection was done. Old underground storage tanks, fire hazards, electrical violations, and illegal dumping areas were uncovered, and government officials were pressured to correct the problems.

Target: Lewcott Chemicals & Plastics Corp.
Inspected by: Quinsigamond Village Health Awareness Group (Worcester, Mass.)
Date: April 16, 1986

This chemical processing plant located in a residential area had been a concern of the neighborhood since the 1950s. The inspection was seen as just one strategy in the campaign against the plant, but it succeeded in creating a "prevention mentality" in contrast to the "compliance mentality" of adding emission controls to the existing plant (since these controls would not prevent a devastating fire, explosion, or spill). Direct negotiation between plant management and the community group led to the signing of a "good neighbor" agreement and relocation of the plant. (See Appendix B, below, for details.)

Target: Monsanto Corp.
Inspected by: Massachusetts Fair Share (Everett)
Date: May 12, 1987

The issues at this unionized (chemical workers) plant included potential hazards to the community as well as cleanup of past problems. When the union had a strike (in part over safety issues), the community wrote a letter of support.

Target: Chevron Corp.
Inspected by: West County Toxics Coalition (Richmond, Calif.)
Date: March 10, 1987

Although the difficulties of a one-day "inspection" of this huge refinery and chemical plant were obvious, there was positive press coverage of the event and the report was a useful focus for the ongoing campaign. A year later, the community group persuaded the regional Air Quality Board to force Chevron to install vapor recovery equipment on its loading docks to prevent the release of benzene, a known carcinogen, into the air. The installation of this equipment was one of the many recommendations in the community inspection report. Moreover, alliances developed between the community and environmental groups, the Oil, Chemical, and Atomic Workers, and stockholders interested in preventing another Bhopal.

Target: Koppers Co., Inc.
Inspected by: West County Toxics Coalition/Parchester Village (Richmond, Calif.)
Date: October 22, 1987

Not wishing to be considered uncooperative, this unionized chemical plant agreed to be inspected. Plant management was justifiably proud of its operation and the recommendation focused on potential problems and suggestions for reducing toxics use.

Target: Walsh Chemical Co.
Inspected by: Delaware Valley Toxics Coalition (Philadelphia)
Date: May 13, 1988

Although the inspection was aborted due to management's lack of cooperation, this plant illustrates why neighborhood inspections are important. Many hazardous chemicals are used in a densely populated urban neighborhood of rowhouses with little concern for their impact on the community. A major spill and evacuation have prompted ongoing concern.

Target: Dynasil Corp. of America
Inspected by: Coalition Against Toxics (Berlin, N.J.)
Date: May 14, 1988

This small, specialty glass manufacturer has a relatively simple operation but, surprisingly, had the potential for a major impact on the community in case of a spill. Management was very cooperative and responsive to report recommendations. Several other inspections are planned and in progress with this group.

APPENDIX B: REPORT OF PLANT INSPECTION BY THE QUINSIGAMOND VILLAGE HEALTH AWARENESS GROUP

INTRODUCTION

The Lewcott/Sandman Company, makers of resin-impregnated fabrics, has been located in this mostly residential Worcester, Massachusetts, neighborhood since 1957. Since that time, there have been numerous complaints of odors, health effects, and property damage connected to emissions from the plant. In recent months, political and regulatory pressure initiated by the Quinsigamond Community Organization has resulted in some operations being moved to a sister plant in Millbury, Massachusetts, changes in the plant's emission control technology, health studies by the community and the Massachusetts Department of Public Health, and generally closer scrutiny of plant operations by outside groups.

Despite the successful and widespread activity the community has generated around the issues of concern, they are not satisfied that the problems in the neighborhood have ended. One aspect of the situation—how the operation of the plant can potentially affect the surrounding community—has not been systematically addressed. When an inspection of the plant by the community was arranged with the Lewcott management, I was called in to provide technical assistance in evaluating the company's health and safety efforts and recommend prevention-oriented changes.

WHY SHOULD THE COMMUNITY BE INVOLVED?

When considering many environmental issues such as air and water pollution, hazardous waste dumps, and health effects from exposure to chemical agents, the role of the workplace is often overlooked. In almost all situations, the source of the pollution is one or more workplaces and the ultimate solution is to eliminate the problem at the workplace—that is, source reduction. One consequence of this approach is recognition that the answers to many worker health and safety problems are ultimately the same as the answers to the community's environmental problems. Seeing the connection between the workplace and the environment is not always easy, and this broad view is not always shared by regulatory agencies. Each regulatory group has responsibility for only a particular area and tends to look at situations in terms of compliance with regulations rather than a holistic preventive approach. Combining a narrow regulatory approach with often inadequate regulations (regulations are always a trade-off between protection and cost) and profit-motivated business interests may leave the community with inadequate protection. The conditions that led to the Bhopal, India, disaster in December 1984, the worst industrial accident in history, would not have violated any U.S. health, safety, or environmental regulations.

When a situation can affect the community, the community must get involved: They have the most to lose (their families' health) when something happens; they are the experts where their interests are concerned; and their organization can push the system to work for the society it is supposed to serve. In situations like the Lewcott plant, the plant's location makes it easier to see the connections: What happens in the plant will clearly affect the community. Being involved in what the plant does is therefore appropriate and necessary.

CONCLUSIONS/RECOMMENDATION

1. The plant on Greenwood Street is inappropriately located in this residential area. It is clear that a processing plant like this would not be sited here today even though the plant has been operating here for the last twenty-five years. The basic regulatory and political approach has been to treat the odor problem as a public nuisance and to require that it be controlled. Although the Massachusetts Department of Public Health (DPH) has tried to look at the effects of past exposures, other regulators tend not to look at the past failures or to consider potential problems.

2. The potential problems with this plant in this location will not disappear with more emission controls, just as the community's resistance will not disappear. Issues to consider include:

- A great deal has been done because of the community's concerns, but surveillance will not continue at this level of intensity as time goes on.
- Lewcott's management has a typical compliance mentality. Health, safety, and environmental responses are generally one-shot efforts in reaction to regulatory pressures.

- As much as 50,000 gallons of flammable liquids are transported, handled, processed, and stored each year. Many of these substances are "dangerous fire hazards" or "moderate explosion hazards" that require special firefighting techniques. Many of these materials are incompatible with various chemicals and require special storage.
- Many of the chemicals used are suspected to cause serious health effects—for example, phenol (skin cancer), formaldehyde (lung cancer), ethylene glycol monomethyl ether (birth defects). When exposed to heat or fire, other highly toxic materials may be produced. The DPH reports that the incidence of cancer is elevated.
- The community's fears that something will happen are legitimate. It has happened in the past: In 1960, two employees were burned in a drying operation fire. Today's production levels are two to three times what they were in 1960. Also, the basic process utilized in the plant includes all the ingredients for potential fires and explosions: heat, flammable vapors, and ignition sources.
- Accidents in the plant can also lead to process upsets, spills, and other incidents. Lewcott's lost workday injury rate of more than twice the private-sector average suggests that accidents are more likely in this plant. The high turnover rate reported at the plant would further indicate more accidents. Statistics show that almost half of all injuries happen to workers on the job for one year or less.
- Business decisions that could increase the chance of upsets or accidents—such as reduced maintenance, increased production, or even process changes—are not evaluated by the community or regulatory authorities before they go into effect.

3. Given the current situation, the question is what can and should be done. Although moving the plant to another location would eliminate the existing and potential problems, significantly reducing the amount of hazardous material used here would greatly reduce the risk of fire or adverse health effects. This could be done by moving the phenol-formaldehyde line (and mixing room), plus the existing and proposed controls, to the Millbury plant. Although I have not visited this plant, it is reported that the nearest resident is much farther from the plant than at the Greenwood Street location. Of course, controls would have to be installed at the Millbury location (and the community there should get involved in what happens), but if something did happen, the increased distance would provide increased protection. An alternative to moving the phenol-formaldehyde line

to Millbury would be moving it to some other more suitable location. Arguments for the move include:

- This move would, of course, involve costs to Lewcott, but the Worcester Industrial Finance Authority has supported Lewcott with almost a million dollars in bonds in the past and could do it again.
- An important consideration for such a move is the possible loss of jobs in the plant. The Millbury plant is only 15 minutes from Greenwood Street, however, and most employees work in other areas of the plant, not on the coating line.
- Most or all of the material coated at Millbury is die-cut in the Greenwood Street plant. This arrangement could continue.
- Moving the coating line would allow enlargement of the Greenwood Street office space. Material flow considerations could be evaluated and other less hazardous operations could be moved to Greenwood Street. (At present, for example, resins are mixed at Greenwood, moved to Millbury for coating, and moved back to Greenwood for die-cutting.)

4. Whatever action is taken, health and safety in the plant need to be improved. Such areas as maintenance, housekeeping, fire protection, accident investigation, hazard evaluation for incoming new materials, and emergency procedures must be reviewed. Written procedures should be established. A cooperative, responsible, ongoing relationship needs to be established by management with neighbors in the vicinity of the plant.

5. The underground storage tanks, because of their age and proximity to residential housing, need to be evaluated carefully. Accountability for the tanks' contents is inadequate, and they may already be leaking. The attached "LUST risk assessment" model proposed by Clayton Environmental Consultants or a similar procedure should be used.

6. A community right-to-know request should be initiated to obtain the material safety data sheets (MSDSs) for all materials stored or used in the plant. These should be evaluated carefully for flammability, incompatibility, storage requirements, and so forth.

7. The emergency contingency plan submitted to the fire department should be obtained and reviewed. What is the nature of the "periodically inspected by company officers as part of their routine duties" statement made by the fire chief? Are the actions contemplated by the company, fire department, and police adequate in light of the hazards in the plant and proximity to residences (limited time to respond to emergencies)?

[The report also includes a brief history of the plant highlighting inspections by regulatory agencies; a detailed report of the walkaround inspection; and background information including material safety data sheets (MSDSs) on materials used at the plant.]

APPENDIX C: COSH GROUPS— A LABOR-BASED RESOURCE FOR COMMUNITY ACTIVISTS

COSH (Coalition for Occupational Safety and Health) groups are nonprofit, labor-based organizations concerned about workplace safety and health. Since the workplace is a major source of pollution for both workers and the community, source reduction strategies are a necessary component of every community campaign. Community activists can link up with workers and unions through COSH groups to work together for clean environments inside and outside the workplace.

The oldest COSH groups have been around for more than fifteen years: CACOSH in Chicago, PhilaPOSH in Philadelphia, and MassCOSH in Massachusetts. About forty organizations across the country have been established by volunteer workers, unions, doctors, lawyers, scientists, industrial hygienists, journalists, organizers, students, and others. Most COSH groups have minimal funding to support a small staff, although workers' compensation reform in states like New York and Michigan have provided more funding for COSHs in these locations.

COSH groups have been called a "grassroots public health movement" devoted to the prevention of occupational disease and injury. Although COSH groups are mostly involved with workplace problems, some groups have become involved in community and environmental issues. In some areas, important links have been forged between occupational and environmental health activists through community fights for right-to-know laws and attempts to deal with hazardous waste problems. In all cases, COSH groups can be a technical resource for information and a political resource for liaison with unions and workers. Specific services provided by COSH groups include:

- Materials about specific hazards and specific methods of hazard control and worker protection. COSHs have useful files, libraries, and research capabilities.

- Workshops, conferences, and courses designed to train and educate workers and others in subjects ranging from specific hazard recognition and control to coalition-building strategies.
- Technical assistance for hazardous waste, workers' compensation, OSHA, contract language, source reduction, and other issues.
- Referral services to occupational health doctors, labor lawyers, scientists, and other experts.
- Liaison with workers and unions located in areas where community groups are active.

For a list of COSH groups across the country, see the Resources section at the end of the book.

APPENDIX D: A PRIMER ON UNIONS

Unions are under attack by the same forces that fight strong environmental laws and ignore community concerns about toxic hazards. Unions are often seen by environmentalists as "part of the problem," but, in reality, union workers are people with the same fears, concerns, and desires as other community residents. These workers also care about their jobs, and the conflict over this question has kept neighbors and workers apart on many toxic hazard issues. With cooperation and understanding of the issues, unions and their members can be a significant addition to the campaign.

Unions exert a big influence on the economy that is on the whole positive. Their most important functions may be to provide a voice for working people and to counter arbitrary decisions by company management. Less than 20 percent of the U.S. work force belongs to a union, although about half of all workers work for companies that have unions in some locations. The basic organizational structure involves the local union at a workplace or particular geographical area. There are about 65,000 local unions in the United States with an average membership of 200 workers.

Above the local union level there are larger organizations of the same union, called district or regional offices, and of different union locals, called labor councils. At the national level there are national unions (many are called internationals because they represent Canadian and Puerto Rican workers) and the AFL-CIO (American Federation of Labor–Congress of Industrial Organizations).

The AFL-CIO, the largest national organization, includes about 100 of the 168 national unions. The Teamsters (the largest U.S. union, with 1.8 million members) and the United Mine Workers (UMW) were recently added, but the National Education Association (NEA) does not belong to the AFL-CIO. The AFL unions are grouped along skill or trade lines— carpenters, machinists, electricians, and so forth—and represent a different approach from the CIO unions, where all workers are in one union on a plant-wide or industry basis. Although the AFL and CIO merged in 1955, the distinctions represented by their different organizing approaches remain in many unions.

Each local union represents workers in its bargaining unit and operates within a wide range of independence or cooperation in their larger organizations. Generally there is one union (bargaining unit) at a location, although in larger companies several unions may represent different groups (production, clerical, and technical workers). In addition, amalgamated local unions have workers from different workplaces in the same local union.

Unions operate in a general way as follows. By a process of collective bargaining between the union and management, a written statement called a contract is established that details agreement on wages and working conditions. Conflicts—alleged violations of the contract—are resolved through a grievance procedure. This process involves several steps up to and including arbitration (resolution by an outside party) and the strike (stopping work until the conflict is resolved).

The leadership in a local union ranges from one or more part-time people up to a fully staffed office, depending on the size of the local. There is usually a president of the union, but the most powerful position may be called business agent, business manager, or secretary-treasurer. In the shop or worksite there are stewards who bring the issues raised by union members in their jurisdictions to the first line of management.

There are references that list the local unions in a particular area, although the Yellow Pages (under "Labor Organizations") can often give you the information you need. In working with a union, it is essential to start with the leadership of the local. Better yet, contact someone the union has worked with before—a COSH group, professionals who work with unions, or the national union's health and safety department can be helpful. This contact is likely to be a new experience for the local union as well as for your community group, so go slowly. The reward for your efforts may be a mutually beneficial alliance that lasts for a long time.

APPENDIX E: BHOPAL

The 1985 Trade Union Report on Bhopal, an international mission to study the causes and effects of the catastrophic gas leak, stated: "None of the factors that caused or contributed to the Bhopal accident were unique to the Union Carbide plant in Bhopal, India. Indeed the causes we identified are common to many chemical manufacturing and other industrial processes throughout the world. These conditions were not the inevitable result of technological progress, but discrete and well-recognized problems that could have been controlled."

In 1985, the Environmental Protection Agency released a five-year report based on limited data and limited areas: In 6,928 accidents involving released toxic chemicals, 135 people had been killed, nearly 1,500 injured, and 200,000 evacuated. Seventy-five percent of the accidents (nearly five each day since 1980) occurred in plants. If the entire nation had been included, the report stated, the number of accidents would have been nearly three times higher.

This was not the first accident at the Union Carbide plant, nor was it the first incident involving methyl isocyanate (MIC):

- 1978: A huge storage area fire raged out of control for ten hours.
- 1981 and 1982: Phosgene leaks killed one worker and severely injured twenty-eight others.
- 1982: MIC leaked from a broken valve and injured four workers and nearby residents.

In May 1982 a safety team from Union Carbide (USA) toured the Bhopal plant. Among the ten major concerns they noted was the potential for release of toxic materials in the phosgene/MIC unit and storage areas.

The word Bhopal has entered our vocabulary. For the Union Carbide Company, the chemical industry, and other businesses, Bhopal is an unfortunate chain of coincidences, a freak accident, a regrettable loss of lives. It was a losing gamble that the inadequate or nonexistent safety procedures, preventive maintenance, and surveillance would not result in tragedy. It was a business setback to be dealt with in the courts and through the media. With little evidence, Union Carbide has, for example, blamed the accident on Indian terrorists and even singled out a disgruntled employee as the cause of the accident.

For the people affected by the accident, Bhopal began as a terror-filled night that has persisted long after the event faded from the front page. At least 2,500 people died that night (some suggest a much higher toll), and evidence of the continuing tragedy is beginning to come to light:

- 100,000 people have been permanently injured.
- Fifteen percent of the 1,400 families surveyed in the devastated neighborhoods have psychiatric problems.
- People in Bhopal continue to die from their exposure at the rate of about one per day. Despite the rhetoric of Union Carbide, it appears that there are long-term health effects from exposure to the chemical released at the plant.
- Children born to gas-injured mothers have been seriously affected: Stillbirths and infant deaths are two to four times the national average.

For most people, an event like Bhopal is hard to translate into action. Our sympathies go out to the victims and we want to help the survivors, but we can't undo what has already happened. Few would dare to say that the tragedy at Bhopal is simply the cost of society's progress, although some have pointed out how important the pesticides produced by Union Carbide are to our food production. Some have argued that the "little Bhopals"— the exposures, accidents, and diseases—that happen every day are the price we must pay for prosperity. That price is too high. Bhopal must become the rallying cry to make prevention and industrial accountability our most important priorities.

In the aftermath of the worst industrial accident in history, everyone wanted to know if it could happen here. And, more important, can such accidents be prevented? The answers, very simply, are yes. It *could* happen here; in fact, it already has happened many times. And, yes, it *could* have been prevented. Other Bhopals will be prevented when people organize and demand changes.

The National Toxics Campaign is using the neighborhood inspection and direct negotiations with industry to pressure companies into "Bhopal Prevention" planning. Moreover, the new Superfund requires states to set up state commissions and local committees to plan in advance for potential chemical accidents. To find out how you can get involved in the process or demand Bhopal Prevention in your community, see Chapter 9.

APPENDIX F: TOXICS PREVENTION REPORT AND REQUESTS FOR EXXON CHEMICALS PLANT, BAYTOWN, TEXAS

FINDINGS

Information obtained by Baytown Citizens Against Pollution (Bay-CAP), Texans United (TU), and the National Toxics Campaign (NTC) indicates the following concerns regarding the Exxon Chemicals plant in Baytown.

Air Toxic Emissions

Air emissions data filed by the Exxon Chemicals plant with the USEPA indicate that, among other things, the Exxon Chemicals Baytown plant each year emits at least 45,000 pounds of benzene, 56,000 pounds of ethylene, 538,000 pounds of propylene, 42,000 pounds of toluene, and 560,000 pounds of xylene. (See Table F-1 for more details on the plant's emissions; see the discussion below on underreporting of environmental discharges.)

Chronic exposure of the community to these chemicals, especially emitted at these enormous levels, is cause for serious health concern. For example, xylene's effects include kidney and liver damage. Benzene causes cancer, birth defects, and lung and reproductive damage. Toluene causes lung and reproductive system damage.

Chemical Discharges to Waterways

Emissions data filed by Exxon as well as data gathered by the Texas Water Commission, Harris County Pollution Control District, and the National Toxics Campaign Environmental Laboratory indicate that large quantities of benzene, toluene, petroleum, chromium, and zinc are being discharged to waterways. Additional tests by NTCEL show high quantities of these compounds in San Jacinto River sediments directly adjacent to wastewater outfalls operated by Exxon. These included samples showing up to 38 percent total petroleum hydrocarbons in the sediments.

Underreporting of Environmental Emissions

The figures reported by Exxon to the EPA, as noted in Table F-1, are an underestimate of actual chemical releases by the company. For instance, while the company has had a number of accidental release incidents, according to Exxon's environmental director the chemicals released in these incidents are not included in the discharge data. This is contrary to the EPA reporting requirements.

Other data, on fugitive emissions and stack emissions, are based on EPA models rather than on actual sampling data. Water discharges reported

TABLE F-1

Exxon Chemicals Plant Emissions Based on Reporting Under §313 of the Superfund Amendment and Reauthorization Act

Chemical	Fugitive	Stack	Water	Land	Total
Acetone	4.8	2.3			7.1
Ammonia	53	5.02	2.8		60.82
Benzene	11	34	0.32	0.26	45.58
t-Butyl alcohol	8.8	140			148.8
Chlorine	0.75				0.75
Chromium	3.8		0.81	0.41	5.02
Cumene	2	0.01			2.01
Ethyl benzene	31	17	0.01		48.01
Ethylene	56	0.06			56.06
Methanol	44	1.3	0.02		45.32
Methyl chloride	59	370			429
Methyl ethyl ketone			0.03		0.03
Methyl t-butyl ether	18	15			33
Naphthalene	3.5		0.05		3.55
Phenol	0.39		0.25		0.64
Propylene	520	18			538
Sodium sulfate solution			14,000	180	14,180
Toluene	36	5.6	0.9	15	57.5
1,2,4-Trimethylbenzene	21				21
Xylene	243	331.3	0.02	23.06	597.38
Zinc		0.6	6.6	3.6	10.8

NOTE: All figures are in thousands of pounds per year.

include direct discharges to waterways and discharges to public sewerage systems, but they do not include any groundwater discharges. The water discharge data reported show large variations from sampling conducted by the NTCEL.

Chemical Accidents

Reports of the Exxon Chemicals plant from February 1987 to December 1988 indicate twenty-two chemical release incidents during that time span. The cause of the accidents included:

Instrument or machinery failure	9 incidents
Operator failure	7 incidents
Leaking seals, lines, or valves	6 incidents

While no serious injuries are reported, some of these accidents apparently exposed the community to harmful levels of toxic chemicals. For instance, on June 6, 1987, "less than 15,000 pounds" of xylene were released. July and December 1988 releases involved an estimated 2,405 and 2,900 pounds of methyl chloride, respectively.

The releases of methyl chloride are especially a concern because methyl chloride is an odorless gas which can have very dramatic effects and possibly delayed effects from exposure. See Table F-2. The Exxon Chemicals file report of methyl chloride indicated "no injuries, community concern, or loss of production." Such language gives us concern that an attitude of complacency or inevitability in regard to chemical accidents may exist among some employees of the chemicals plant.

Need for a Preventive Program

The incidents and emissions reported are an indicator that massive amounts of chemicals are being dumped into the environment, and that chemical accidents can and do happen at the Exxon Chemicals plant. The plant needs a program to ensure that in the future emissions and accidents will be prevented, not tolerated as inevitable or written off when there is no immediately visible health or economic damage.

TABLE F–2

Methyl Chloride Health Effects

Symptoms following exposure: Inhalation causes nausea, vomiting, weakness, headache, emotional disturbances; high concentrations cause mental confusion, eye disturbances, muscular tremors, cyanosis, convulsions.

Fire hazard: Flammable. Poisonous gases are produced in fire. Flashback along the vapor trail may occur. Vapor may explode if ignited in an enclosed area. Wear goggles and self-contained breathing apparatus. Stop discharge if possible. Cool exposed containers and protect men effecting shutoff with water. Let the fire burn.

IDLH value: 10,000 parts per million (ppm). The immediate danger to life and health (IDLH) is the maximum concentration from which one could escape within thirty minutes without suffering escape-impairing symptoms or any irreversible health effects.

SOURCE: U.S. Coast Guard.

Other health effects: Pulmonary congestion and edema. Mild exposure is akin to inebriation. Symptoms of exposure can continue for hours or, with chronic exposure, for several months. Mutagenic in laboratory studies. Damages brains, lungs, kidneys, and livers. Excitation and convulsions; paralysis of the extremities at threshold response level.

Detection: No odor or other warning properties. Methyl chloride is a gas at normal temperatures.

Protection: Gas masks and charcoal absorbents are not effective.

SOURCE: *Patty's Industrial Hygiene & Toxicology,* 3rd rev. ed., vol. 2B, edited by George D. Clayton and Florence E. Clayton (New York: Wiley-Interscience, 1981), pp. 3437–3536.

The best solution to toxic chemical hazards is one that, wherever possible, minimizes the use of toxic chemicals. It is not enough to stop putting the chemicals into the air, because the worst chemicals typically present fire and explosion hazards on the ground as well as air pollution risks. For instance, of the four chemicals emitted to the environment in the largest quantities, these are all considered "high" or "medium" hazard chemicals by the authoritative book *Dangerous Properties of Industrial Materials.*

If the most dangerous chemicals can be eliminated, this leaves no danger of these same chemicals being emitted to the environment by any pathway. In the absence of this preventive approach, Exxon can simply shift the problem from one medium to another. For example, scrubbers installed in the plant's smokestack may wash the xylene out of the stack only to send it to the nearby river. This would not be a good solution to the xylene emission problem. A better solution would be to avoid turning xylene into waste material in the first place or, better still, to use a safer substitute for xylene if one is available. It is well known that substitutes exist for many of the most toxic chemicals. It is also apparent that Exxon Chemicals lacks a systematic program to identify and use these substitutes.

SUMMARY OF ACTIONS SOUGHT

In view of the above findings, BayCAP, TU, and NTC request the following actions and programs from the Exxon Chemicals plant. In general, we request that the company begin to truly "manage" all chemicals in the plant, from the loading dock to the point of production to the point where chemicals go out as products. We realize that some chemicals may have to be discharged into the environment, but we do not believe that this is at all appropriate unless the company is doing all that it can to prevent this. Therefore, we are requesting that Exxon use the management approach described here toward a goal of *zero emissions* to all environmental media. We are requesting, as detailed in the following document, that the company take the following measures:

1. Establish a toxics reduction program to reduce chemical waste production, as well as the presence of the most dangerous chemicals at the facility.
2. Establish an emissions reduction program to study and reduce the emission of toxic chemicals to air and water.
3. Establish an accident prevention program to prevent future chemical accidents.
4. Provide certain information and clarifications regarding material you have previously given us, as well as an informational tour for members of our organizations.

We recognize that some of this will be a major undertaking. We anticipate that certain things can be accomplished immediately, and that other tasks may take some time. We request that Exxon Chemical show its good faith by signing a Good Neighbor Agreement in which it will commit to completing all of the tasks, as detailed below, within the coming year and to work with our organizations to ensure that these tasks are satisfactorily accomplished.

DETAILS OF THE ACTIONS REQUESTED

Measures to Reduce the Usage of Toxic Chemicals by Exxon Chemicals

We request that the managers of the Exxon Chemicals plant work with the community to demonstrate that maximum efforts are being made at the plant to reduce the unnecessary usage of toxic chemicals and the unnecessary production of toxic wastes. We request that the company commit to a systematic review of available measures to reduce the usage and production of the most dangerous chemicals and to reduce the production of chemical waste streams. This review should include:

1. Auditing chemicals used and wastes produced in each production line
2. Identifying toxic chemical reductions to date
3. Reviewing available opportunities to reduce chemical usage and waste production for each production process or operation in which a targeted toxic or hazardous substance is used:
   - Substituting the use of less toxic chemicals for the ones that are used
   - Changing the formulas of final products or even changing the types of products that are produced, so that less toxic chemicals are needed for the Exxon Chemicals plant
   - Changing production processes, such as revising the methods by which chemicals are combined so as to produce less waste in the process
   - Improving operations, such as employing better housekeeping techniques, switching to nontoxic cleaning methods that generate no chemical wastes, or using fully enclosed operations that emit no fumes
   - Recycling products in-house so that chemicals are reused instead of being disposed or shipped off-site
4. Implementing cost-effective options out of the alternatives reviewed
5. Ensuring that personnel are constantly considering the reduction alternative as a result of ongoing chemical and cost accounting methods and training in reduction options

Other Emissions Reduction Measures

Fast-Track Program to Reduce Emission and Discharge of Problem Chemicals. We request that a plan be adopted within thirty days to sharply curtail the emission of the chemicals that are being discharged to the environment in the largest quantities.

Eliminating Open and Vented Storage Containers. Storage containers that are either open or vented to the atmosphere are a major source of emissions from the Exxon Chemicals plant. It is apparent that floating roofs or other enclosures would eliminate much of the toxic emissions. We request that the Exxon Chemicals plant present us with a plan to eliminate storage containers that are open or vented.

Preventive Maintenance of Valves, Seals, and Instruments. In the past two years, the most frequent cause of accidental emissions reported at the Exxon Chemicals plant has been valve and seal failures. Other emissions were due to instrument failures. We request that the Exxon Chemicals plant develop and present to the community a plan for timely review and replacement of valves, seals, and instruments. This should include more frequent review and replacement of valves, seals, and instruments used for particularly caustic chemicals and processes.

Plan to Reduce Problem Flares. We request that Exxon Chemicals prepare and provide to us a concrete plan to identify and reduce problems at flares that tend to release particulate matter into the environment. Vent gas volumes should be minimized during offloading and filling operations. Volatile organics should be condensed or recycled wherever possible to minimize flare use.

Under no circumstances should inorganic chemicals be flared, since these emissions are not effectively controlled through flaring. Sulfides, metal-containing fumes, and acidic compounds should be recovered by packed tower absorption or similar methods and destroyed by chemical treatment. Wastewater generated by these measures must be chemically treated before primary or other conventional treatment or discharge.

Review and Remediate Water Quality Impacts. Study the water impacts of the Exxon Chemicals plant on nearby waterways, through a chemical quality survey of San Jacinto River sediments adjacent to Exxon operations. Reduce toxic water emissions and enter negotiations for remediation of these areas. Route all process and drainage water through a wastewater treatment system. Minimum treatment should include oil and water separation, primary settling, and granular activated carbon treatment.

Accident Prevention

Accident Prevention Plan. We request that Exxon provide us with their risk reduction work plan. Such a plan should identify:

- The quantities of extremely hazardous substances generated, stored, and handled by Exxon, including those that could be produced in an accident. Chemicals quantified should include, at a minimum, the acutely toxic chemicals identified by the U.S. Environmental Protection Agency under Title III of SARA and any other chemicals that either pose similar toxic hazards or pose fire or explosion hazards.
- The nature, age, and condition of all equipment involved with these extraordinarily hazardous materials and the schedules for their testing and preventive maintenance.
- Measures taken to control against external intrusions, to control discharges within the facility, and to prevent "knock-on" incidents in which an explosion or fire caused by one chemical results in a release of other toxic chemicals to the environment.
- Circumstances that would result in a chemical release and measures taken to prevent such a release.
- Alternative methods of production that might prevent such releases and why they are not employed.

Accident Containment Measures. In several cases where hazardous materials have been released from the Exxon Chemicals plant, emissions could have been prevented by double-walled tubing or other containment technology. We request a plan to ensure that such containment will be employed at every possible location where such chemicals are utilized. Contingencies for containing spill-contaminated runoff and drainage should be made. Systems should be in place for containing such drainage in at least a 100-year precipitation event.

Employee Training. Operator failure was reported to have been responsible for about a quarter of the chemical incidents reported at the Exxon Chemicals plant. Please provide information on employee training for handling hazardous materials and other health and safety issues such as fire hazards and accident prevention. Please include the written Hazard Communication Program required under the OSHA hazard communication standard. Also describe staffing and corporate responsibilities for health and safety training and capabilities on-site—including the number of environmental engineers, industrial hygienists, etc. who are on-site. Also, we request that you identify the portion of the work done by outside contractors. How is adequate training of these personnel ensured, given their temporary status at the facility?

Clarifications and Additional Information Requests

Reported Durations of Chemical Releases. Some of the release reports filed by the Exxon Chemicals plant with the State of Texas and the USEPA state that the duration of chemical releases were "zero" hours. This appears to imply that employees are not keeping track of the duration of releases or that the duration of releases is being misreported. Please clarify these reported durations and policy regarding the timing of releases.

Flare "Smoke"

1. Characterize the content. Please identify the chemical content of "smoke" reported in incident reports as being emanated from smoking flares. Particulates and volatile organic compounds from smoking flares should be sampled and characterized by USEPA certified broad-scan GC/MS methods.
2. Determine the mass weighted average destruction efficiency of flares in use. USEPA certified broad-scan GC/MS methods should be used to characterize the actual destruction ratio efficiency (DRE) of the flare as well as to determine the measurable products of incomplete combustion. We request the results of such testing and analysis.
3. Identify the remote sensing approach. What systems are being utilized to regularly sample air emissions from areas of the plant? We are aware of the "Snuffy" system outside the plant; but we are also aware of high-technology measures that allow widespread monitoring throughout a facility. For instance, in one laser-based technology a laser beam can scan a whole facility for unusual emissions released from the facility at various spots. Another approach is to have air tubes dispersed throughout the facility, which simultaneously capture

emissions from several locales. How many sites are being monitored simultaneously at the Exxon Chemicals plant and what technology is being used?

Insurance Coverage Information. In the event of an accident at the Exxon plant, there could be severe personal injuries and property damage in the vicinity of the facility. In addition to the enormous suffering this could impose on the community, it could also inflict disastrous financial consequences on the public and the company. Please provide complete information on pollution liability coverage and accidental incidents insurance coverage at the Baytown complex, including insurers' name, parameters of liability coverage, and copies of the policies.

Citizen Tour. We request that Exxon Chemicals provide a walking tour of all parts of the Baytown plant to members of BayCAP, NTC, and TU and to any experts these groups designate to accompany them.

Written Agreement and Ongoing Review

We request that the manager of the Exxon Chemicals plant commit to the foregoing requests through a written agreement enforceable by BayCAP, Texans United, and the National Toxics Campaign. This agreement should include assurances and funding for the citizens' groups to hire their own experts to review actions taken by Exxon Chemicals under this agreement. Such an agreement will serve as the cornerstone of future working relations between our groups and the Exxon Chemicals plant and will ensure that these tasks are satisfactorily accomplished.

6

Working with the Media

PETER OBSTLER

Why should toxics activists care about developing and executing good media strategies? The benefits of good media coverage are an essential factor in winning your campaign and building your organization. Good media coverage can project the message that your organization and its leaders have power in the political arena. Moreover, good media coverage gives your organization credibility with the public and allows you to define the debate about issues on your own terms. Finally, good media can project your organization's program and solution to the problem. It can give you power by raising public consciousness around an issue. Tactically, it can give your organization an opportunity to press your adversary publicly and effectively. Whatever your organizational issues and political objectives, good media coverage can help you get there.

Getting media coverage is no accident, however. It takes more than good luck. Media coverage is not a right bestowed on your organization because you are morally correct or because you are fighting for justice. Getting good media is much like getting good results in any other organizing task. There are do's and don'ts. There are basic themes that work and those that won't. You will get the desired results when you execute the fundamental nuts and bolts tasks within the context of a thoughtful and well-defined strategy. This strategy, in turn, will fit into your overall organizational program. Of course, media coverage is never a shortcut or substitute for developing a

147

successful campaign and building an organization. It is, rather, an essential part of the process.

This chapter draws on our experience in working with the media on both local and national toxics issues for organizations across the country. It delineates the basics of media coverage, discusses useful tips gathered from different campaigns around the country, and concludes with some thoughts about more complex and long-term media strategies. With these insights you can develop your own media strategies and thereby strengthen your organization, whatever its focus and scope.

DEFINING YOUR MESSAGE

The first step in developing a successful media strategy is creating a central message or basic theme. Before your organization can execute the necessary steps to get media coverage, you need to define exactly what you want to *say* through the media. A well-defined message has two key components. First, it is simple, direct, and concise. Second, it defines the issues on your own terms and in your own words. An example of a well-defined message can be found in the slogan used by Ronald Reagan's presidential campaign in 1980. The central theme projected by the Reagan campaign at every media opportunity was the slogan: "Are you better off today than you were four years ago?" The simplicity of this message is obvious. But the message also allowed the Reagan campaign to control the terms of the 1980 presidential election debate at every turn, regardless of the nature or complexity of the situation in which it was used.

Obviously, pollution prevention campaigns differ dramatically from a presidential election campaign. Toxics issues often contain a great deal of highly technical information. Reducing your campaign to a single slogan may seem next to impossible. It may not do your issue the justice it deserves. Nonetheless, grassroots toxics organizations often make the issue too complex and technical. The result is that the general public and the media are unable to understand what all the concern is really about.

An excellent example of a simple, direct, and concise media message was in the Lowell Fair Share's campaign to win timely and effective cleanup of the Silresim Chemical Corporation's hazardous waste site in Lowell, Massachusetts. Citizens from this organization relentlessly hammered home a media message that controlled the terms of the debate in the media and also built support for the organization's agenda and goals. Fair Share began all its media activities by projecting variations on a basic theme the general public could easily understand. Slogans such as "Health and Safety First," "No Price Tag on Our Lives," and "Who Pays and How Much for Safe Cleanup?" allowed the organization to present its own agenda through the media by making the issue essentially a political one, rather than a technical one.

Apart from projecting these slogans, Fair Share presented a list of demands along with the names of the key industry or government players. Any time the organization did anything media-oriented, the public knew exactly what they wanted, why they wanted it, and who could give it to them. The organization's ability to project a simple and direct message allowed them to dominate media coverage on the issue for years. Government officials and industry executives involved in the issue were almost always responding and reacting to the organization's activities and agenda. Fair Share also made the issue easy and enjoyable for the media to cover. The story of a neighborhood fighting to guarantee its health and safety was, as one TV correspondent put it, "very, very sexy." As a result, the organization not only got good coverage that advanced their issue, but got it consistently whenever they wanted it.

Defining a good message, then, is the first step in your successful media strategy. Remember to keep it simple, concise, and direct. Put it in terms that you, your organization, and the general public can understand and identify with. Then add information on your basic agenda or program—say in simple language what your organization wants, who can give it to you, and why you're demanding it. If you follow this strategy, you are well on your way to creating an excellent foundation on which to build a winning media campaign.

COMMUNICATING YOUR MESSAGE

Now that you've decided what to say to the media, it's time to execute the basic steps of how to say it. The first step in this process is designing a press advisory or press release—the fundamental means by which virtually all news is communicated to the media.

THE PRESS ADVISORY

Essentially, the *press advisory* is a bare-bones press release which simply notifies the media that your event is taking place. You should send it to media outlets about three to five days before the scheduled time and date of your event. It should be typed, double-spaced, on paper that will stand out

National Toxics Campaign
29 Temple Place
Boston, MA 02111
Telephone: (617) 482-1477

For more information:
Press Advisory: June 30, 1990   Eddie Stookems
   FOR IMMEDIATE RELEASE   (617) 779-3654

TOXIC HAZARD CAMPAIGN TO HOLD PUBLIC MEETING
WITH EPA, INDUSTRY OFFICIALS

On Monday, June 30, 1990, at 7:30 P.M., member organizations of the
Anytown chapter of the National Toxics Campaign (NTC) will hold a
public meeting with officials from the Environmental Protection Agency
(EPA) and representatives from toxic waste generating industries in Mas-
sachusetts. *The meeting will be held at Calvary Baptist Church, 26 Extoll
Street, Anytown, Mass.*

At the meeting leaders from grassroots toxics organizations will present
a detailed list of cleanup requests concerning abandoned toxic dumpsites
around the Anytown area. EPA regional administrator Travis Cowles and
Frank P. Snow from Excelsior Products, Inc., will be among several
officials who will respond to residents' concerns about toxic waste
cleanups.

The meeting will serve as a public forum to give local residents the
opportunity to present alternative proposals for site cleanups to those
already proposed by EPA and industry officials. There will also be an
opportunity for members of the public at large to question officials.

The Anytown chapter of NTC is a nonprofit coalition of citizen organizations fighting for timely, effective, and safe cleanups at hazardous waste
sites in the Anytown area.

—30—

Figure 6–1. *Model Press Advisory*

from the hundreds of other press advisories and releases the media may receive every day. We suggest a brightly colored paper such as "golden red," an almost "radioactive" shade of yellow paper, or a blue or off-white shade to distinguish it.

The press advisory achieves its goal by providing only the basic information needed to assure the media's attendance. Don't offer any detailed information since that can be obtained at your event. In fact, presenting too much information in an advisory may actually fail to get the media to cover the event. If you say too much, the news editor may cut corners on a busy news day and allow a reporter to write up your story without actually attending the event.

Information provided to the media in a press advisory should answer the five basic questions that all media require. These five questions, often referred to as the five "W's", are the cornerstones of your press release or press advisory:

- *Who?* Who is doing the event? Who is your organization?
- *Where?* Where is your event taking place? At least include the address where you're holding the event. (It may also be helpful to attach directions so reporters will know exactly how to get there.)
- *When?* The time and date of your event should be clearly readable on your advisory so reporters don't show up on Thursday afternoon for a Wednesday morning event. We suggest underlining this information on the advisory so that even the most overworked and distracted reporters will notice it.
- *What?* What is the nature of the event? You may want to include a few details about your event to entice the media into covering it. But don't provide too much detail—you want to keep the media hungry for more information.
- *Why?* Explain why you are doing your event and what you hope to achieve. Again, keep this explanation to a bare-bones minimum in a press advisory.

Apart from organizing your press advisory around the five "W's," you should provide several other key pieces of information to complete the structure of the advisory:

- Use an organizational letterhead at the top of the page listing your organization's name, address, and phone number (if there is one)—the same as you'd use for a letter.

- In the top left-hand corner, just under the letterhead, the paper should be clearly marked "Press Advisory: 20 June 1990 (the date of the event)."
- Just under the advisory notice, you should mark "For Immediate Release" (if you want the outlet to release the story in advance) or "Embargoed Release" (if you would like announcement held until the date of the event or any other particular date).
- In the top right-hand corner you should list a contact person with his or her phone number so that outlets wishing additional details have someone to contact.
- The advisory should contain a heading or title, much like a newspaper headline. This is the lead-in to the basic information.
- Every advisory should conclude with a tag—a brief descriptive background paragraph about your organization.
- Your press advisory should have a "—30—" symbol at the bottom of the page to inform the outlet that the advisory has ended. If the advisory is more than one page, the first page should end with "—more—" to let reporters know there is another page; the last page, as always, should conclude with "—30—".

THE PRESS RELEASE

A *press release* follows the same format and structure as a press advisory. But the release is different from the advisory. It is more than a notification to the press that an event is taking place. The press release answers the five "W's" in much greater detail. Its goal is to communicate to the media the entire story of what is happening at your event. In short, your press release is the complete story you'd like the media to report about your event.

While its format and structure parallel that of the advisory, the press release contains specific details you want highlighted in the media's reports. It is the fundamental means by which your entire message is committed to reporters and ultimately the public. Anything relevant to the expression of that message needs to be included in the press release.

Not only are the details of your program delineated in your press release, but the release should be laced with sharp quotes from your organization's representatives, much like the quotes found in any newspaper article. In fact, your press release should read as if *you* were the reporter writing an article about your issue and organization. Note the comparisons between the sample press advisory and sample press release in Figures 6-1 and 6-2.

National Toxics Campaign
29 Temple Place
Boston, MA 02111
Telephone: (617) 482-1477

For more information:
Press Release: June 30, 1990   Eddie Stookems
   FOR IMMEDIATE RELEASE   (617) 779-3654

CITIZENS PRESSURE GOVERNMENT AND CORPORATE OFFICIALS TO CLEAN UP TOXIC SITE IN ANYTOWN

On Monday, June 30, 1990, in the Calvary Baptist Church, more than 200 citizens from the Anytown chapter of the National Toxics Campaign (NTC) presented federal EPA officials and corporate executives with a list of 10 demands to clean up Anytown's toxic waste problems. Anytown citizens also presented corporate officials with a barrel of toxic waste that citizens said came from the Excelsior Products Company.

Mrs. Ruth Murray, a leader of the community group, said, "We are sick of being told we have nothing to worry about in Anytown. We have sick children, and many other health problems. If we don't get action on these problems within a month, we will pay a visit to EPA and stay there until they address the problem."

At the meeting, the citizens presented Frank P. Snow, president of Excelsior Products, with a barrel of toxic waste and challenged the company to reduce its toxic discharge by 50 percent over the next year. James Woods, of Anytown, in presenting the toxic barrel to Mr. Snow, said, "We don't need Excelsior using our local community as its private .mping ground. If your company wants to stay in Anytown, then you must become a 'Good Neighbor' and reduce your toxics discharge and your use of toxic chemicals."

The Anytown chapter of NTC is a nonprofit coalition of citizen organizations fighting for timely, effective, and safe cleanups at hazardous waste sites in the Anytown area.

—30—

Figure 6–2. *Model Press Release*

Unlike the press advisory, which is basically a notification to the media, the press release can be used in several ways:

- It can be used as a handout to the media at the event itself. This is important since even the best reporters will miss certain key details of your event in their efforts to cover the story. Reporters will appreciate the release. It makes their job easier. If they miss key information in their coverage, they can fall back on the release when they prepare the story for their media outlet.
- It can be sent to media outlets or reporters who fail to show up at your event. If there's a key media outlet that fails to show up but wants to cover your story anyway, they can create a fairly decent story of your event from your press release. We suggest sending a press release to every media outlet you want coverage from. You'll be surprised how much good coverage a well-written press release can generate from outlets who missed your event. (You'll be even more surprised when your press release shows up verbatim in a newspaper article with a reporter's byline above it!)
- It can stand on its own as a news item even if you're not doing a "media event." This can be particularly helpful if your organization wants to respond to a specific item, report, or decision. Let's say, for example, a company presents the results of its water test, which shows that there is no well contamination. You can immediately write a press release criticizing their finding and demanding an independent water test—a low-tech, high-yield method for getting media coverage.

Often the difference between a press advisory and a press release is slight or even nonexistent. In this chapter we have delineated the fundamental differences to demonstrate the basic aspects of both pieces. But organizations have used detailed advisories as press releases and have used press releases as advisory items. Despite the technical differences between "release" versus "advisory," it's important to understand how these basic communication items are used and to choose the one that fits *your* goals.

THE PRESS CONFERENCE

Beyond the occasional press release, most citizen groups communicate their message through a variety of "news-oriented" events. Actual events, demonstrations, press conferences—all offer grassroots organizations several distinct advantages over the isolated press release.

First, events are much more likely to make your story newsworthy. They offer reporters something spontaneous and interesting. Usually, you need to *do* something to make the news. Second, events offer reporters an opportunity to question and clarify your community's concerns. They can get more of the feeling of your message from an event than a press release. Third, unlike the press release, an event gives reporters (particularly from TV and radio news) a chance to interview your spokespersons in a setting (the local toxic dump, for example, or city council meeting) that makes your story interesting.

The media event used by most citizens' organizations is the basic *press conference*. The press conference, or the news conference, is an event that is exclusively oriented to the media. It allows your organization to speak directly to reporters at a setting and time of your choosing. Beyond answering reporters' questions, the press conference allows you to develop the event as you choose. Plan carefully so the event goes as smoothly as possible. If you cover the basic steps and divide up the preconference work in your group, your efforts will almost always result in a successful press conference.

The first component is choosing a *place* to hold the news conference. This site will depend on your goals for the event. If you're releasing technical information that includes detailed reports, charts, and maps, you may want to schedule it in a room with tables and chairs, sound equipment, and blackboard space. We recommend public buildings, particularly the statehouse or city hall, for this type of news conference. Not only do they have the necessary facilities, but they are familiar and convenient places for reporters to cover stories. To use a public building, you'll need to reserve a room at least several days in advance. It's helpful to have a friendly city councillor, state representative, or state senator request the room in his or her name. If you're holding a press conference that is more action-oriented, choose a site that adds good background to the message you want to communicate. Holding a press conference outside the factory gates or company headquarters, for example, is a good place to draw attention to a company's negligence. Sometimes a toxic victim's home is a good setting for a conference. You might also consider places like abandoned hazardous waste sites, outdoor settings with good natural scenery, or outside an unresponsive public official's office or home.

The second component of a press conference is the *timing* of the event. You want to hold your event at a time that is convenient for reporters and does not conflict with other news events. Generally, weekday mornings are good times. But a little research on what a particular "news week" looks like will be very helpful to your cause. Obviously, you don't want to schedule your event on a day when the president of the United States is scheduling a press conference. Avoid huge news events like elections, disasters, and strikes at all costs. These "fast" news days are not the best days for you to tell your story. Of course, you can never be absolutely sure your event is scheduled on a "slow" news day. One airplane crash or a surprise jury ruling can change a good news day to a very, very bad one. If you're concerned about the pace of coverage for a specific week but want some press anyway, you could try a Saturday morning event. Although there are fewer reporters awake then, Saturday is almost always a slow day. Local TV, radio, and newspapers are usually starved for newsworthy items on Saturdays.

The third key component is the *substance* of the press conference itself. What do you say when the microphones get turned on? Some of your delivery will derive from your goal and your message. Even so, there are still a few tactical matters to keep in mind. First, there should be a moderator or host, played by somebody in your organization. The moderator can deliver a short introductory statement, set the tone of the event, introduce the speakers, and control the flow of the event. Second, the other speakers should have clearly defined roles so they don't become repetitive. Each speaker should have a different angle on the issue: a mother, a factory worker, an organizer, and so on. And don't have so many speakers that the event drags on. If your event is longer than a half-hour and it's not really a hot issue, you will inevitably lose the press. Remember: A reporter's time is just as valuable as your time.

It's a good idea for speakers to type their statements (double-spaced) before the event. Not only will these statements help them with their presentations, but they can be given to reporters as part of the "press packet" they receive at the event. The press packet provides background information to reporters. It should include:

- The press conference's agenda (including the speakers' names, titles, and so on)
- Short biographies of key speakers
- Double-spaced typed statements of speakers
- A press release
- Background reports and research reports
- Any other background information such as charts, graphs, and voting records

- Other relevant news clips about your issues
- A list of all requests the organization is making

There are several other key details to remember. An organizational banner is a good visual aid that projects your group's name into the public eye. If your organization doesn't have one, you should get one for all media events. If you plan to have TV coverage and you want signs, charts, and slogans at your event, remember to do them on any color posterboard but white. If you're holding a sit-down event, remember to leave an area in front for the TV people to set up their equipment. Finally, you should have a press sign-in sheet for all members of the press to sign if they attend. This list can serve as a good contact sheet the next time you plan an event. (For guidelines on other media events, see Chapter 2.)

THE PRESS SECRETARY

Good relations with the media are essential if your organization is to receive good coverage. It's essential, therefore, to designate a press secretary in your group who can cultivate good contacts with reporters, assignment editors, and photographers from the various outlets. Virtually every organization with a media strategy has a press secretary. If you don't already have one, it's time to appoint one.

Apart from developing contacts and relationships, the press secretary keeps a comprehensive list of all media contacts, their names, addresses, phone numbers, and so on. This list gives your group a systematic way to mail press advisories and releases to all outlets in advance of a media event. You can compose this list by using a media directory.

Whenever you hold an event and want media coverage, make sure you give timely notification to the various outlets. If you contact them too far in advance, they may well forget about your event in the blitz of contacts and notifications they get during a regular news day. If you mail the release too late, reporters may already have their coverage schedules in place.

A good media strategy usually employs a mailing or dropoff of the press advisory so that the outlets receive it three to five days in advance. The press secretary should follow up by calling the outlets the day before the event, even the morning of the event. Always check to see that they've received your advisory. You can also ask them if they're planning to cover the event. There is a fine line between pestering them and failing to inform them adequately about your event. When in doubt, give them the extra reminder.

It's always a good idea to have a pocketful of change at the event itself so you can make media calls in a hurry.

THE THREE BASIC MEDIA OUTLETS

In the previous sections we looked at the nuts and bolts of media strategy. No media event, however, can be considered newsworthy or successful if the media don't show up to cover it. In this section we'll discuss media turnout and suggest ways to get the three basic media outlets (TV, radio, and print) to cover your campaign.

TELEVISION

When dealing with your local TV news station, remember that it's the assignment editor and not the reporter who decides whether or not they will cover an event. Always mail the press advisory to the attention of the news assignment editor. At most local TV news outlets there is a daytime and an evening assignment editor. Depending on which news slot you desire (6:00 P.M. for daytime events or 11:00 P.M. for evening events), you need to contact the appropriate editor. We suggest a call around 8 to 11 A.M. to a daytime editor.

Always ask to speak with the assignment editor, not to an assistant or intern. Even if a reporter says she is going to cover your event, be skeptical, since it's ultimately the assignment editor who decides what local TV news reports. This doesn't mean that developing good relationships with TV reporters is not beneficial. But all reporters have to check with the assignment editor before they can cover a story.

Local TV news is known for its snap decisions about coverage of certain events. Never count on TV to show up, even if they promise to do so, but never count them out, either. Local TV news is the most unpredictable news outlet. They often make their scheduling and coverage decisions minutes before an event. (They are also notorious for losing press advisories or telling you, after the fact, that they didn't show up because they didn't know about the event.) The extra call to the assignment desk before your event never hurts when dealing with local TV.

TV news is visually oriented and generally thin on substance. Events that promise good visuals and background are more likely to attract TV coverage than a more substantial event. TV crews are also notorious for breaking up agenda-oriented press conferences. Since they often have room for only one to three minutes of story, they prefer ad hoc interviews to give the appearance of spontaneity (rather than covering the event you had planned). A good method to counteract this helter-skelter style of coverage is to have your press secretary greet the TV people when they arrive and explain what's going to happen at the event. They in turn can let you know if they have special coverage requests you can accommodate without sabotaging your planned event. (This is a good strategy with radio and other media as well.)

Should you be lucky enough to attract its coverage, national network news is generally a different game entirely from local TV news. Their coverage decisions are usually made by the bureau chief. The bureau chief is your key contact for press advisories, mailings, and so forth when dealing with network TV news. A press advisory is rarely enough to get these folks out to your event unless it is a *very* hot story. It's a good idea for your press secretary to meet with the bureau chief at least three days before your event. Network news is usually far more dependable than the local TV news. If they plan to cover you, they usually let you know far in advance and spend a fair amount of time (by TV standards, anyway) for research and preparation.

Another type of TV coverage useful to your media strategy is the editorial slot. Editorials usually appear twice a day, several days per week. They generally precede prime-time national news and are seen by many people. To get an editorial slot, you need to schedule a meeting with the station's editorial director. A meeting may be easier to get than you think and is always worth a try.

Public affairs shows, public service announcements, talk shows, and TV magazine slots are also good bets for TV coverage. Your press secretary should always be alert for chances to get slotted into these segments and should keep a detailed list of shows and appropriate contacts. And don't forget the local cable TV outlets. While they may not have the audience of network TV, they are generally easy outlets from which to get coverage. As more and more people get cable, it will become an increasingly effective way to get your media message out.

RADIO

As in local TV coverage, it's the radio station's assignment editor or news director who makes the final decision about what goes on the air. Always mail your advisory or release to the appropriate assignment editor. Many radio stations, however, don't have reporters who leave the office to cover events unless it's an "all-news" station or has a large news staff. To get radio coverage, your organization's spokesperson has to call the station for a phone interview immediately before or after your event. Despite this problem, radio stations are an effective form of news coverage. Many people use radio stations to get their daily news.

All-news radio stations are one of the most desirable forms of media coverage. They generally send reporters out to events for on-the-spot coverage. Don't despair, however, if they fail to send a reporter to your event—it's always worth the effort to phone in your story. These stations are often equipped to give you good coverage via a phone interview.

Be careful with "embargoed" releases to radio stations. If they do a phone interview with a representative of your organization before your event and you don't want the story released until the event takes place, you must clearly request that the station *hold* the story until that time.

Like TV, radio stations may have editorial, talk show, or public service segments that are well worth investigating. Again, your organization's press secretary should make an effort to get coverage in these slots.

PRINT

Perhaps the most available form of media coverage for citizens' groups is the print media. The press includes everything from tiny weekly suburban papers to medium-sized dailies, trade publications, magazines, and large regional and national daily newspapers. Unlike TV and radio reporters, print reporters often have a fair amount of freedom to cover what they want—provided it's within their "beat" or topic area. Developing good personal contact with such reporters, as well as editors, will result in more frequent and better media coverage.

When cultivating relationships with reporters, citizens' groups often make mistakes that result in misleading or unwanted reporting. To avoid this, several rules should be observed when talking with reporters, particularly those from the print media:

- If you say something to a reporter, the general rule is that it's fair game to be used in a story. The moral: If you don't want it in print, don't say it.
- If you want to leak information but don't want to be quoted or have the information attributed to your group, tell the reporter that the information is "off the record." But be sure to tell him the statement is off the record *before* you say it. Most good reporters will honor your request.

In general, you should use off-the-record statements only with reporters you know and trust. Another way to leak information to reporters is to give them news that is "not in attribution." This means the reporter can use what you tell him without independent confirmation, but cannot give the source of the information. You see examples of this all the time in national news coverage when an article quotes a "senior White House official" or an "unidentified source." Again, use this type of statement carefully.

• If you want to cultivate relationships with reporters, provide them with information about good stories that may not be directly associated with your issue or organization. The help you give them will enhance the coverage you receive.

When you mail press advisories or releases to newspapers, send them to various people depending on the nature of the story—the city desk editor, the relevant topic or department editors, and the reporters who cover related topic areas. Don't put all your eggs in one basket.

Your press secretary should develop a good understanding of how each publication operates. Urban dailies have different assignment channels than a small suburban weekly. There are no rules on whom to contact when dealing with the print media, except to understand that each publication has its own modus operandi. The better you know your publication—its proper channels, the right contact people, its particular quirks—the better your chance for consistent coverage.

Don't forget the editorial, public service, and calendar departments of your newspaper. The business sections of major newspapers have also been covering hazardous waste issues recently. Moreover, a good number of trade publications may provide surprisingly good coverage of your campaign. One final piece of advice on the press: The more media people you contact, the better your chance of good coverage.

PART II

Toxics and the Law

7

Federal Statutes

SANFORD LEWIS

This chapter describes where our toxics rights stand today. How are the courts, agencies, and legislatures responding, or failing to respond, to the public's call for such rights? Our strategy here is to cover the range of laws affecting government and industry and suggest how to use these laws to help win your campaign for toxic cleanup and prevention. This overview of legal approaches to toxics is not a substitute for hiring a lawyer, although it may help you to converse on a more equal footing with any lawyer you hire. The laws vary from state to state. Find out where the law in your state stands on any given point. The notes at the end of the chapter will give you or your lawyer a head start in finding the law that applies to your case.

THE RELATION BETWEEN FEDERAL, STATE, AND LOCAL ENVIRONMENTAL LAW

When citizens confront a potential environmental problem in their community, they usually assume that the law will protect them. They say, "There must be a law against this." As soon as they start reviewing the laws on the books, however, they find a confusing patchwork of laws that apply to the local, state, and federal levels. They learn that the laws are not strong enough and, moreover, deal with environmental problems in a piecemeal way. They also find that even where the law appears to be strong, it is not being enforced. When reading the following chapters on the law, be forewarned that sometimes you'll need to become outspoken just to get the law enforced, and even enforcement will not necessarily protect you from

165

toxics. The law is not the ultimate solution, but only another tool in a citizen's organizing toolbox.

FEDERAL LAW AS A MINIMUM

Most federal environmental laws prescribe only the minimum requirements for control of toxics. State agencies typically implement the federal law in each state and may be stricter or require more than the federal law requires. Federal laws prohibit weaker state regulations that would allow more pollution than a federal standard. Under the Clean Water Act, for example, the EPA administrator can allow a state agency to run the federal water pollution permit program, issuing permits to each company that discharges pollutants into waterways. The federal minimum blocks states from competing for business by becoming havens for firms to operate cheaply with no pollution controls. A state water pollution agency operating a federal water pollution program cannot legally authorize activities that would violate the federal minimum. It is also supposed to ensure adequate inspection and prosecution of violators in order to maintain its authority to operate the federal program.

The federal/state framework of pollution laws allows local activists to seek enforcement of the federal minimum through different levels of government. First, you can turn to the state agency designated to enforce the law and encourage it to undertake full enforcement against a violator. This could mean issuing an order against a firm to comply with the law, seeking penalties against a firm, or even attempting to shut it down.

If the state agency refuses to enforce the federal minimum, you can turn to the federal agency that oversees state implementation (EPA most of the time) and demand action against the state. A nonenforcing state agency may risk losing its administration of the federal program. If this happened, the federal agency would assume the program's administration in the state and any federal funds going to run the state's program might be cut off. Most state bureaucrats don't want to see this happen. Even without taking away full program administration from the state, the federal agency may sometimes enforce federal minimums directly against polluters, issuing orders or penalties, or suing polluters in the courts.

Finally, in many instances, federal environmental laws allow citizens to sue for a court order to force certain actions by state or federal officials. For example, a state agency cannot legally write a permit weaker than the federal standards. If the federal standard says that no more than one part per million of benzene may be dumped into waterways, but a state agency writes a permit allowing a company to dump two parts per million, you might sue to invalidate the permit or require the state to tighten it up. (See Chapter 8 for your legal recourse.)

FEDERAL OVERRIDES OF STRONGER LAWS

While federal law is generally only a minimum requirement, often industry will object that the state or local law is either unconstitutional or preempted by a federal law. The one constitutional argument that causes problems is the violation of the Interstate Commerce Clause. Where a state restricts the import of items of commerce across state lines, the courts tend to strike these statutes down as a violation of the commerce clause. This includes restrictions on chemicals or waste passing over state lines. States can overcome this objection by treating waste and chemicals in their own state with the same degree of stringency they apply to waste from other states. Instead of banning all waste imports (which would likely fail the interstate commerce test), for instance, a state might limit the import of hazardous waste or garbage that has not been regulated or reduced to the same extent that they require within their own state.

Other constitutional arguments are generally easy to overcome. The Constitution does contain a few elementary restrictions on state and local government action. For example, it requires regulation to protect the public interest, rather than only private interests, and it blocks arbitrary discrimination in applying the law. It requires officials to respect businesses' "due process rights" by giving firms a chance to argue their case before being judged guilty. Most of the time these restrictions are carefully met by state and local regulators, so that constitutional arguments are generally unfounded. Preemption issues—arguments that local or state laws are invalidated by related federal statutes—are often more difficult to dismiss. Whether or not a state or local law is preempted can be difficult to predict. For certain subject areas, federal laws explicitly preempt state and local activity. For example:

- The Toxic Substances Control Act (TSCA) provides that where EPA requires some testing of a substance, or partially regulates certain activities related to the substance, states and localities may not adopt their own stricter rules. The law provides exceptions, however. There is no preemption under TSCA if a community bans certain uses of an EPA-regulated substance (other than in the manufacture or processing

of other substances) or if a community adopts and enforces a rule identical to the EPA rule.
- Most nuclear industry regulation has been preempted by federal statutes. Federal law blocks most local regulation of nuclear power plants, for instance, and sets forth the ground rules for states to join together in regional agreements, called "compacts," to site disposal facilities for nuclear waste.
- Many states block local regulation of the siting of new hazardous waste facilities in order to prevent local opponents from stopping such facilities.

Knowing whether local or state activity is preempted is more difficult if the statute in question says nothing about preemption. Courts often find that Congress and state legislatures have intended preemption even though they didn't explicitly say so. Preemption may be inferred where a comprehensive state or federal law occupies the field, or where an agency enacts sweeping rules that leave little room for states or localities to act.

THE LAWS

Since 1970, Congress has enacted a variety of laws to control the amount of pollution in the environment. This section summarizes these laws and describes how they may be useful tools for citizens fighting toxics.

YOUR RIGHT TO KNOW

Congress enacted provisions in the federal Superfund Amendment and Reauthorization Act (SARA) on October 13, 1986, establishing a nationwide public right to know about local chemical usage and releases and establishing community-by-community preparedness for chemical accidents. While many aspects of SARA may aid citizens in their attempts to clean up dumpsites, the provisions in Title III of the act will revolutionize the way people view toxics problems.

By October 13, 1987, any facility that is required to have material safety data sheets (MSDSs) available to its employees under OSHA regulations had to provide to a local emergency planning committee either a list of each chemical used and its hazardous components, by category of health or physical hazard, or an MSDS for each chemical. Each MSDS must contain the following information:

- Chemical or common name of the substance (or the name of its hazardous component if it is a mixture)
- How the substance is identified on its label
- Physical and chemical characteristics
- Physical hazards
- Health hazards, signs of exposure, medical conditions it might aggravate
- Primary route of entry to human body
- Threshold exposure limit
- Whether it has been found to be carcinogenic
- Precautions for using the chemical or risking contact with it, including recommended engineering and work practices
- Emergency first aid procedures for exposure to the chemical

This MSDS information was previously available only to employees or where state or local law provided it. With implementation of this rule the information will become available to anyone who seeks it from the local emergency planning committee. If the committee does not have the MSDS you are looking for, they must request it from the facility and then make it available to you.

CHEMICAL INVENTORY FORMS

Beginning March 1, 1988, facilities were required to quantify their chemical usage by submitting inventory forms on categories of hazardous chemicals. These forms indicate both the average daily amounts and the maximum amounts present at a facility during the preceding year. The forms also include the general location of the chemicals at the facility. This information, known as a "Tier I" inventory, must be submitted to the local emergency planning committees, state commissions, and fire departments and must be made available to the public through the committees and commissions.

Firms are also required to complete "Tier II" inventory forms. These contain the exact chemical or common name of each hazardous chemical and its manner of storage and location. This Tier II form may be requested from a facility by a local committee or state commission and provided to the public. If you seek this Tier II information and the local committee or state commission has it in their files, they must give it to you upon your written request. Only the exact location of a substance in the facility may be withheld from you (at the facility owners' request). If the committee or commission does not have this information, then it must, within forty-five days of your inquiry, at least request from the facility Tier II information on any hazardous substance that was present at any time in the last year in an amount over 10,000 pounds.

ANNUAL ACCOUNTING OF TOXIC RELEASES

Starting July 1, 1988, additional information was made available to the public quantifying the toxic chemicals entering the environment. Under this Section 313 requirement, facilities with more than ten employees who manufacture, process, or use certain chemicals are required to specify the following for each toxic chemical:

- Whether it is manufactured, processed, or used, and the manner of use
- Estimated maximum amount present at any time during the preceding year
- Treatment or disposal method for each waste stream carrying the chemical and an estimate of the method's efficiency
- Quantity of the toxic chemical entering each environmental medium

The toxic chemical release form containing this information (also known as an industrial survey) will be required to be submitted annually until at least 1993. The EPA administrator is authorized to reduce the frequency of reporting after that date.

OTHER INFORMATION ON CHEMICAL HAZARDS

The first step in assessing a company's accident hazards is to obtain an analysis conducted by the firm in question. Under Title III of SARA, Local Emergency Planning Committees (LEPCs) are clearly empowered by the broad authority of Section 303(d)(3) to ask facility owners or operators to disclose any information that may be useful to the emergency planning process. This should be construed to include chemical accident hazard assessments. While the law does not specify what should be included in such an assessment, experts note that it should include sufficient information to determine:

- Evacuation distances or lethal dosage distances based on frequent and adverse weather conditions (using dispersion analyses) for each extremely hazardous substance

- All plausible types of accidents and the extent of damage likely from them
- All assumptions used in the assessment

TRADE SECRETS

The new federal right-to-know law permits certain circumstances under which firms may withhold from the public the specific identity of chemicals that would otherwise be disclosed. Even if the specific name is withheld as a trade secret, the facility must disclose all other information required, substituting the generic class of chemicals for the specific chemical's name. In order to claim this privilege, a facility owner or operator must be able to show that:

- The specific identity has been treated and will be treated confidentially.
- The identity is not required to be disclosed by other law.
- Disclosure would likely cause substantial competitive harm.
- The identity could not be discovered by reverse engineering.

To claim secrecy, at the time a company submits a form or report that would have contained the secret information it must substitute the generic class name; it must explain in the submittal the specific reasons why the preceding four points justify withholding the information; and it must submit the omitted information itself to the EPA. Later the company may be required by the EPA to provide more detailed information to back up its secrecy claim. If its assertion of trade secrecy is found by the EPA to be inaccurate and frivolous, EPA may assess a penalty of $25,000.

Initiating a review of a claim of trade secrecy is a relatively simple matter. You simply submit a petition to the EPA in opposition to a secrecy claim. The receipt of your petition triggers a requirement for EPA to review the claim. Within thirty days EPA must determine whether the assertions made to support the claim of the privilege would, if true, meet the legal tests to justify confidentiality. If so the EPA must request from the claimant detailed information to prove the truth of the assertions. Based on this information, EPA is required to make a determination as to the truth of the secrecy claim within nine months of your original petition. If the EPA fails to reach a final decision on your petition within that time, you can bring a civil suit against the agency.

GUIDELINES FOR ACTION

- Use your right to know in order to obtain information needed to determine what chemicals are used by local facilities and the hazards they may present. Consider going beyond the basic information provided by the right-to-know law to obtain more information that you need to assess the facility and to call for reduced toxics usage and emissions, as well as an on-site inspection of conditions at the facility. (See Chapter 9 for strategy ideas; see Chapter 5 on neighborhood inspections.)
- Tap the federal right-to-know database, which contains all the company-by-company chemical release information reported under Section 313 of SARA. With a computer and a modem, you can gain direct access to find out how much of what chemicals are being emitted into your local air and water. Contact TOXNET at 1-800-638-8480 for more information. You can write to them at Medlars Management Section, National Library of Medicine, 8600 Rockville Pike, Bethesda, MD 20894.
- Petition the EPA in opposition to trade secrecy claims if access to a specific chemical name might be useful. Frequent petitioning by citizens helps to ensure that facilities do not assert the privilege lightly.
- Participate in EPA's decision making. In contrast to triggering an EPA review of secrecy claims, participating in the process of deciding whether a chemical identity is secret may be much more cumbersome. Much of the information submitted in defending the claim of trade secrecy is guaranteed to the public. Yet no formal process is provided for the EPA to invite public participation in its decisions on secrecy. A strong effort by your organization may help get your concerns considered in the decision.
- Use your right to sue to know. The new right-to-know law gives citizens the right to sue facilities and agencies who are not in compliance with the right-to-know provisions. Sixty days prior to commencement of your suit you must notify the party being sued; in a suit against a facility, you must also notify the EPA and the state. The court may order your expenses to be paid by defendants, including attorney's and expert witness fees.
- Seek enforcement action. As of January 1989, the EPA estimated that as many as 15,000 companies were in noncompliance with at least one component of the right-to-know requirements. The federal right-to-know law (Section 326) grants citizens and LEPCs the power to bring

civil suits to force information disclosure. Section 325 provides EPA with the power to assess penalties administratively (without prior court action) for violations of the federal right to know. You can bring a suit yourself or call on officials to act.

CLEANUP OF HAZARDOUS WASTE DUMPS

There are more than 30,000 hazardous waste sites littered across the American landscape. Most of them are not being "cleaned up," despite the fact that there are laws in place to accomplish this. This section describes the laws and explains why they have failed to protect the public.

THE LAW

Two federal laws are focused on the cleanup of hazardous waste dumpsites. The Comprehensive Environmental Response Compensation and Liability Act (CERCLA, also known as Superfund) establishes a broad federal/state program for cleanup of hazardous waste dumps.[1] EPA has broad authority to clean up dumpsites listed on the National Priority List (NPL). Parties responsible for creating the sites, including waste generators, transporters, and dumpsite owners and operators, are held strictly liable for cleanup of their sites. EPA can clean up a site and assess the costs against these parties afterward. The Superfund allows up-front expenditures by EPA to pay for cleanups and to cover costs where "responsible parties" fail to do so.

In addition to CERCLA, the Resource Conservation and Recovery Act (RCRA) also can apply to cleanup. While RCRA primarily regulates safety precautions at hazardous waste facilities that continue in operation today, it also has strong provisions potentially relevant to cleanup, if any part of a facility was in operation during the 1980s.

THE SUPERFUND PROCESS

CERCLA sets forth a procedure for assessing and cleaning up potential hazardous waste sites. First, results of a preliminary assessment (PA) and a site investigation (SI) determine if a site presents a serious enough threat to be put on the National Priority List of hazardous waste sites upon which EPA will take action. Sites on this list undergo testing and monitoring, referred to as remedial investigation (RI), to evaluate the dangers they present. The RI report sets forth the threats presented by the site that will be addressed in the remedial schemes to be developed.

The next step is the feasibility study (FS), which sets forth the cleanup goals (preventing contamination of groundwater, for example, or making the site usable) and discusses alternative strategies for achieving those goals. The FS report recommends one or more of the alternatives, based on feasibility and cost. A public comment period follows the publication of the FS, and significant comments must be responded to by the EPA.

From the outset, EPA's management of Superfund has been riddled with scandal and disappointment. During the early years, EPA administrator Ann Gorsuch and Superfund chief Rita Lavelle were implicated in attempts to allow waste generators to conduct quick, "bargain basement" cleanups and evade liability for any further cleanup. Later the faces changed, but the results did not markedly improve. The program continued to move slowly and accomplished little permanent cleanup. Of the 880 sites on the National Priority List, fewer than 10 had been deemed cleaned up by the EPA as of mid-1986. And even at the sites that were "cleaned up," the EPA had largely taken only temporary measures to contain the toxics at the sites or move them from one site to another.

A comprehensive study of the Superfund program conducted by the National Toxics Campaign in December 1985 found that in about 85 percent of the instances where the EPA had made final decisions on cleanup plans, the plans either called for containment or movement of waste from one site to another. As a result of grassroots action following this study, the law was strengthened in 1986 with provisions to help bring about faster and more effective remedial action at sites. These new provisions can make a difference if citizens continue to use proven tactics and build strong local organizations to press for action on their sites. Here are the key provisions:

- Funding of Superfund shot up from $1.6 billion for the first five years to $9 billion in the second five years.
- The EPA is required to begin cleanups at no fewer than 375 sites over five years. Remedial investigations and feasibility studies must be done at no fewer than 650 sites.
- Technical assistance grants are to be made available to community groups.
- The new Superfund corrected certain defects in EPA's public participation approach. For example, in the past the EPA tended to publish and seek comments on a "laundry list" of possible technologies for cleanup of sites. This practice never gave citizens an opportunity to focus their comments or to criticize the details of a single proposal. The 1986 amendments require the EPA to state its proposed solution and to allow

public comment on that proposal. The new law also requires the EPA to respond to all significant comments received.[2] Although these provisions constitute a stronger tool for activists to force effective action, they are only a tool, not a self-executing solution to the shortcomings of the Superfund program.

- Superfund as amended requires permanent cleanup wherever it is feasible. But the EPA has not rushed to comply with this mandate. According to a study of EPA activities conducted by the congressional Office of Technology Assessment (OTA), 42 percent of remedial actions approved by EPA during 1987, the year after the amendments were enacted, involved land disposal and containment, not permanent cleanup. Moreover, the EPA justified these inadequate cleanup strategies unlawfully. By law, EPA is allowed to consider cost only after having chosen effective permanent alternatives and solutions that will adequately protect health. The EPA is never justified in selecting a short-term remedy (like landfilling or capping) simply because it is cheaper than a permanent alternative.[3] But this approach was not being followed. Also contrary to the law, EPA seldom analyzes the risks of future failures, damages, and cleanups when it recommends containment or landfilling. A typical EPA "remedial action" may dig up wastes at one site and then rebury them in another landfill. Often the new landfill does not even meet hazardous waste management requirements under RCRA, such as liners and groundwater monitoring.
- The amendments authorized $15 million to begin the removal of lead-contaminated soils in the worst-contaminated urban areas. The problem of lead in soils is one of the nation's most serious urban toxic problems.

GUIDELINES FOR ACTION

Monitor and participate in negotiations between government and responsible parties at Superfund sites. Use the deadlines under the Superfund law's settlement process in dealing with negotiations between EPA and responsible parties. The law blocks the EPA from taking certain actions for a designated period of time after giving notice to responsible parties of its intention to negotiate. The EPA cannot commence a remedial investigation or feasibility study for ninety days after giving responsible parties notice and cannot commence remedial action for six months after giving such notice. While the law does not strictly block the agency from negotiating longer than that, your group can create a public demand that these deadlines be viewed as the time by which negotiations must end. Moreover, responsible parties have sixty days after receiving a notice of negotiation from the EPA to propose to undertake or finance a solution (for a remedial investigation and feasibility study or for remedial action).[4] The EPA has discretion to accept or reject the proposal. If no proposal is made by the sixty-day deadline, or no agreement is reached within these ninety-day or six-month time frames, then the EPA has waited long enough. The passing of one of these deadlines is an appropriate occasion to call for immediate EPA action—to call on the EPA to begin spending Superfund money to correct the problem. This would leave the responsible parties with liability to repay the agency possibly three times the costs incurred by EPA.

Consider calling for local health studies funded under Superfund. Use the law's requirements for the Agency for Toxic Substances and Disease Registries (ATSDR) to monitor health effects in the community from toxic exposure. At every National Priority List site, ATSDR is required to assess the potential health impacts of exposure. It can recommend exposure reduction measures, such as relocation of residents, and can also recommend and fund data gathering, studies, and periodical medical screening of local populations for disease risks created by exposure.

Petition to get the site reviewed and listed on the NPL. The amended Superfund law gives citizens the right to petition for assessment of a site. You can file a petition with the EPA for site assessment. If the release of chemicals noted was not previously reviewed, EPA's assessment must be completed within one year of the petition and, if appropriate, an evaluation must be conducted for NPL listing. Usually a site is placed on the NPL according to its score on the Hazard Ranking System (HRS), which incorporates data on population, quality and quantity of waste, evidence of contamination of soil and water, and other parameters. Your group can examine the scoring sheets for omissions of important data (such as failure to monitor air quality) or errors in analyzing them (such as choosing a substance that is not the most toxic material present). Even if the site does not qualify under the HRS, your group can exert pressure on the EPA, via your state governor's office or members of Congress, to use its power to place the site on the list.

Get immediate dangers eliminated immediately. Whether your site is listed on the NPL or not, if it presents "imminent and substantial dangers" you can request the EPA or your state to take immediate remedial action. If a simple request does not seem to be enough, try triggering a response with a demonstration at the EPA or state offices, a press conference with a concerned physician or health official, and a media event, such as a mock "hazardous waste cleanup day." The National Toxics Campaign may be able to assist you by using its Environmental Laboratory to conduct sampling on or near the site.

Get long-term action on your site by using Superfund. Let the EPA know from the start that you are serious about demanding an effective permanent cleanup. Choose the issues that are most critical to you, develop your position, organize around it, and get your proposals in before the decisions are made. Help your EPA officials shape a community relations program that will maximize direct interaction with community groups. Urge them to set up formal hearings at several critical points in the process. Learn how to use the cleanup information center (for example, your library) that is required to provide public access to key Superfund documents.

There are a number of points in the Superfund process where community action can be valuable:

- When the remedial investigation is completed, examine the report. Make sure that it covers every potential threat from the site and demand additional testing and monitoring if any potential hazards have not been adequately examined.
- Comment on the feasibility study. Make your point of view known both at public meetings and through written comments. Make sure the plan meets the legal environmental standards and that sensible alternatives are not eliminated without adequate reason.
- Examine the remedial design to assure that the plan minimizes health threats to the community during any excavation or construction. Insist that there is an emergency plan in case of accident.
- During the cleanup, make sure that work is progressing as planned.
- During maintenance and operation phases, keep informed. Get cleanup reports from the state and ask to be notified if there are any problems.
- Apply for technical assistance funds. Make your participation in the Superfund process effective by applying for a technical assistance grant. These federal grants are provided so that those who are directly affected by a Superfund site can make an independent evaluation of the actions taken by EPA. Grants are available for community groups to hire experts in interpreting information relating to a local Superfund site and its cleanup. One grant of up to $50,000 can be made for each Superfund site, though a group might obtain more than this by requesting that its grant be renewed or by gaining a waiver of the limitations by EPA. The community must provide 20 percent of the amount granted (in funds or services), but this requirement too can be waived by the EPA in compel-

ling cases. Although the grants may not be used to finance legal actions, the information obtained with grant funds can be used in legal actions.
- Use RCRA closure requirements to clean up existing dumpsites. RCRA may be useful in cleaning up your local dumpsite if the site was receiving wastes during the 1980s. RCRA authorizes EPA cleanup enforcement without the cumbersome Superfund process of either declaring a site an emergency or placing it on the National Priority List.

The three key ways to bring a site's cleanup into the RCRA process are:

1. Direct disposal or treatment of hazardous waste on land after July 1982. If land disposal or treatment of hazardous waste has taken place on the property after July 26, 1982, RCRA cleanup requirements for that area are likely to apply.
2. Operation of any hazardous waste activity that requires a RCRA permit after November 8, 1984. If any part of the facility obtained (or legally should have obtained) a permit after November 1984, the firm must clean up hazardous waste in "land disposal units" on the site, regardless of whether they are located in the designated RCRA activity.
3. Failure to completely clean up a hazardous waste land treatment or disposal unit operating after November 1984. RCRA facilities failing to clean up closed hazardous waste surface impoundments, landfills, and the like are required to obtain a postclosure permit, and this requirement triggers the mandate for corrective action.

If RCRA requirements apply, cleanup of the site may include the following elements.

Closure Plan

If the facility disposes or treats hazardous waste on land, it must submit closure plans either 180 days before closure or within 15 days after ordered to do so by EPA. The closure plan must include:

- A description of how and when the facility will be closed and meet applicable closure standards
- An estimate of the maximum amount of waste in the facility at any time during the life of the facility
- A description of the steps needed to decontaminate facility equipment

- The total time required for closure (for a landfill, for example, the time required to treat and dispose of all waste inventory and to place a final cover)

Questions for Reviewing a Closure Plan

- Does the closure plan consider all the contaminants and all the environmental and health problems this contamination could cause? Is off-site contamination addressed?
- Does the plan for testing the environment include appropriate substances and locations given the history of the site?
- Will cleanup, especially of soil and groundwater, be adequate? Will the contaminants be cleaned up to meet federal drinking water standards or background level? RCRA presumes that hazardous wastes will be cleaned up to background (precontamination) levels or at least to drinking water standards. However, the EPA or the state frequently attempt to establish an "alternative concentration limit," a higher level of contamination that, legally, must be justified by the agency. Thus citizens often find themselves at loggerheads with agency officials proposing to undermine this RCRA presumption of full cleanup.
- Will the facility remove all of the hazardous waste? (If not, see the postclosure requirements described below.)

If EPA is persuaded that a company's proposed closure plan is inadequate, the agency can order a closing facility to do more cleanup, rewrite the plan, or conduct more testing. You should be prepared with maps, photos, a history of the uses at the site, and any other evidence that will show the flaws in the cleanup plan. If the closure plan approved is inadequate, financial assurance levels based on the plan may also be inadequate. The site could one day compete with thousands of other sites for state or federal Superfund money to pay for cleanup.

Postclosure Plan and Permit

One of the key questions to ask in reviewing a closure plan is: Do they plan to "close clean"? Land disposal and treatment facilities including surface impoundments and landfills closing after the early 1980s must leave no contaminated subsoil. To avoid the law's rigorous postclosure requirements, a land disposal facility that received hazardous waste as defined under

RCRA must (1) have closed in accordance with state or local law before November 19, 1980, when federal RCRA regulations became effective or (2) have stopped receiving hazardous waste by July 26, 1982, and certified closure to the EPA by January 26, 1983. Otherwise the facility must meet extensive postclosure requirements:

- Prepare a postclosure management plan with groundwater monitoring, leachate collection, and full facility maintenance plan.
- Obtain a postclosure permit with full public review.
- Comply with financial responsibility requirements to ensure the availability of money for postclosure care of the site.
- Ensure the safety of the site and describe the monitoring and maintenance planned.
- Clean up all waste areas on the site, not just current hazardous waste handling areas. Toxics in any previous or current waste handling area at the site must be cleaned up regardless of whether that area is itself considered a hazardous waste treatment, storage, or disposal facility.

Old Dumpsites at RCRA Facilities

One of the most powerful legal handles under RCRA is the requirement for broad facility cleanup—far beyond what is mandated under other federal laws. Any RCRA permit issued for the treatment, storage, or disposal of hazardous wastes after November 8, 1984, must include requirements for corrective action for releases of hazardous waste from any solid waste disposal area at the facility, regardless of when that area received waste. This means that old landfills, even though they existed on-site before RCRA took effect, must be controlled and cleaned up where RCRA wastes continue to be treated, stored, or disposed of in a manner requiring a permit. To ask EPA questions about these applications of RCRA, call the RCRA hotline at 1-800-424-9346.

REGULATION OF HAZARDOUS WASTE

The Resource Conservation and Recovery Act (RCRA) regulates the treatment, storage, and disposal of hazardous wastes that are generated today.[5] This law is intended to prevent today's wastes from winding up in tomorrow's Love Canals. The materials regulated as "hazardous waste" are defined in detail in EPA regulations.[6] Generally the material must be a waste—a material that is either discarded or being stored or treated prior to discarding—or a material that has served its intended purpose. It is considered a hazardous waste if it meets any of the EPA characteristic tests for hazardous wastes (ignitability, reactivity, corrosivity, or toxicity) or if it is specifically named by the EPA as a hazardous waste or is a mixture that contains such "listed" wastes.

The definitions include numerous loopholes in which certain materials that would otherwise fit into one of these categories are not considered hazardous wastes. Materials excluded from "hazardous wastes" include many dangerous substances that are so prevalent they were excluded largely to reduce the burden on government of regulating them. These substances, which include incinerator ash and arsenic-treated wood wastes, can still be very dangerous and should be tightly controlled at the state and local levels. Other materials excluded from RCRA regulation include wastes regulated under other federal laws (such as certain radioactive materials and pollutants covered by the EPA water pollution program) and wastes produced by "small generators," those producing less than 220 pounds of waste per month.

EPA regulations cover many aspects of handling hazardous wastes—from the point of storage at the site of generation to the disposal site. Under this law, firms must prepare detailed facility plans for waste treatment, storage, and disposal; prepare emergency preparedness and facility closure plans; obtain insurance to demonstrate their financial responsibility; and comply with facility safety specifications. RCRA regulations also pertain to cleanup of sites that have been in operation since the rules took effect in the early 1980s. Congress recognized that the operation and siting of new facilities would depend heavily on community acceptance. Therefore, RCRA cleanup provisions are geared to ensuring that facilities operating today will not become tomorrow's Superfund sites. The law makes it tougher for a firm to abandon or ignore a site than it was in the past. Even after an RCRA landfill is closed, for example, the law specifies legal obligations for the owner to continue to care for the site and maintain financial backup to ensure that care.

Amendments to RCRA enacted in 1984 contain waste minimization provisions that require every generator of more than 1,000 kilograms/month of hazardous waste to file reports with the EPA every two years to demonstrate that:

- It has a program to reduce the volume or quantity and toxicity of this waste to the degree determined by the generator to be economically practicable.

- The proposed method of treatment, storage, or disposal minimizes the present and future threat to health and the environment.[7]

Moreover, the EPA is required by the 1984 RCRA amendments to prohibit the land disposal of untreated waste unless the dumper can show that there will be no migration from the disposal unit for as long as the waste remains hazardous.[8] Any waste that might migrate must be treated so that its toxicity and mobility are minimized prior to land disposal.

PROGRESS

There has been some progress under RCRA. Many of the worst facilities have been closed or are in the process of being shut down and cleaned up. The 1984 amendments contain the key waste minimization and land disposal restrictions. The amendments also include requirements for a large number of disposal sites to close beginning November 8, 1985, if they were out of compliance with groundwater monitoring or insurance requirements. According to David Lennett of the Environmental Defense Fund, as much cleanup occurred under RCRA in the late 1980s as under Superfund.

Nevertheless, the facilities that will remain open can continue to cut corners on safety by reliance on numerous regulatory loopholes:

- Land Disposal and Underground Injection: Despite strong provisions of the law to virtually preclude landfilling and underground injection of wastes, these environmentally hazardous waste disposal methods continue to be used and condoned.
- Storage Tanks: The location of storage tanks is not adequately regulated in relation to residences and water supplies.
- Recycling/Reuse: Exemptions from regulation are given for recycling of wastes. Beware of sham recycling!
- Incineration: The emissions from the smokestack of a hazardous waste incinerator are not fully regulated. For example, EPA has failed to set rules controlling the by-products of hazardous waste burning, even though these by-products may be more toxic than what is put into the incinerator. A facility may put in PCBs and get out dioxin, but the EPA doesn't require dioxin monitoring.
- Insurance: Facilities are required by EPA regulations to prove their financial responsibility to ensure compensation of the public in the event that a facility causes property damage or sickness. Yet no cover-

age is required after a facility's closure, even though environmental contamination or illness may emerge many years after closure. The amount of coverage required by the EPA is low ($1 million per incident). Incinerators and underground storage tanks are not required to hold insurance for slow leaks and slow public exposure, even though these are the biggest risks at these facilities. Hazardous waste insurance policies are legally allowed to have loopholes excluding birth defects, cancer, and depressed property values from coverage. Companies with substantial assets are even allowed to use them as their proof of financial responsibility. This "self-insurance" is allowed by the EPA even though a firm that is in good financial shape today might make a mess next week and then quickly go broke.

- Waste Minimization: The waste minimization provision in the 1984 RCRA amendments was only a small step toward bringing serious waste reduction. Under the provision and the EPA regulations that implement it, companies that refuse to do any waste reduction are largely shielded against enforcement action by the EPA. Waste generators need only submit a vague report of their progress every two years. It appears from the EPA's comments thus far, and from the legislative history, that generators will be free from EPA pressure to reduce their wastes. (For a detailed local strategy to move companies to reduce toxic chemical usage and waste, see Chapter 9.)
- Waste Exclusion or Nonenforcement: Some wastes that should be regulated are not. Some dangerous wastes have been expressly excluded by the EPA from regulation under RCRA; others, such as toxic ash from municipal waste incinerators, have not been expressly excluded. But the law is honored more in the breach than in compliance. The EPA and most states have chosen not to block placement of these toxic wastes in ordinary landfills, despite the dangers posed to the environment and the clear violation of the law that is involved.

GUIDELINES FOR ACTION

- Campaign locally and statewide for company toxic reduction programs.
- Review and challenge RCRA permits for facilities in your area.
- Find out when permits or renewals are due for local facilities. For many facilities a detailed "Part B" RCRA application is likely to be reviewed for the first time within the next few years. Call for a hearing and testify.

- Noncompliance can be addressed at any time; file formal complaints if you know of existing violations.
- In many cases, it may be possible to open a permit to changes at any time. Find out whether a "reopener" clause is included in the facility's permit to allow you to force immediate changes in the conditions for its operation.
- Many states have special regulations or siting laws in addition to their state RCRA program. Find out whether local regulation of hazardous waste facilities is allowed in your state; consider possible uses of fire code regulations and water supply rules.
- See the suggestions on page 178 as a guide to using RCRA for cleanup of dumpsites that were operational during the 1980s.

SAFE DRINKING WATER

Until recently Americans took for granted the guarantee that the water coming out of their taps was safe. This belief has changed during the past decade as hundreds of toxic chemicals have been detected in public water supplies nationwide. Unfortunately, the laws designed to protect our drinking water are weak and poorly enforced.

THE LAW

The Safe Drinking Water Act (SDWA) is geared to protecting public water supplies—those supplies serving at least fifteen locations or at least twenty-five people.[9] A short list of water contaminants and the maximum contaminant levels (MCLs) legally permitted for each has been set by the EPA. The EPA can order water supplies to shut down or to meet a timetable for reducing contaminants if a contaminant exceeds an MCL. In addition to the list of substances with legally binding MCLs, the EPA has designated certain other substances to be tested:

- Organic Chemicals: The EPA requires certain water supplies to be tested for organic chemical contamination.[10] Each supply system covered in this requirement is given a schedule for testing water sources and treated water.[11] While the EPA has not set MCLs for most of these chemicals, it has issued legally nonbinding guidelines on acceptable levels of organic contaminants. Many states have adopted their own standards for such substances.

- Sodium: Annual testing for sodium is required for surface water supplies; testing every three years is required for groundwater supplies.[12]
- Corrosivity: Sampling for corrosivity characteristics is required twice each year for supplies drawn from surface waters, once each year for supplies drawn from aquifers.[13]
- Toxic Plumbing Materials: Community water systems are required to identify whether the following materials are present in their distribution system and report to the state: lead from piping, solder, caulking, and home plumbing; copper from piping, service lines, and home plumbing; galvanized piping, service lines, and home plumbing; asbestos cement pipe. In addition, a state may require water suppliers to report other materials present in the distribution system such as vinyl-lined asbestos cement pipe and coal-tar-lined pipes and tanks.[14]

YOUR RIGHT TO KNOW

Consumers have a right to know if their tap water is contaminated with toxics. Under the Safe Drinking Water Act, community water suppliers must include a notice with consumers' water bills or send another written notice to each consumer within three months after the public water system:

- Fails to comply with an applicable MCL
- Fails to comply with applicable testing or monitoring requirements
- Is granted a variance from an MCL
- Fails to live up to a schedule of water supply improvement imposed by the EPA or the state

If the system fails to meet an MCL, water suppliers must also publish a notice in the newspaper within fourteen days after discovery of the failure and submit copies of the notice to local radio and TV outlets.[15] The only exemption to these public notice rules is if the state finds that the public health threat was eliminated promptly after discovery.

PROTECTING THE WATER SUPPLY

Wellhead Protection Areas

By June 19, 1989, each state had to adopt and submit to EPA a program for protecting areas around all wells supplying public drinking water systems. At a minimum, each state program must:

- Specify the duties of state agencies, local entities, and public water supply systems.
- For each wellhead, determine the wellhead protection area based on available hydrogeologic information.
- Identify all potential man-made sources of contaminants that may have an adverse affect on health.
- Set forth any needed technical and financial assistance, control measures, education, training, and demonstration projects to protect the water supply.
- Include plans for the provision of alternative drinking water supplies should contamination occur.
- Consider all potential sources of contaminants within the expected wellhead area of a new water well that is to provide drinking water.

The states must encourage the public to participate in developing these protection programs—through citizens' advisory committees and notice and opportunity for public hearings. A state program developed under these requirements will be deemed adequate unless the EPA administrator determines, within nine months of receipt of the program, that it is inadequate for protecting public water systems from contaminants. EPA must provide the states with a grant of 50 to 90 percent of the cost of developing and implementing an approved program.

Sole-Source Aquifers

The EPA can designate an area where the underground water is the principal drinking water supply as a *sole-source aquifer*.[16] This designation means that no commitment for federal financial assistance (grants, contracts, loan guarantees) may be granted if the administrator determines that a project may contaminate the drinking water. This ban on threatening activities is not absolute, since proposed projects may be modified to eliminate the threat to drinking water. Nevertheless, since many forms of development rely on federal assistance, this provision may help to protect local water supplies against toxics.

Once an area has been designated as a sole-source aquifer it also becomes eligible for federal funding of a "critical aquifer protection area" demonstration project. To qualify for such funds, a state or locality must develop a comprehensive management plan for protecting all or part of the aquifer area against contamination. This plan may include limits on projects assisted financially by federal, state, and local governments; protective actions to prevent damage to water quality and recharge capabilities; and innovative measures (such as the transfer of development rights) sufficient to protect the aquifer. The EPA has 120 days after submission of an application by a state or locality to approve or disapprove the project based on such considerations as the number of people using the groundwater and the benefits of the proposed program. A sole-source aquifer demonstration project may receive up to 50 percent federal funding (up to $4 million per aquifer per year).

PROGRESS

As of early 1986, approximately twenty-five areas had been designated as sole-source aquifers. Amendments to the SDWA in 1986 gave the EPA a stronger mandate for drinking water protection. While the list of substances with legally binding MCLs was small in 1986, the EPA was mandated by the reauthorization to regulate more than eighty contaminants by 1989 and more than a hundred by 1991. Under the new law, EPA is required to issue rules for monitoring wells in the vicinity of underground injection of wastes. The amendments granted the EPA substantial new enforcement authority and increased civil and criminal penalties for violations.

GUIDELINES FOR ACTION

Participate in wellhead protection programs in your area. Urge state or local government to map the critical recharge area for your local aquifer and establish a groundwater protection program mandated by the 1986 SDWA amendments. Participate in the program's development. Insist on the passage of strong new legal requirements to limit toxics in the wellhead protection area such as:

- Banning new land uses that would involve the use of toxics
- Imposing stringent reduction requirements for toxics users in the area
- Imposing stringent accident prevention and spill control requirements for any toxics that remain in use after reduction efforts

Enforce SDWA notice requirements. You can enforce the requirements that water suppliers must notify the community of water contamination as well as other requirements of the Safe Drinking Water Act. If you suspect contamination, you can threaten to sue the supplier, the state, and the EPA.

A letter threatening a suit over, for instance, a failure to issue legally required consumer warnings should prompt some response from these parties within sixty days. The law blocks your civil suit until sixty days after your letter. The letter itself, if publicized in the local media, can bring public attention to the water system's lack of safety. If you pursue a suit, the court that issues a final order may award costs of litigation including reasonable attorney and expert witness fees.

Pursue other options for citizen enforcement in the EPA's regulations under the Safe Drinking Water Act. If the state is the primary enforcement authority but inadequately enforces the law, the EPA administrator may take enforcement action directly against a water supplier.[17] Notify the EPA if the state is failing to correct a water supply violation and request that it notify the state of the violation. If the state abuses its enforcement discretion for more than sixty days after the EPA notice, the EPA can act directly against the water supplier.[18] The state risks losing its authority for enforcement of the drinking water act by repeated nonenforcement.

Petition the EPA to designate your area as a sole-source aquifer. Your petition should cover at least the following points:

- Explain why you are interested in the EPA's determination. State who you are (for instance, local residents concerned about toxic contamination) and why the drinking water supply is important to you.
- Explain why you believe contamination of the aquifer would result in a significant hazard to public health (for example, why toxic contamination could occur and violate SDWA standards).
- Describe the aquifer and its location, as well as the recharge and streamflow source zones for the aquifer and their locations. If this information has not been mapped by the U.S. Geological Survey (USGS) or a state agency, EPA may insist that this information be developed before deciding on your petition. In this case the first phase of your campaign will be to ask the USGS to provide this information in cooperation with state and local officials.
- Describe the location of the area for which the aquifer is the sole or principal drinking water source, as well as the public water systems using water from the aquifer. This information may be available from local water companies.
- Give the population in the area. (See the most recent U.S. census.)
- List alternative sources of drinking water for the area, if any.
- Describe projects that might contaminate the aquifer through the recharge zone (for example, a proposed hazardous waste facility).

If EPA finds your petition reasonably complete, it will publish a notice in the *Federal Register* soliciting public comment on the proposal to list your area. Generally EPA's decision may take a year or more (unless underground injection wells are threatening water supplies and there is no state program in place to regulate underground injection; see SDWA sec. 1424(a)).

Regardless of the EPA's decision, your petitioning may sharpen the public's awareness of the importance of local groundwater. In Warren, Massachusetts, where the petition for sole-source aquifer designation was part of a campaign to stop a major interstate hazardous waste facility from being built, the petitions were carried from door to door in the community to gather names and addresses. If your area is in fact designated as a sole-source aquifer, you can propose an ambitious demonstration project to protect the area against toxic contaminants.

CLEAN WATERWAYS

An integral part of America's heritage is the mighty rivers that water the rich agricultural states, provide drinking water to millions of people, and offer recreational enjoyment to fishermen, boaters, and others who love the outdoors. American industry and corporate agriculture, however, have taken our rivers and lakes away from us and turned them into their private toilets for dumping toxic chemicals. In 1987, industry reported that they dumped 9.7 billion pounds of toxic chemicals into surface waters. The law designed to protect our waterways from this toxic assault is the Clean Water Act.

THE LAW

The Clean Water Act (CWA),[19] originally enacted in 1972, set ambitious goals for cleaning up the nation's waterways. We were to have fishable and swimmable waters by 1983, toxic pollution was to be banned, and all pollution discharges were to be halted, by 1985. To reach these goals a complex system was established. The act required EPA to set pollution discharge standards defining the levels of pollution allowed based on the technology available to each type of industry. The *best conventional technology* (BCT) was to be applied to a short list of previously regulated pollutants. The *best available technology* (BAT) was to be applied to toxic pollutants, with less cost/benefit balancing by the EPA than on BCT. In addition to these technology standards, EPA was also required to set standards related to water uses—for example, how much pollution is acceptable for waterways used for fishing or swimming or recreation? The states were required to designate the uses of each waterway.

The EPA standards are applied to specific companies through National Pollution Discharge Elimination System (NPDES) permits. Any company that discharges pollutants to a waterway must apply to the state or to EPA for an NPDES permit. The permit sets limits on pollutants based on the technology standards (BCT and BAT) or, if necessary to protect local waterway uses, based on customized local water-quality limits.

Much of industry's toxics pass into waterways and the ocean by way of sewers and sewage treatment plants. The Clean Water Act contains a pretreatment program to regulate industrial toxics in sewers to prevent harm to both the treatment plants and the waters that receive their effluent. Sewage treatment plants designed to receive more than 5 million gallons of sewage flow per day are required to set and enforce limits on industrial dumping.

Other parts of the Clean Water Act have had noteworthy results:

- Requiring regional water quality plans for every part of the country is probably the closest the federal government has ever come to national land-use planning. These plans specify management of both *nonpoint* pollution sources, such as storm runoff over parking lots, farms, and construction sites, as well as *point* sources, such as effluent pipes.
- Water of very high quality is protected against deterioration.

PROGRESS

The ambitious goals of the Clean Water Act have not been met. Control of pollutants has been particularly disappointing. The EPA has been slow to implement toxic standards—primarily in response to lawsuits by environmental groups. Many industrial NPDES permits do not specify numerical limits on the full range of toxics actually discharged by the permit holder. By default, those that go unmentioned are generally allowed to be discharged in virtually any amount. This huge gap in regulation exists because state and federal regulators ignore these toxic pollutants rather than face the time-consuming task of setting case-by-case limits on pollutants unaddressed by EPA's standards.

As other avenues of toxics disposal such as hazardous waste dumpsites become less available, industrial dumpers are taking to the sewers. Today, dumping of toxic chemicals into sewage treatment plants is one of industry's favorite "out of sight, out of mind" toxic disposal tactics. At least 1.9

billion pounds of hazardous pollutants enter publicly owned treatment works (POTWs) nationwide each year.[20] Forty to sixty percent of these toxics end up in the environment—by passing through treatment plants into receiving waters, by bubbling into the air during treatment, or in treatment plant sludge residues that are ultimately disposed of in the environment. Enforcement of pretreatment has been lax. Local sewage officials, who have prime responsibility to regulate toxic sewer discharges, are reluctant to impose any costs on local businesses. Until recently, the EPA and the states, who are supposed to oversee local pretreatment programs, made little effort to force POTWs to control toxics in the sewers.

GUIDELINES FOR ACTION

- Press your state to regulate toxic water pollutants according to their impact on water uses, rather than relying only on EPA standards.
- Obtain copies of all permits for a local firm's water pollution discharges. Review them for the toxic substances covered and compare this list with all available information on chemical usage and releases at the plant. Use your right to know, monitoring records, and any available information on the chemicals generally employed by this type of industry. (Chapter 4 explains how to develop a list of chemicals likely to be used by different industry types.) Many firms discharge numerous toxic pollutants that are not listed or restricted in their permits. Call public attention to the government's failure to restrict these discharges and begin a campaign to get them reduced and regulated.
- Walk or boat down local streams to find out which businesses discharge pollutants into local waters without federal or state permits. You can obtain a guide to this process of "streamwalking" by contacting NJPIRG at 609-393-7474 or MASSPIRG at 617-292-4800.
- Estimate the total amount of toxic water pollutants discharged by a firm or by all firms in your area. Publicize the health and environmental harm that could result.

CLEAN AIR

Perhaps nowhere has the government failed more miserably to protect the public than in the area of clean air. Our cities have become choked with automobile and industrial air emissions. In some cities where petrochemical plants are located, like Baton Rouge, Louisiana, and Texas City, Texas, residents have to repaint their cars each year because the chemicals in the air rust the paint off. There are even days when EPA tells us it is dangerous to go outside. Although clean air seems like a basic civil right to most of us, we are deprived of it in many regions of the country.

THE LAW

The Clean Air Act (CAA) authorizes EPA to establish a comprehensive program of air pollution regulations.[21] The EPA prepares minimum pollution standards, and the states write implementation plans detailing how they will attain these standards. The legislation requires permits for emission sources and calls for monitoring the state's ambient air.

The act's National Emissions of Hazardous Air Pollutants (NESHAP) provision is a broad mandate for the EPA to regulate toxic air pollution.[22] EPA is required to keep an up-to-date list of industrial pollutants that are hazardous to human health. Within one year of adding a pollutant to the list, the EPA is supposed to set an emission standard for it to protect public health with an "ample margin of safety."

PROGRESS

The EPA has moved painfully slowly to control air pollution, often taking action only when under court order to do so. According to health experts, the public health threat from routine air emissions of toxic pollutants is even more damaging than from hazardous waste dumpsites, because the cumulative human exposure is greater. Yet by 1990 emission standards on chronic environmental exposures had been set for a mere six hazardous pollutants from industrial sources: asbestos, mercury, lead, beryllium, vinyl chloride, and benzene. A few others have been listed as hazardous, but the EPA still has not set any emission standards. Another thirty-seven compounds have been under review for over eight years; about a third of these have already been named as carcinogens by another federal agency. The EPA has decided not to regulate certain known toxic air pollutants, including toluene and polycyclic organics.

These figures on unregulated chemicals are most appalling when considered in context. In a congressional survey, for example, the nation's largest chemical manufacturers submitted the names of 196 compounds emitted from their facilities that are "extremely hazardous" according to Union Carbide's own criteria. Regulation to prevent one-time releases of very dangerous chemicals is even more lax. In late 1985, the EPA published a list of acutely toxic chemicals—those that may cause serious sickness or death if released in a spill or leak. Rather than issuing preventive regulations, EPA called for voluntary local programs to address such hazards.

One reason for the EPA's poor record in regulating air pollution is that, contrary to Congress's mandate, crude cost/benefit analysis has been substituted for the Clean Air Act's standard of public health protection in making regulatory decisions. Some cost/benefit decisions are being challenged in the courts; even if these challenges are successful, it will be many years before toxic air pollution is adequately regulated by the EPA.

In the reauthorization of the federal Superfund law, some progress has been made toward stronger air toxics laws. A community right-to-know provision was included, along with requirements for emergency plans for toxic spills. But there is still no national regulatory program to reduce the use of extremely dangerous chemicals or to ensure extra security against spills. Federal regulation of routine emission of air toxics remains on a slow track.

GUIDELINES FOR ACTION

- Press your state to adopt a policy to regulate toxic air pollutants beyond those regulated by the EPA.
- Obtain copies of all permits for a local firm's air pollution emissions. Review them for the toxic substances covered and compare this list with all available information on chemical usage and releases at the plant. Use your right to know, monitoring records, and any available information on the chemicals generally used by this type of industry. (Chapter 4 explains how to develop a list of chemicals likely to be used by different industry types.) Many firms discharge numerous toxic pollutants that are not listed or restricted in their permits. Call public attention to the government's failure to restrict these emissions and begin a campaign to get them reduced and regulated.
- Find out which businesses discharge pollutants into the local air without federal or state permits.
- Estimate the total amount of toxic air pollutants discharged by a firm or by all the firms in your area. Publicize the health and environmental harm that could result.

PESTICIDES AND HERBICIDES

During the 1950s, the chemical industry persuaded American farmers to use exotic new pesticides and herbicides to increase their crop yields and wipe out common pests. Forty years later, after the chemical saturation of our farmland and groundwater contamination throughout the country due to pesticides, farmers are still addicted to chemicals that are not only costly but do not solve their pest problems. Meanwhile, the rest of us continue to eat fruits and vegetables that are grown with known or suspected carcinogens, endangering our health and that of future generations.

THE LAW

Pesticides and herbicides are probably the only group of toxic chemicals that are produced with the primary intention of dispersing them into our environment.[23] Herbicides, fungicides, and insecticides are handled by large numbers of agricultural workers and are an unwelcome addition to much of our food. Although they were among the earliest chemicals to be regulated by federal law, there remains a surprising lack of public protection.

Both the Federal Insecticide, Fungicide, and Rodenticide Act (FIFRA)[24] and the Federal Food, Drug, and Cosmetic Act (FFDCA)[25] regulate pesticides. Originally requiring mere registration of pesticides, FIFRA was amended in 1972 to require testing for short-term and long-term toxic effects prior to registration. For pesticides used on food crops, EPA establishes an upper limit on the amount of residue that can remain on food, based on human tolerance levels. The FFDCA requires the Food and Drug Administration (FDA) to enforce these residue limits by monitoring and seizing foods whose residues are in excess. Health and environmental data submitted by manufacturers in registering pesticides can be publicly disclosed by the EPA.

PROGRESS

Federal pesticide laws are not being adequately enforced. Under FIFRA, pesticides existing prior to the 1972 amendments were supposed to be tested and reregistered. But out of 40,000 pesticides on the market, fewer than 100 have been reregistered. Some of these pesticides, as well as some newer compounds, were registered based on fraudulent tests by one commercial lab.

The EPA generally takes regulatory and enforcement action under FIFRA only when pressed. Ethylene dibromide (EDB), for example, a soil and grain fumigant, was reported to have serious health effects in 1965 and again in 1973. It took a major water contamination outbreak in 1983 to get the EPA to finally suspend its use. The federal record in setting residue limits and protecting farm workers has been equally weak. The FDA's enforcement record under the FFDCA is also unimpressive. Three-quarters of FDA food inspections are for the food's appearance only. The agency's laboratory techniques as of 1985 didn't even look for over two-thirds of the pesticides used on food crops.

In 1988, Congress enacted amendments to FIFRA. Environmental and public interest advocates called the new bill "FIFRA Lite" because it only partially rectified problems under the law. The amendments, which were supported by the chemical industry, partially eliminated industry subsidies under the law and accelerated reregistration of 600 old pesticides within eight to ten years. They failed, however, to meet other important needs:

- To establish a program to protect groundwater from pesticides
- To restrict the export of banned or restricted pesticides
- To allow citizen suits that would be available under most other federal environmental statutes
- To require labeling of long-term health effects on pesticide products

The problem of pesticide usage extends beyond regulatory laws into the realm of agricultural economics and the present system of federal research and support for farmers. As of 1988, for instance, the United States farm system was structured to drive family farmers off the land and to encourage ever greater reliance on farm chemicals. The 1985 Farm Bill limited the number of acres that farmers could grow their crops on, but it encouraged them to maximize their yield on each acre. Since there was no guarantee of a fair price for each bushel produced, family farmers were being driven to pump the land with chemicals to make ends meet.

An alternative system based on bushels rather than acres has been proposed to allow farmers know how much of a crop to grow and to assure them of a fair price in the marketplace. Such a program would not only help save the family farm but would allow farmers to put land back into production with lower chemical usage. The result would be a dramatic decline in the use of farm chemicals.

GUIDELINES FOR ACTION

- Find out which pesticides are most widely used in your area. Examine FIFRA registration records to learn of health effects and any health testing inadequacies.
- Press for a local ordinance to regulate significant local pesticide uses such as lawn care and aerial spraying.
- Sponsor forums or an information exchange on integrated pest management—agricultural practices that control pests while minimizing the use of chemicals. Ensure that your area's agricultural extension service provides this kind of information.
- Ensure that organically grown produce is available in your local stores. And buy it.
- Lobby for stronger state regulation, greater appropriations for enforcement, and a national bushel-based supply management system for agriculture.
- For pesticide strategies and up-to-date information on pesticides, contact the National Coalition Against the Misuse of Pesticides at 202-543-5450.

WORKPLACE SAFETY AND HEALTH

Workers have led the way for citizens in the fight for a clean environment. Throughout the 1970s, workers fought for and won the right to know about chemicals used in the workplace that could be hazardous to their health. The law designed to protect workers from environmental threats on the job is the Occupational Safety and Health Act of 1970. But like many of our other environmental laws, this law is weak and hardly enforced.

THE LAW

Approximately 11 million workers are exposed to known carcinogens in the workplace. Some 100,000 workers die each year from occupational diseases caused by hazardous exposures, and 340,000 more are disabled. The Occupational Safety and Health Act was enacted in 1970 "to assure so far as possible every working man and woman in the nation safe and healthful working conditions."[26] The Occupational Safety and Health Administration (OSHA) is required to issue basic safety and health standards, inspect workplaces, and force plant managers to reduce or eliminate job hazards.

The act generally governs health and safety protection in firms employing more than ten people. For chemical substances, OSHA sets standards on:

- Chemical levels above which worker exposure is prohibited
- Exposure levels that trigger actions such as medical surveillance of workers
- Labeling
- Protective equipment and control procedures
- Access by OSHA and employees to company records and to chemical hazard information in material safety data sheets (MSDSs) provided by chemical manufacturers to employers
- Employee training on safe handling of chemicals

OSHA allows employees to file complaints with local OSHA offices alleging violations or requesting inspections. The act sets forth safeguards against employers firing workers for filing complaints.

PROGRESS

OSHA was very hard hit by the Reagan administration's deregulation program. Without ever changing a word of the law, the government gutted the OSHA program. OSHA citations dropped sharply. A 1983 study found that citations for willful violations of OSHA decreased by 92 percent below the Carter era. Citations for serious violations declined by 47 percent. Fines collected fell by 78 percent.

A variety of policies were responsible for these declines. In the 1980s, three-quarters of the nation's workplaces were exempted from on-site inspections. In the old days OSHA inspectors used to tour workplaces looking for dangerous conditions, even without a workers' complaint. Now, in routine inspections, the inspector is required to stop off at the front office first to review records of lost work days due to injuries. If this self-reported rate is less than the national average for the industry, the inspector leaves without ever setting foot in the work area. This policy may have resulted in the death of a worker from cyanide exposure at the Film Recovery Systems plant in Chicago. OSHA inspectors had visited the plant two and a half months before the incident, but never went into the work space due to this rule. The employers were later convicted of murder.

Follow-up on health and safety violations has been minimized. Violations discovered in a workplace used to result in follow-up inspections by OSHA to ensure that the firm had come into compliance. These days an OSHA inspector merely makes a follow-up phone call, taking the plant manager's word that the violation has been corrected. Moreover, workers have been discouraged from inspecting their own workplaces, a right they are granted by law. Previously workers had a right to continued on-the-job pay while they conducted the inspections. This right to "walkaround pay" has been eliminated.

Formerly the employer's legal obligation to provide a safe workplace was enforced by OSHA. Even where no specific standard covered a dangerous condition, an inspector would issue a citation if a workplace contained a recognized hazard. These days the "general-duty" citations have all but ceased, buried under an impenetrable pile of red tape.

Standards for chemical exposures in the workplace are based largely on data and standards of 1970, when industry's voluntary standards were made mandatory under the new OSHA law. These standards were based on the immediate, acute effects of toxic exposure. They have not been updated to take account of current scientific knowledge of long-term effects, such as reproductive damage, birth defects, and cancer. What is worse, only about 500 of approximately 100,000 workplace chemicals are covered by any standards.

GUIDELINES FOR ACTION

- Join workplace and community antitoxic efforts. Many of the rights sought today by workers may also benefit you, as a plant neighbor, by leading to reductions in toxic releases and usage. Be sure to include local unions and workers in your strategy for community campaigns.
- Support local union efforts for health and safety protection.
- Organize citizen inspections of industrial plants to evaluate their toxic chemical management practices. (See Chapter 5 on neighborhood plant inspections.)
- To ask the federal government questions about OSHA, call the OSHA hotline at 1-800-392-6454.

GENERAL TOXICS CONTROLS

While almost all federal environmental laws deal with the problems of toxics once they are created, Congress passed one law—the Toxic Substances and Control Act—that was meant to address the production of dangerous chemicals before they entered the marketplace. This law has been a failure. While more than 60,000 chemicals are in commercial use, more than 95 percent of them have never been tested for their contribution to birth defects, cancer, and other long-term health effects.

THE LAW

The Toxic Substances Control Act (TSCA) was enacted in 1976 to fill the gaps left by the many other federal laws on toxics. It also addresses toxics at the point of production rather than only after they've entered the market or the environment.[27] Basically the act authorizes EPA to require chemical producers to test for health and environmental effects of chemicals before or after they enter the market and to ban or restrict chemical uses where "manufacture, processing, distributing in commerce, use or disposal of a chemical substance or mixture . . . presents or will present an unreasonable risk of injury to health or the environment." Among other things, the law requires chemical producers to notify EPA before manufacturing new chemicals and to notify EPA if they are aware of information that may indicate significant risks of the chemicals they market.

PROGRESS

Is it reasonable to expose the public to risks from highly toxic substances when safer substitutes exist? Most Americans would say "no way." Yet even though safer substitutes exist for many highly toxic chemicals, few of the roughly 65,000 chemicals covered by TSCA have been regulated for unreasonable risks. The limited use of the law's regulatory authority is due in part to government policies that narrowly interpret EPA authority under TSCA and favor information gathering over regulation of chemical usage, production, or handling. Only five previously existing chemicals were regulated under this law from 1976 to 1986.

The EPA's testing authority is also used narrowly. For example, the agency receives 1,500 premanufacture notices of new chemical compounds being produced each year. Unless EPA or another agency specifies otherwise, the manufacturers who submit these notices may market these substances without further assessment of their toxic effects. The agency asks the notifier to do some form of testing or provide further information in only about 10 percent of these cases.

The publication of a list of acutely toxic chemicals amplifies the peculiar defect of TSCA in leaving new chemical testing largely voluntary. Even though federal, state, and local concerns are turning to acutely toxic chemicals, makers of new chemicals can legally decide not to test substances in relation to acute toxicity criteria—to avoid bringing adverse attention to their new substances. Under current EPA regulations, irresponsible firms have the option of deciding that it's "better not to know."

YOUR SHRINKING RIGHTS TO PETITION

TSCA allows citizens to petition EPA to:

- Require companies to test the chemicals they manufacture or use.
- Prohibit the introduction of a new chemical.
- Regulate existing chemicals or prohibit their manufacture, processing, or distribution for certain uses.
- Require companies to report information about toxics.

The EPA may hold a public hearing or conduct an investigation to decide whether to grant such a petition. If the petition is granted, the EPA administrator must promptly initiate a proceeding. If the petition is denied, he must publish his reasons for denial in the *Federal Register.* Petitioners then have sixty days to sue.

If the petitioners want information submitted to the EPA or want chemical testing done, they must prove in the suit that EPA's information is insufficient to evaluate the effects of the substance. They must also show that, in the absence of such information, the substance presents an unreasonable danger or is produced in high enough quantities to lead to major environmental releases or human exposure. If the petitioners are seeking a rule or order controlling a substance, their suit must demonstrate why EPA's action is needed. If the petitioners meet these hurdles, the "court shall order the administrator to initiate the action requested by the petitioner."

The EPA has made it as hard as possible for petitioners to jump through the hoops of this petition process. From the time the law was first passed, the agency began formulating excuses for refusing to fulfill petitions. Most of the petitions granted to date relate to asbestos. The agency was already examining issues related to asbestos, but these petitions forced the agency to place asbestos on the top of its agenda. In January 1986, the EPA instituted a two-phase ban on asbestos. One other petition was partially granted. This petition by the Environmental Defense Fund and National Wildlife Federation requested EPA to regulate dioxins and furans in air emissions, solid waste disposal, and product contents. The petition was filed in 1984, denied in January 1985, and still pending in court as of December 1989.

In contrast, dozens of petitions have been denied by the EPA. For example:

- Requests for regional control of pollution problems in southeast Chicago and central Michigan—denied because EPA was concerned about not setting a precedent for using TSCA to solve regional pollution problems.
- Requests to ban substances that had already been examined by the Consumer Product Safety Commission—denied because EPA found no reason to question the judgment of that agency.
- A request to ban the active ingredient in tear gas—denied because the agency concluded there were no safer substitutes.

Even though EPA seems to have no shortage of reasons for denying petitions, in 1985 the agency issued a "guidance" on what should go into a petition. These guidelines could make it even harder for petitioners to win. While the guidance does not change the legal requirements for petitions, it suggests what will constitute a complete petition to the agency. Petitioners are told to provide information:

- On "the nature and severity of harm (toxicity) to humans or the environment from the chemicals of concern. . . . These findings are usually made on the basis of laboratory tests on animals, studies of human populations (epidemiological studies), medical case reports, or by analogy to similar known toxic chemicals or relevant studies."
- On exposure levels, "typically based on monitoring data, simulation model estimates, or other measurements."
- Allowing the agency to conduct a risk assessment.
- Describing actions by state or local government that could be used to provide the desired relief and explaining why federal action is needed.

In addition, the agency states that it will evaluate petitions "relative to existing regulatory priorities."

A draft EPA memorandum warned that the resource demands placed on petitioners by the new guidelines are so severe that future petitions are more likely to be filed by companies than by citizens. According to the EPA memo, petitions may be merely "a weapon that corporations can add to their arsenal of . . . legal procedures . . . to perpetuate their own interests. . . . Citizens' petitions might then evolve into . . . corporate petitions."

While the EPA cannot legally alter the law's petition requirements, the new guidelines show how its discretion will be used. Courts are reluctant to second-guess the EPA. Some types of discretion implied by the guidelines may be illegal. For example, if the EPA leans on the role of state and local government or the importance of a risk relative to other regulatory priorities in order to support denial of a petition (as opposed to merely setting a long-term schedule to act), a court might override EPA's action and grant a petition that the agency had denied.

GUIDELINES FOR ACTION

- Support efforts to reauthorize and strengthen TSCA.
- Sign or formulate citizen petitions for action under TSCA.
- To ask EPA questions about TSCA, call the hotline at 202-554-1404.

ENVIRONMENTAL IMPACT ASSESSMENTS

Recognizing that certain projects and facilities can dramatically alter or degrade a local environment, Congress passed a law that requires federal agencies to assess the environmental impact of a project before going forward with it. While this law has been weakened by the courts, it still remains a useful lever for citizens opposing dangerous facilities.

THE LAW

The National Environmental Policy Act (NEPA) requires federal agencies to prepare an environmental impact statement (EIS) for all "major federal actions significantly affecting the quality of the environment."[28] An EIS must study the range of environmental effects that a proposed project will have, as well as alternatives to doing the proposed action.[29]

In general, a specific EIS must be filed for every project. The courts, however, have allowed some exceptions for conflicting and overlapping agency requirements. No EIS is required if preparing it would clearly conflict with other agency mandates—such as a legal requirement to act quickly in an emergency or to consider only certain factors in making a decision. Moreover, if an agency prepares a study that is "functionally equivalent" to an EIS, then no actual EIS may be required. For a study to be equivalent, it must be primarily geared toward examination of environmental questions, fully consider environmental issues,[30] and be presented in a process allowing meaningful public participation in the decision making.[31]

PROGRESS

Since this law was enacted in 1970, court decisions have eroded its ability to force full consideration of environmental concerns. The courts have taken an increasingly hands-off approach to agency compliance with NEPA. Given the widening exceptions to when an EIS is required, federal agencies can evade the study requirements. In other cases, they may comply with the analysis requirements and then move forward with environmentally inferior alternatives.

In April 1986 the Council on Environmental Quality, which administers this law, eliminated the rule requiring a "worst case analysis" in an environmental impact statement.[32] This decision could have serious implications for EISs involving toxics. Instead of considering the worst possible environmental impact, EIS preparers now need only consider the effects that are "reasonably foreseeable" and "supported by credible scientific evidence." Thus the lack of safety studies on many substances could become a standard excuse for ignoring potentially far-reaching environmental impacts.

Despite these shortcomings, NEPA remains a useful tool for sharpening the public's awareness of environmental issues and, at times, delaying harmful government action.

GUIDELINES FOR ACTION

- Use NEPA to demand full evaluation of toxic risks and the alternatives to using toxics in federal projects and approvals. If the projects fail to meet the requirements of the law, consider suing under NEPA to halt the federal action.
- Learn whether your state has a "mini-NEPA" law. Many states' laws require environmental impact statements not only for major state actions but also for state-funded and state-permitted activities. The reach of such a law can be quite broad. Find out whether it can be applied if you are challenging state permits or even state policy.
- Press for an EIS review of alternatives to dumping toxics into the environment, including technologies for reduced toxics usage, in challenging a federal or state pollution permit for a specific company.

CONSUMER GOODS

Human exposure to dangerous chemicals is not restricted to living next to industrial plants or beside farms that spray with pesticides. Many household products and building materials contain toxic chemicals that endanger our health. With just a brief look under their kitchen sinks, citizens can find a wide array of dangerous products that are hazardous to the environment and their health. These hazardous products continue to threaten the public for decades to come—either through leaking landfills or through garbage incinerators that send the toxics into the air or deposit them in the ash that eventually gets dumped in a landfill.

THE LAW

The authority to ensure the safety of foods, drugs, medical devices, and cosmetics is found in the Federal Food, Drug, and Cosmetic Act (FFDCA).[33] The act prohibits the adulteration and misbranding of products.[34] Food and drugs that fail to meet FDA standards are considered "adulterated and/or misbranded." Such products may be seized by the FDA, and sellers or distributors may face criminal penalties.

The FFDCA requires FDA approval of new drugs, certain nonprescription drugs, and food and color additives. Products are approved for certain uses and may not be sold for other uses without FDA approval. Regulation of cosmetics under the act is not as strict as the regulation of other substances but relies more on voluntary industry compliance and product labeling requirements.

Another federal agency with authority to protect consumers is the Consumer Product Safety Commission (CPSC), which regulates other consumer goods. Under the Consumer Product Safety Act[35] and the Federal Hazardous Substances Act[36] the commission develops safety standards for consumer products and does research to protect the public from unreasonable risks. Unsafe products can be recalled or banned. CPSC may require protective labeling, design, or packaging or specify composition of products. For example, CPSC regulations limit the asbestos and formaldehyde content of products and require the labeling of products such as turpentine, antifreeze, and fire extinguishers.

The CPSC also has authority under two other acts. The Flammable Fabrics Act authorizes CPSC to set flammability standards for fabrics used in clothing, children's sleepwear, mattresses, carpets, and vinyl plastic film.[37] Fabrics are tested and rated according to their burning speed. The Poison Prevention Packaging Act requires the CPSC to establish standards for child-resistant containers.[38] Turpentine, most prescription drugs, aspirin, furniture polish, and lighter fluids are among the items that must be so packaged.

PROGRESS

The FDA has developed innovative ways of expanding the consumer's participation in the decision-making process.[39] Periodic meetings between the FDA commissioner and consumer representatives on a national scale, as well as district meetings on a local scale, have enabled the agency to hear what consumers have to say.

But is the FDA really listening? Despite the advances in consumer participation, FDA actions in the 1980s have exposed the public to unnecessary risks, hindered vigorous law enforcement, and stifled dissemination of information. For example, the FDA has attempted to reduce consumer protection from carcinogenic additives. The FDA has not sought the authority it needs to allow it to detain food suspected of containing illegal pesticide residues, nor to levy civil penalties on those who produce and ship such foods. The FDA has opposed efforts to require mandatory labeling on food products, favoring instead a voluntary approach.

Compliance with the FDA's rules and regulations, even when the public health is at stake, is becoming an increasingly voluntary matter. In the 1980s, enforcement actions regarding food, drugs, medical devices, and other regulated products have dramatically declined. The FDA withdrew its proposal regarding the consumer's right to know—abandoning proposed regulations requiring each drug package to inform consumers about such things as the side effects of drugs. Today this information is only required to be provided to the product's distributor, such as a doctor or pharmacy.

CPSC, like FDA, has been greatly altered by the spirit of deregulation and budget cutting of the 1980s.[40] The broad authority CPSC possessed under its 1972 charter to promulgate safety standards was diminished by 1981 amendments.[41] The agency must now invite industry to propose voluntary standards before the commencement of mandatory rule-making proceedings.[42] Any incentive for industry to establish voluntary standards before this official invitation has been removed.[43] The amendments also require additional factual findings by the CPSC in its rule making, thus bogging down an already lengthy rule-making process.[44]

The agency's once broad power to regulate a product's design, construction, finish, and packaging has been sharply curtailed. Product standards must now be expressed in terms of performance or labeling and cannot be expressed in terms of design.[45] Consumer rights to petition for product safety rules have been cut back, so that citizens can no longer obtain a fresh ("de novo") court review of their petition if it is denied by the CPSC.[46] Finally, and most significantly, the CPSA provisions that remain in effect are enforced by commission members who favor industry's self-regulation and whose goal is increasing reliance on voluntary standards in the future.[47]

GUIDELINES FOR ACTION

- Make use of the FDA's consumer inquiry and complaint phone lines in your district if you suspect that a food producer or drug manufacturer is allowing contaminants to enter the marketplace.
- Complain to the CPSC about other products that are hazardous due to composition, inadequate labeling, or packaging. You can use the toll-free complaint line at 1-800-638-2772.
- Press for regulation of consumer products that you think are hazardous. You can petition the FDA or CPSC, contact appropriate officials, or work through consumer groups.
- Make use of the district consumer exchange meetings in your locale to comment on FDA actions and issues important to you. To obtain information on the time and place of these meetings, contact the nearest FDA regional or district office.
- Contact the CPSC's national Program Manager for Chemical Hazards. You can also contact consumer organizations in Washington who attend national consumer exchange meetings, or CPSC briefings, and ask them to express your concerns directly to the appropriate officials.
- Subscribe to the CPSC's weekly public calendar, which informs the public of items to be addressed at their weekly commission briefings.

NOTES

The author gratefully acknowledges the assistance of the following people: David Sapiora, David Hunter, and Sam Boxerman, Harvard Law School; Toni Messina and Laura Gallant, Northeastern Law School; Virginia Vanslyck and Pierre Erville, Tufts University; Nancy Lessin, Massachusetts Coalition on Occupational Safety and Health; Jim Lanard, New Jersey Environmental Lobby; Susan Jeffrey, University of Massachusetts, Boston; Mark van Putten, Clean Lakes Natural Resource

Center; David Zwick and Amy Gluckman, Clean Water Action Project; Marco Kaltofen, Greenpeace; Dr. William Goldfarb, Cook College, Rutgers University; Zyg Plater, Boston College School of Law; Sue Kiernan, Save the Bay, R.I.; David Lennett, Environmental Defense Fund; Pete Sessa, Collier and Sessa; William McDonald; Irene Kessel; Stephen Kolberg; Annette Goodro; Gary Cohen, Richard Bird, Ken Silver, and John O'Connor of the National Toxics Campaign. Thanks also to the New England Community Environmental Education Program for its financial assistance.

1. 42 USC 9601 et seq.
2. CERCLA sec. 117(b).
3. CERCLA sec. 121.
4. CERCLA sec. 122(e)(2)(B).
5. 42 USC 6901 et seq.; regulations at 40 CFR 240–271.
6. See 40 CFR part 261 for detailed EPA regulations on determining whether something is a hazardous waste.
7. The Hazardous and Solid Waste Amendments of 1984, sec. 224, amending secs. 3002, 3005, and 8002 of RCRA.
8. *Ibid.,* sec. 201.
9. 42 USC 300(f) et seq.; regulations at 40 CFR 140–149.
10. See *Federal Register* of 41 FR 5281, January 5, 1976, for water supply systems designated pursuant to this provision.
11. 40 CFR 141.40.
12. 40 CFR 141.41.
13. 40 CFR 141.42
14. 40 CFR 141.42(d).
15. 40 CFR 141.32(b).
16. 42 USC 300h-3(e).
17. 40 CFR 142.23.
18. 40 CFR 142.31.
19. 33 USCA sec. 1251 et seq.; regulations at 40 CFR 260 et seq.
20. EPA Report to Congress on the Discharge of Hazardous Wastes to Publicly Owned Treatment Works; February 1986, p. E-5.
21. 42 USC 7401 et seq.; regulations at 40 CFR 50-8021.
22. 42 USC 7412.
23. This section is based primarily on information from *Pesticides: A Community Action Guide.*
24. 7 USC 136 et seq.; regulations at 40 CFR 162–180.
25. 21 USC 301 et seq.; regulations at 21 CFR 1-1300.
26. 29 USC 651 et seq.; regulations at 29 CFR 1910, 1915, 1918, 1926.
27. 15 USC 2601 et seq.; regulations at 40 CFR 700–799.
28. 42 USC sec. 4332(2)(C).
29. 42 USC sec. 4332(C). Specifically an EIS must address: (1) the environmental

impact of the proposed action; (2) any adverse environmental effects that cannot be avoided should the proposal be implemented; (3) alternatives to the proposed action; (4) the relationship between short-term uses of the environment and the maintenance and enhancement of long-term productivity; and (5) any irreversible and irretrievable commitments of resources that would be involved in the proposed action should it be implemented.

30. *EDF v. EPA*, 489 F.2d 1247, 1257 (D.C. Cir. 1973).
31. *Portland Cement Association v. Ruckelshaus* 486 F.2d. 375 (D.C. Cir. 1973).
32. *Federal Register*, April 25, 1986, pp. 15618–15626.
33. This section is based on information from Mary Devine Worobec, *Toxic Substances Controls Primer* (Washington, D.C.: Bureau of National Affairs, 1983), pp. 60–61.
34. 21 USC 301 et seq.; regulations at 21 CFR 1-1300.
35. 12 USC 2051 et seq.; regulations at 16 CFR 1015–1402.
36. 15 USC 1261 et seq.; regulations at 16 CFR 1500–1512.
37. 15 USC 1191 et seq.; regulations at 16 CFR 1602–1632.
38. 7 USC 135; 15 USC 1261, 1471–1476; 21 USC 343, 352, 353, 362; regulations at 16 CFR 1700–1704.
39. E. Haas, "An Assessment of FDA's Track Record on Issues of Consumer Protection," *Food, Drug, Cosmetic Law Journal* 253 (1985):40.
40. For example, the CPSC budget for fiscal year 1982 amounted to only 30 percent of its funding for fiscal year 1981; M. Lemor, *Consumer Product Safety Commission*, sec. 3.09, 3-13, n. 4 (1981).
41. P.L. No. 97-35, tit. XII, 95 Stat. 703 (1981) (codified in scattered sections of 15 USC).
42. CPSA, sec. 9(a), 15 USC 2058.
43. E. Klayman, "Standard Setting Under the Consumer Product Safety Amendments of 1981—A Shift in Regulatory Philosophy," *George Washington Law Review* 96 (1982):101–102.
44. CPSA, sec. 9(f); see "Standard Setting," p. 102.
45. "Standard Setting," p. 104.
46. Ibid., p. 110.
47. See *Legal Times*, September 9, 1985, p. 10, col. 1; *Los Angeles Daily Journal*, August 28, 1984, p. 5, col. 1.

8

Your Legal Recourse

SANFORD LEWIS

Today's toxics crisis arose during the twentieth century in the face of a legal system that had evolved over hundreds of years. For most of that evolution, the law was written primarily by judges as common law—law made case by case by comparing and contrasting precedents in similar cases. But the slow approach of that system has been unable to deal with vast corporate bureaucracies that have created and distributed thousands of synthetic chemicals. The "state of the art" rule, for example, may have given companies the message that if *everyone* dumps poison in their backyard, no one will be liable.

Reliance on judicial precedent to control corporate environmental abuses has led to a toxic mess from sea to shining sea. Today legislators are struggling to pass statutes that control toxic hazards just as efficiently and comprehensively as big business can churn them out. Yet neither legislatively enacted statutes nor common law effectively controls toxics.

TOXICS AND THE LEGAL SYSTEM

One reason for the law's continued ineffectiveness is the all-pervasive influence of money in our system. The chemical industry pumps millions of dollars into shaping legislation in its favor. In 1986, for example, the chemical industry's Political Action Committees contributed $10 million to legislative campaigns. While many well-intentioned statutes have been passed, industry's lobbying and donation efforts have succeeded in infusing ambiguity and complexity into the language of the laws.

Once the statutes are written, industry's legal maneuvers have just begun. Far more lawyers help industry to delay and cut corners than work to clean up dumps or compensate victims. Moreover, toxics statutes leave many questions to official experts. Yet most of these issues don't really require special expertise. Rather, they are questions of just how much it's worth for a clean environment. Where the laws say that polluters must pay, there is immense pressure on the government to cut industry's costs.

An odd dilemma has emerged. The agencies set up by Congress to solve the problems the courts were too slow to address actually stand between the public and a clean environment! Under the original federal Superfund law, for example, Congress never explained how quickly the nation's dumpsites must be cleaned up or answered the question "how clean is clean enough?" As a result, EPA moves slowly and tends to opt for "bargain basement" solutions—capping sites or carting wastes to other sites rather than eliminating the toxic threat.

Only citizens who have organized to exert political pressure have made EPA do the job right. Even though opinion polls show that the public wants a cleaner environment, little is really done until public opinion is translated into public pressure. It is united citizen action that makes the system produce results.

DO I NEED A LAWYER?

Your decision whether and when to hire a lawyer is a strategic choice that *you* are in the best position to make.[1] Never let a lawyer make that decision for you. Remember: You don't need a lawyer to solve most local toxics problems.

You don't need a lawyer to read the laws and regulations applicable to your case. But you may want a lawyer who's familiar with the law to help you find your best avenues of leverage and avoid legal pitfalls.

You don't need a lawyer to talk to politicians for you. Hiring a lawyer to deal with politicians would be a waste of your money. You can say it better than them—from the heart and from your own experience. But you may want to get the advice of a lawyer if the government claims that legally they cannot address your concerns or meet your demands. Often officials hide behind the law. A competent attorney may help you to rip through such arguments. But before you rush to hire a lawyer, check behind the scenes to see whether the legal issue is really preventing results or is merely a flimsy excuse to avoid action.

You don't need a lawyer to get the EPA to clean up your dumpsite or to sit at the bargaining table with EPA and responsible parties on a dumpsite cleanup. You can organize for a strong cleanup and press your way to the bargaining table. But if you decide to intervene formally in the case to gain veto power over any proposed agreement between the government and polluters, you'll probably want to seek a lawyer's advice.

You may need a lawyer if legal documents are involved in your case. A lawyer can help you review the details of any agreements, legislation, and contracts that emerge as a result of your efforts to clean up or prevent toxic hazards. Too often industry's lawyers undermine the public's apparent victory with ambiguity, fine print, and loopholes. An environmental lawyer with a keen eye for detail can help you recognize such tactics and prevent you from losing in the translation.

Even though you may decide to represent yourself in a lawsuit, consult with a lawyer if you're contemplating a suit or want to preserve your ability to file a suit later.

HOW TO FIND A LAWYER

Don't allow yourself to be overwhelmed by the mystique of lawyers and the legal profession. Shop around. Plan to talk with two or three different lawyers to see the different styles, attitudes, and rates of attorneys in your area. Remember that when you speak with a lawyer on your first visit, you are interviewing *them*. While they will want to learn about your case, you'll also want to learn who they are and what they can do for you. You may want to ask them:

- What would their services gain for you? If a lawsuit is contemplated, what are the chances of winning? What do you get if you win?
- How much would it cost and when? If the lawyer doesn't know how much it would cost, can he or she find out?
- Does the lawyer have enough time to put into your case?
- Will the lawyer you spoke with supervise your case or will the case actually be handled by someone else?
- Does the law firm have any conflicts of interest in your case or relations with the defendants that you should be aware of?

Lawyers should be looking for possibilities, not roadblocks. If you talk with a lawyer who takes the whole time telling you what won't work rather than exploring what might work, try another lawyer.

Talk with lawyers with different kinds of expertise. If you're dealing with an environmental problem, for instance, talk with at least one environmental lawyer. A lawyer who's ignorant of environmental law may end up billing you for his education while preparing the case.

GETTING FREE LEGAL HELP

It doesn't always have to cost a fortune for you to get legal advice or services. Here are a few pointers for getting free or low-cost legal help.

Enlist public-interest groups and firms. Look for an environmental advocacy group or public-interest law firm in your area. Some national groups may provide consultation or help you to find a lawyer with the expertise you need:

- National Toxics Campaign
- Citizens Clearinghouse on Hazardous Waste
- Environmental Defense Fund
- Environmental Action
- Natural Resources Defense Council

Talk with law schools. Some law schools have an environmental law society or faculty-supervised environmental law clinic to provide advice and handle cases at no charge.

Obtain free ("pro bono") assistance. Some law firms that ordinarily charge high fees also take a few cases each year on a "pro bono" basis. A community toxics problem is an attractive issue for some lawyers. It can be far more interesting than drafting wills or doing divorces. In some communities, however, it may be hard to find a firm that doesn't represent local polluters or local government; these firms may be unwilling to get involved in cases that make waves.

Bring compensation cases on contingency. Most compensation suits are brought on a contingent-fee basis, which generally means that you pay the lawyer nothing unless you get a recovery in the suit. In the event of success, you pay the lawyer 30 or 40 percent of the amount won (after expert witness fees are subtracted off the top). Later we'll see what makes a good compensation suit.

Put government lawyers to work. If you can enlist state or local prosecutors on your behalf, you may not need to hire your own lawyer. For example, you might pressure the county prosecutor to prosecute a local polluter, thus avoiding the need to file a suit of your own. Since county and state prosecutors and attorneys general are often elected officials, they are subject to your political pressure. Similarly, if you can press town officials to pursue the community's interests in blocking an environmentally unsound activity, they might put their own attorney on the job. Beware, however, of lawsuits by state or local government that are merely window-dressing to persuade you to stop organizing or arranged to cut the best deal for the local polluter. Winning the support of a government attorney may be helpful, but your group must keep the pressure on.

Streamline your case for cheaper litigation. Can your case be shaped so that no factual questions are in dispute? If so, you may reduce your litigation costs dramatically. It takes much less time and expense for a lawyer to prepare a case when there's a clear-cut legal violation and no experts are needed. Suppose an agency writes a permit that violates the agency's own standards. A lawyer can take the permit and the standards, set them side by side, and file a lawsuit without much other homework. But if your lawyer must prove that a local dump is endangering your drinking water, hydrogeologists and toxicologists might be needed—taking more time and costing you more in lawyers' and experts' fees.

Use laws with attorney fee provisions. Many federal and state environmental laws allow a judge to award fees for attorneys and experts to citizens who win a suit against an agency or a polluter.

Do some of your lawyer's work. You might reduce your legal fees by doing some of the legwork for your lawyer. Discuss with your lawyer the possibility of assisting in sorting files, gathering data, and so forth.

Consider taking prelitigation action yourself. You can take some pre-lawsuit actions without hiring a lawyer. The citizen suit clauses of the federal environmental laws, for example, allow you to sue the EPA, the state, or polluters to clean up local pollution violations. They require you to send a letter to polluters and government a certain number of days before you can file a suit. If you have documentation of lawbreaking or imminent public health threats, you might carefully read the relevant citizen suit clause and send this letter yourself. We'll discuss the issue of citizen suits later.

You can represent yourself in court. Most states allow citizens the right to "pro-se" representing—that is, the option of representing themselves in court. There are different ways this rule might be used to your advantage in a toxics case. You might have a lawyer advise you on the law, for example, but argue the case in court yourself. Be sure to think through the pros and cons of representing yourself before trying this strategy.

I'VE GOT A LAWYER—NOW WHAT?

If you finally do select and hire a lawyer, be sure to draw up a clear contract. What is the lawyer expected to do and by when? What are you expected to do and by when? Here we'll consider a few things to keep in mind—and discuss with your lawyer from the outset.

You should control the key decisions on your case. Use your lawyer for advice. Some lawyers automatically discuss the handling of their case with their clients; others do not. If your lawyer seems to be making important decisions without consulting you, it may be time to get another lawyer. Remember: You hired the lawyer—you are the boss.

If there are several people in your group, it may be wise to select a key person to deal with the lawyer. This will make it easier for the lawyer to work with your group and vice versa.

Your lawyer's help or legal action can be a useful complement to your local organizing. But don't let your lawyer decide your organizing strategy. Most lawyers are not experts on organizing. They may even see your organizing as a threat to their efforts. Make it clear from the outset that you'll continue to exercise your own judgment on organizing strategy.

Establish a clear plan to keep your organization together while your legal strategy proceeds. Many people think that once they've hired a lawyer they no longer need to participate in the local group because the lawyer has the problem under control. Nothing could be further from the truth. If your group brings a compensation suit, for example, this may be a good time to seek new members and plan some events that have nothing to do with your legal strategy.

Your lawyer may instruct you not to speak to other parties in your case—not even to the press or anyone else—about the case. You must make your own decision about such advice. Lawyers have ethical rules that prevent them from talking with your opponent without the opponent's lawyer present. But unless you are under court order, no strict legal or ethical rule prevents *you* from talking to other parties or the press. If you're planning to talk publicly or privately with others about your case, do ask your lawyer what kinds of statements you should avoid.

SHOULD I SUE?

There are only a limited number of circumstances in which it makes sense to sue. You'll have to decide with your lawyer whether a lawsuit is reasonably likely to help accomplish any of the following:

- Result in a court order for an agency or a polluter to take a specific action.
- Help to win the delays or leverage your group needs in combination with other strategies. (Suits about inadequate environmental impact statements are usually most helpful in getting a delay of agency action. Ultimately the agency can correct the inadequacies and move forward with the challenged action unless you've taken other action to stop them.)
- Win compensation to help people who have suffered personal injuries or whose property has been damaged or devalued and to punish polluters or other wrongdoers.

The next section details some of the grounds on which you can bring a lawsuit against the government. But first we should take a look at the fact-gathering process known as discovery.

THE FACT-GATHERING PROCESS

After you file a suit, both sides begin an extensive information gathering called *discovery*. Lawyers have broad powers at this time to demand any information that may be relevant to your suit.[2] Written lists of questions, called *interrogatories*, are filed by each side for the other to answer. Live hearings, called *depositions*, are held with a stenographer (but no judge) to ask extensive questions of potential witnesses in the case. In toxics cases, extensive research through company files can also be done. Thus the discovery process can help you and your group to find out what's really going on beyond the factory gates. Defendants may be required to give you information they were unwilling to turn over before the litigation.

Some defendants may try to force you to treat all information that emerges in the course of discovery as secret. Such confidentiality could stifle your ability to make public statements and take public action. To prevent this, be sure your lawyer insists on limits on confidentiality agreements or rulings.

The discovery process is sometimes used by industry lawyers to harass citizen plaintiffs by asking endless questions designed to upset or intimidate you. A judge can issue an order to protect you against harassing or irrelevant questioning. But judges don't like to hear about the discovery process, so lawyers usually try to work out such problems among themselves. If bargaining between lawyers isn't working, insist that your lawyer protect you against harassment.

LEGAL RECOURSE AGAINST AGENCIES

Everyone knows that bureaucracy moves slowly. Across the country, therefore, citizens have been perfecting techniques for getting bureaucrats to address local toxics issues more quickly. These methods are described throughout the book, but here are a few thoughts from the perspective of a lawyer who works with community groups.

When officials tell you they have too much work and not enough staff to do it with, it may not be just a line to get your group out of their hair. The truth is that federal, state, and local agencies are seldom given the resources they really need to do their jobs effectively. In the 1980s, the shortage of resources reached scandalous proportions. In 1985 the EPA had double the duties to protect the environment and public health compared to 1975. But the level of funding, adjusted for inflation, was the same at the start and end of the decade. There are simply too few agency personnel to deal with the tasks before them.

This doesn't necessarily mean you should give up entirely on getting action. Instead, you should be thinking about how to get an official to act. It may help to picture him at his desk with a pile of papers three feet high. One of those papers has your name and your problem on it. Some of the papers have meaningless bureaucratic routines on them, but many have situations in other people's neighborhoods. Each community group faces the same challenge: to get their papers to the top of the pile! Here, then, are a few tips on getting action by bureaucrats.

Remember that many, perhaps most, environmental officials went to work for their agencies because they wanted to protect the environment and health. Once they get into the government, however, they're hampered by overwork, by well-financed pressure from industry, by the political appointees that head their agencies, and by plenty of red tape. Well-meaning bureaucrats often look to the public's actions to provide the justification they need to cut through the obstacles. If you sense that an official wants to help but is being frustrated by someone or something, try having an informal, off-the-record conversation with them. When they're relatively relaxed, ask whether they think your group could do anything that would make it easier for them to take the action you seek. They might tell you who to write to or suggest where the pressure is needed or . . . You never know unless you ask.

If the official seems less well meaning, remember that the last thing this person wants is to be given still more work. Any action that threatens to create additional work can help move your problem to the top of the pile. Continued inquiries and pressure are one tactic to keep the official aware of your problem. He may finally give you the information or action you need just so you'll disappear.

You can also mobilize lawyers, politicians, and the media to create a threat of added work for a bureaucrat—to ask questions and create an overwhelming sense that the problem will not go away until it is dealt with.

Look for specific legal deadlines to impose on bureaucrats. For example, you can file a notice of intent to sue the EPA, as the law requires a specific number of days before a citizen's suit can be brought—giving the agency a limited time to head off a lawsuit. In this way you can force the agency's attention before the sixty or ninety-day deadline runs out.

Never put all of your eggs in one basket. Use a complementary strategy of governmental and nongovernmental tactics when attacking a pollution source. Chapter 9 explains how to pressure local companies directly for action. By exerting pressure directly on a firm (by threatening their financial stability, for instance), you may actually move the polluter to ask the government to take enforcement action so the case will be closed and your pressure tactics will end.

USING A LAWSUIT TO FORCE ACTION

Your ability to use a lawsuit to force agency action is limited. Most judges are reluctant to tamper with a government agency's decision making. Given their overloaded court dockets, they're often unwilling to delve into toxics problems and defer to agency experts on the complex matters before them. On top of this judicial reluctance, our legislatures have tied judges' hands on many issues by granting agencies sweeping discretion. Under most toxics laws, agencies have great latitude to decide what constitutes a legal violation—and even more latitude to decide whether and how to take enforcement action against violators.[3]

As a result, some environmental officials believe they have the same kind of "prosecutorial discretion" that policemen have. Just as the cop on the beat doesn't arrest every drunk for loitering, so these officials insist that they should only go after the most serious toxics lawbreakers. Yet when it comes to protecting public health, one polluter can be the spoiler for all of us. "Prosecutorial discretion" is not the way to prevent polluted drinking water or a potential Bhopal in your backyard. Yet the unwillingness of the courts to force stronger prevention and enforcement sometimes seems to support this weak view of toxics laws.

WHEN CAN I SUE TO FORCE ACTION?

Because bringing a lawsuit is difficult and litigation is slow and costly, strong political organizing and public pressure are necessary to bring about improved controls of toxics. Fortunately, you have several opportunities to back up your local political clout with legal recourse to force an agency to act. In this section we'll explore the exceptions to broad agency discretion—situations where lawsuits may help force action.

Violation of a Statute or Regulation

First, a court may stop an agency from acting beyond its legally prescribed powers.[4] You can sue an agency that takes a weak or damaging action related to toxics if the action is outside its powers or jurisdiction. If a health agency passes weak air pollution rules but has no authority to regulate air pollution, you might bring a suit to overturn the rules.

Second, under most toxics laws, agencies write standards and rules spelling out how the law will be applied. Often these standards are applied through permits or licenses. Unless agency regulations or laws allow waivers from these standards, an agency may not legally give an applicant permission to violate them. If an EPA standard flatly prohibits air emissions of more than one part per million of dioxin, for example, an agency may not authorize a company to emit two parts per million.

Finally, where a law requires an agency to take an action by a given date, citizens may sue for a court order to force such action. Also, in general, if an agency unlawfully withholds or unreasonably delays action, a court may force it to act.

Abuse of Discretion

When an agency acts within its discretion, it still must have a reasonable basis for its decisions. If it acts "arbitrarily and capriciously"—that is, if a decision appears to be random or based on inadequate information or inappropriate factors (such as racism)—a court may overturn the decision. Courts can also require an agency to put its reasons for a decision in writing so the decision can be evaluated in accordance with this standard.[5]

Violation of Decision-making Procedures

An agency must obey certain basic procedures—for example, hearings to protect individual rights. The Fifth Amendment guarantees that no person can be deprived by the government of "life, liberty, or property without due process of law." Thus an agency may not make a decision regarding someone's rights—such as revoking a company's license—without a formal or informal hearing to allow that person to argue his or her side of the case. Typically a formal "adjudicatory" hearing is provided when a person's rights are at stake. This proceeding is similar to a court hearing, each party having the right to cross-examine witnesses and present evidence in their favor. Members of the public may assert that their legal rights are affected by an agency's decision, thus entitling them to a hearing. If the government proposes an action that would render your property valueless, for example, you might seek an agency hearing or even a court review to reverse the decision or seek compensation.[6] A creative attorney might also argue for a hearing as due process for denial of "life" due to serious pollution risks that the government will impose on a citizen exposed to toxics.[7]

Moreover, in most cases an agency cannot conduct a major project such as cleaning up a dump without soliciting public comment. Federal and state laws and regulations prescribe the minimum requirements for public comment:

- Notices published a designated number of days before a major decision will be made
- Public access to relevant documents
- Opportunity to submit written comments
- Opportunity to request a hearing for the agency to hear the public's comments (but not necessarily allowing cross-examination of witnesses)
- Sometimes a written record of the agency's response to comments received from the public

It should be noted, though, that agencies are legally permitted to evade or vary their procedural compliance with the Administrative Procedure Act under certain circumstances. For example, if an action is needed immediately to protect public health against an imminent hazard, the government can order companies to take immediate action without a right to a hearing before they take their action. Similarly, if the need is urgent enough, and the fairness questions are minimal, an agency can put into effect a temporary regulation without public comment and then, afterward, receive public comment to revise the rule for its final form.

Violation of Normal Agency Practices

Even if an agency is technically in compliance with the law on procedures for public input, a court may still overturn a decision if the procedure is inconsistent with the agency's normal practices. In Virginia, for example, a landfill for ash from Philadelphia's municipal incinerator was licensed without a public hearing within a two-week period. Although no public hearing was technically required by state law, the issuance was rushed and inconsistent with normal procedure. Citizens then organized and pressured the county commissioner to bring suit challenging the license. Ruling that the license was improperly granted, the court blocked operation of the landfill.[8]

Violation of EIR Requirements

Federal law and some state laws require the environmental effects of government-approved activities to be studied before an agency reaches its final decision. An environmental impact report must contain a careful review of possible environmental impacts and alternative actions that might be less environmentally harmful. The public must be given an opportunity to review it. If an agency neglects any of these requirements, you may be able to sue to halt action until a proper study is done.

THE MECHANICS OF YOUR LAWSUITS

What Do You Win in Court?

Individuals who file lawsuits against government agencies usually want to obtain a court order, called a *writ of mandamus,* for an agency to take a specific action. In too many instances, however, judges are reluctant to prescribe the exact action an agency should take. There may be facts still outstanding, or the court may not want to second-guess the agency's experts as to how to address a problem. Thus after a judge decides against an agency's action, he or she typically *remands* the decision—sends it back to the agency for reconsideration.

The court's reliance on remands can mean that an agency has another shot at finding a way around what you want done. Suing an agency can be a long, frustrating, and expensive fight. Lawsuits are never your only clout. If you rely on lawsuits without organizing, you may spend huge sums on litigation and still not get the agency to do what you want.

The Statutory Basis of Your Suit

A key weapon in challenging an agency's actions is the ability to sue them and have them pay your lawyer's fee if you win. There are several legal means by which you can sue an agency to do the right thing:

- Citizen suit provisions in most environmental laws give you a legal right to sue agencies who violate such statutes or create an imminent hazard to the public or environment. Most provisions require you to notify the agency and any other defendants in writing a certain number of days or months prior to filing the suit. Most clauses also allow a judge to order defendants to pay the plaintiff's attorney fees (and, sometimes, expert witness fees).[9]
- The Administrative Procedure Act generally allows suits for review of an agency's decision if you can demonstrate that it harms your interests. Unlike citizen suit provisions, there is no specified right to recovery of fees.

THE QUESTION OF TIMING

Your suit to challenge an agency's action must be correctly timed. Generally it must come after a "final agency action" but before the legal deadline for a court challenge runs out. A court ordinarily allows a suit against an agency only if you've first gone through available agency channels—"exhausted your administrative remedies." If an agency has a hearing process available for review of a decision you disagree with, for example, generally you must make at least a minimal effort to go through that process first. If you haven't even requested a hearing, a court might reject your suit.

Similarly, a court will usually reject a citizen suit if the agency has not yet taken a "final action" on the matter. Generally an EPA action is final once they determine how they will act in a situation. Under the Superfund amendments of 1986, a challenge regarding the extent of cleanup on Superfund sites generally will not be allowed until the EPA has actually completed the cleanup.[10] Consult a lawyer for the timing of your legal recourse under that intricate law.

One exception to the rules against early lawsuits is where a citizen suit provision allows you to sue an agency to stop an imminent hazard. Under such provisions, the only time limit on suing is the number of days of notice that must be given before such special suits. Many environmental statutes contain deadlines for filing a suit after a final agency decision. If you don't file a suit within the deadline—sixty days under the Clean Air Act and ninety days under the Clean Water Act—you forfeit your rights to challenge the agency's decision.

TAKING PART

Lawyers for the government who are negotiating with industry often try to convince the public that they have no need to be at the bargaining table. But without the public's participation, one-sided agreements are likely to be reached between bureaucrats and polluters. While public involvement may complicate the bargaining, the end result is far more likely to protect the public's interests.

In dumpsite cleanup negotiations, for example, the EPA's policy is to exclude the public from settlement discussions with responsible parties.[11] An official comment to the National Contingency Plan even states that "EPA does not require and is not suggesting that the public be allowed to participate in the actual negotiation sessions."[12] Not only the substance of talks, but also negotiation and litigation positions, are held in strict confidence.

In defending its public lockouts, the EPA claims that secrecy is needed to induce responsible parties to negotiate. Company officials might not discuss payments or cleanups so freely, the argument goes, if the discussions were public. Moreover, government lawyers sometimes claim that their closed-door discussions with industry relate only to who will pay and how much. The public can express its views on levels of testing and cleanup elsewhere—through public comments on draft studies, for example—or so it is argued.

Yet many issues that may be discussed in the closed-door sessions are of great concern to the public. While the public may be given an opportunity to comment on a proposed settlement with responsible parties after it's agreed upon, such eleventh-hour comments are too late to affect the outcome of negotiations. Thus you have a strong interest in being at the bargaining table. Let's look at some of the issues that may be addressed there.

Long-Term and Permanent Cleanup

There are several critical aspects of cleanup that are worked out in the negotiating sessions between EPA and responsible parties. Issues such as monetary amounts, liability, long-term monitoring, and choice of cleanup method are key components of the plan to restore or protect your community. If you're not at the bargaining table, EPA is likely to cut a deal with the polluters that will not adequately address the long-term health of the community.

- The settlement process may lead to releases from liability for responsible parties—limiting the money available to clean up the site completely. Under 1986 federal Superfund amendments, EPA may agree to pay for part of the cleanup out of the Superfund. Not only may responsible parties gain liability releases, but the share that EPA agrees to pay in such settlements may actually limit future federal liability for cleanup at the site, in case the remedial measures fail.[13]
- Even when no releases are provided, the sums of money discussed behind closed doors may limit cleanup expenditures. According to Joel Hirschhorn of the congressional Office of Technology Assessment, responsible parties and the EPA sometimes reach explicit or implicit agreement on the amount to be spent on site cleanup even before they determine the appropriate technology. The amount they decide to spend then limits the choice of technologies. If this approach is taken at a site, environmental and public health protections suffer a massive setback before the site cleanup discussion even moves into the public eye.
- A settlement can determine the long-term efforts to maintain or restore a site and to provide further remediation in the event of later toxic leakage. Long-term public monitoring may also be affected.
- Many elements of the technical cleanup plan may be discussed and formal or informal agreement reached. Even though these technical issues may "officially" be left open to public comment, by that time the issue may already be decided.

Informational Issues

Apart from the issues mentioned above, all relevant information about a cleanup site or a company should be available to the public. There are two major informational issues:

- Government lawyers may fail to demand key information to assess the adequacy of a cleanup plan.
- Government might agree to keep secret certain information discussed in the negotiations.

Other Issues

Government policymakers and attorneys ordinarily view the objectives of settlement in the narrowest way possible. With citizen involvement, however, the settlement process might yield a more complete solution to a local hazardous waste problem. Suppose, for instance, that citizens near a site have continuing concerns about their health. The settlement could require studies to address these concerns. A truly complete settlement might also ensure that polluters are doing all they can to reduce the toxic chemicals they use and then release in the environment.

Without the public's involvement in negotiations, major concerns may be overlooked or even overrun at the bargaining table. Instead of helping to shape the issues, you may be handed a "draft settlement" that is essentially final. While you may be given thirty days or more to provide your comments, nothing more than fine-tuning is likely. The lawyers who participated in the negotiations have already invested too much of their time and energy. Clearly they'll defend their painstakingly negotiated product, rather than renegotiate any dramatic changes you claim are needed. If you're only given a say at that late point in the process, you may also lack the clout to block a weak agreement.

GETTING TO THE BARGAINING TABLE

In view of the government's policy to exclude the public from negotiations with polluters, joining in on the discussions is not easy. Nevertheless, there are a few strategies at your disposal.

Elbowing Your Way In

When an agency negotiates with a polluter for legal compliance or cleanup without bringing a lawsuit, you ordinarily have no legal right to participate as an equal at the bargaining table. Getting into the negotiating room under such circumstances is strictly a matter of organizing. Your group must exert enough pressure on the agency that they feel compelled to let you in. It may even help to literally jam your foot in the door!

By organizing in such circumstances, some citizens have succeeded in getting to the bargaining table. A representative of the Ayer City Home-owners in Lowell, Massachusetts, for example, meets periodically with the EPA and responsible parties for the local Silresim dumpsite. These meetings were finally arranged after years of criticism and organizing by the residents.

Suing Your Way In

If a government agency has sued to force a company to take a specific action, however, such as to clean up a site or repay the government's cleanup costs, you may be able to intervene. This procedure involves a formal legal process allowing an additional party to join a lawsuit between two or more others. Courts require you to show that:

1. You have an interest relating to the case.
2. The decision in the case may impair your ability to protect that interest.
3. The government agency does not adequately represent your interest.

If you meet all three of these tests, you may win the right to intervene.[14] You also must petition to intervene early enough in the case. Never wait till the last minute when government and polluters are preparing to sign an agreement. Courts will be most reluctant to permit intervention when lots of money and time have been spent by the parties attempting to reach an agreement. In fact, a judge may shut you out if you try to intervene late in the negotiations or after a settlement has been proposed.

Your group's biggest obstacle to intervention may be to prove that an agency does not adequately represent the community's interest. If an agency's job is to protect the environment, a court may presume that the agency is pursuing the public's interest. Yet, given the EPA's national cost-cutting agenda, you know that your interests don't necessarily coincide with those of the EPA.[15]

In 1986, two important victories occurred that will make it easier to meet this inadequate representation test. In Glen Avon, California, a group called Concerned Neighbors in Action (CNA) petitioned to intervene in the suit between the EPA and the thirty-one responsible parties at Stringfellow Acid Pits. In considering whether EPA would make all of the citizens' arguments, the court observed that EPA and the dumpers "certainly have an interest in attempting to place the blame on each other, [but] it does not necessarily follow that CNA's claims will be prosecuted as vigorously as they would be if the CNA were granted leave to intervene." In allowing the intervention, the court noted that allowing citizens into the case could lead to a more rigorous discovery process and prevent the government from bargaining away the public's interests.[16] This recognition of the need for citizen involvement sets an important precedent for future cases.

This development was then reinforced by the passage of the Superfund reauthorization in 1986. A provision of that law shifts the burden of proof to the government, under both Superfund and RCRA, to show that an intervening party is adequately spoken for by the other participants in the suit.[17] These two developments may give strong support to your intervention case. But try to develop your own proposals that go beyond what the government has shown it is willing to accept. In this way you can bolster your argument that the government will not adequately advocate your interests.

Weaker Forms of Participation

If you can't intervene, a second-best option is to become an amicus curiae, or "friend of the court." This allows your lawyer or citizens' group to submit briefs for the court's consideration. This option is much weaker than intervention, because it doesn't allow you to take depositions of witnesses, sit at the bargaining table, or veto proposed settlements. Finally, remember that federal regulations give citizens thirty days to comment on proposed settlements.[18] Your state may have similar rules.

RECOURSE AGAINST GOVERNMENT FOR DAMAGES

The principle of "sovereign immunity" has traditionally shielded government agencies and officials against lawsuits for damages by citizens harmed by their actions. But in recent years state and federal legislatures have made exceptions to this blanket exemption from liability. In the federal government, and in some states, statutes allow you to bring a lawsuit for damages against officials whose wrongful actions were not justified by their legal authority.[19] The federal law bars suits against officials who were exercising a discretionary function, however, regardless of whether they abused that discretion.[20] Even so, suits have been won even where agencies seemed to be using their discretion.[21]

Damage suits are also allowed where an agency or official violates a citizen's constitutional rights. Both federal and state activities are subject to such suits. Again, some special immunity is offered to officials, particularly where an official acted with a reasonable belief that his or her conduct was lawful.[22]

LEGAL RECOURSE AGAINST POLLUTERS

Although in general the cards are stacked against citizens in the fight with polluters to clean up their act, there are situations when you *can* sue a polluter to clean up a site or pay damages to victims.

CLEANUP ORDERS

Most judges are reluctant to order firms to clean up the pollution they caused. Rather than issuing court orders, called *injunctions,* they are inclined to estimate the damage and order the defendant to compensate for that harm. Under these traditional principles of equity, to get a court order you must show that money damages clearly could not provide adequate relief and that you will suffer irreparable harm if an injunction is not issued. Even after you prove this, judges engage in a thinking process called "balancing the equities," in which they compare the relative interests and harms of plaintiff and polluter. If the plaintiff would suffer more harm from the continuing pollution than the defendant would suffer from stopping, the court may order the pollution stopped.

This test, however, favors big companies rather than citizens affected by toxic pollution. You stand the best chance of winning an injunction if:

- The defendant has done little or nothing to control the pollution.
- The government has done little or nothing to halt the pollution.
- Your damage from the pollution is apparent.
- The cost of halting pollution is minimal compared to the harm caused.

Some judges, though, see the equities differently from others. If you get the right judge, even with these principles of equity, a defendant may be ordered to stop polluting regardless of the relative economic interests.[23]

Today, federal and state environmental laws allow citizen suits for injunctions against pollution without needing to meet the tests of equity.[24] Instead, you need only prove that a defendant is violating the law or, under some laws, is creating an imminent danger. Most of these provisions require you to give an agency and polluter written notice sixty or ninety days prior to filing a suit. A judge can order defendants to pay plaintiff's attorney fees (and, in some cases, expert witness fees). Attorney fees are not generally recoverable in lawsuits to force polluters to clean up. Citizen suits are an exception. Some of these provisions also block court action if an agency is actively prosecuting the matter.

You can file a lawsuit to pay for costs that you incur or plan to incur in regard to a local dumpsite. Citizens are authorized by CERCLA to file suits to recover "response costs" from contributors to any site that has been the source of a release of hazardous substances. The site need not be listed on the National Priorities List in order to use this provision. Your response costs may include alternative water supplies, relocation, cleanup costs, expert witness fees, medical monitoring of your family's health, and, in some courts, your attorneys' fees. The law requires that you undertake some level of expenditure prior to filing the suit (for example, conduct some of your own sampling). Also, you need to comply with the EPA regulations known as the National Contingency Plan. See section 107 of CERCLA for other prerequisites to the filing of such suits.

EMERGENCY ORDERS

In an emergency—where a toxic source is presenting an immediate danger to people's health, for example—you might attempt to obtain an emergency court order, temporary restraining order, or preliminary injunction. Given the complexity of most environmental toxics cases, however, it's tough to persuade a court that an issue is so significant that court action is necessary prior to litigation that will take months or years to complete. These orders are only likely to be given when:

- The potential pollution damage that would result without an order is very clear and irreparable.
- It seems likely that you will ultimately win your case after a full trial.
- Issuing an order in the meantime is in the public's interest.

In general, it's difficult to obtain an emergency order in a pollution case, because the facts are usually too complex to meet these tests.

COMPENSATION

In seeking compensation for toxic pollution, victims find substantial obstacles in their way. Perhaps one out of a hundred toxic pollution incidents will meet all the tests needed to make a viable compensation suit, known among lawyers as a *tort suit.* If you're seeking compensation for damage to property or to your health from toxic pollution, you may be able to obtain timely and adequate compensation through the courts if your case meets all of the following criteria:

1. Your monetary needs are not urgent. You must be able to wait until your case is resolved, possibly as long as five years. If you need money now to move out of a contaminated neighborhood, pay immediate medical bills, or secure water for household use, five years is far too long to wait. Government agency action would be more appropriate. Unfortunately, though, government agencies seldom fill all of these needs.
2. Your suit is filed within your state's statute of limitations, a deadline that blocks suits after a certain number of years have elapsed.
3. A toxic dumper can be identified and is able to pay your damages. If you have no idea who created the mess, or where to find them, or the owner is bankrupt, you may be out of luck.
4. The defendant is legally at fault, meaning that his past behavior is viewed by a judge or jury as irresponsible enough to require him to compensate those harmed. The defendant's activities must be found to lack due care, be unusually dangerous, or unreasonably interfere with the enjoyment of another's property (be a "nuisance"). This rule can make it particularly difficult to sue multiple polluters at a dumpsite where wastes may have been sent many years ago with government approval or even under government orders.
5. Your injuries are "more likely than not" caused by the acts of the defendant. This rule can make it difficult to sue where evidence is costly to obtain, nonexistent because of gaps in past environmental monitoring, or statistically complex.
6. Your injuries are of a type that is compensated under your state's court rulings. In most states, damages compensated include:

   • Medical bills and other "out-of-pocket" expenses
   • Lost wages while you were out of work sick

- Pain and suffering (as estimated by a jury)
- Property damage, diminished property values, and lost rent
- Costs of obtaining alternative water supplies or taking other reasonable actions to protect your family's health

In most states, the following damages are not compensated:

- Fears of getting sick in the future, however well justified those fears are, if you are not sick today
- Your risk of getting sick in the future, if you are not sick from the toxics today

In some states, courts also allow punitive damages—an amount assessed against defendants to punish their bad behavior and deter similar acts by others.

7. Either the amount of damage you suffer is considerable or many others have suffered similar, relatively small, but demonstrable damages. To bring your case on contingency—to arrange to pay your lawyer through a percentage of any settlement won—the amount of harm you have suffered as approximated in a monetary amount must be large enough that it is likely to be worth a large investment of time and preparation expenses. Typically a personal injury case must be worth at least $100,000. In a factually complicated case, this threshold may be even higher. For instance, lawyers for the plaintiffs in the Woburn, Massachusetts, hazardous waste case invested more than a million dollars in evidence to build a compelling case. That case was ultimately settled for an estimated $9 million.

An exception to this $100,000 threshold is where you can file a class action suit—that is, where many people have suffered similar damages that can be combined into a sizable class. Some individuals are listed as exemplary plaintiffs and participate fully in the suit. Most of the others are less directly involved in the case, but unless they decide at the outset to file their own suit, they'll share in any award to the class.

To the extent that your case fails to meet these criteria, the court system will probably not meet your compensation needs. This system just doesn't bring justice to most toxic victims. It shuts out those whose needs are too urgent, whose monetary claims are too small, or whose problems are too new for compensation through antiquated legal rules.

If you think you may have a good compensation case, ask a lawyer for an assessment. Since a viable compensation suit can later prove profitable for the lawyer, most attorneys will not charge to take an initial look at your case.

CAN THE POLLUTERS SUE US?

When citizen groups press local companies to clean up their act, company lawyers sometimes file suits against the citizens alleging libel, slander, harassment, or other charges. These suits are intended to scare you off. It's easy enough for the firm to file such charges. But rarely will such a firm prevail in the case. In the event that such charges are filed or threatened, consider the following strategies.

Have your lawyer prepare a memorandum to your group explaining the chances of the company winning the suit. If their case is weak, blast them publicly and consider countersuing.

Tape record your group's conversations with outsiders, and let them know that you're recording. One activist described a situation in which a firm charged members of her group with slander. The company even got false statements in affidavits from five local businessmen to back up its charges. In the end, the citizen group got the charges dropped because of damaging statements they had of company officials on tape.

Contact the local chapter of the American Civil Liberties Union (ACLU) for legal support. The ACLU is concerned about the threat such suits pose to your First Amendment rights to free speech.

Use their lawsuit as an opportunity for sweeping information-gathering on the firm's activities. Remember: The discovery process allows your lawyer to demand any information that may lead to information relevant to the suit. Since the firm's character has been placed at issue by its suit, you are entitled to make broad inquiries about anything that could lead to discovery of unethical or unsafe behavior in the firm.

WHAT CAN GO WRONG: A FINAL CAVEAT

We've just seen many possible ways in which citizens can sue polluters or the government to protect their community. Nevertheless, it's important to reiterate that bringing legal action is never a replacement for organizing your community. The following example highlights what can go wrong when you put all your eggs in a lawyer's basket.

In 1983 a group in a suburban area contacted the Citizens Clearinghouse for Hazardous Waste (CCHW) for guidance on opposing the construction of a solid-waste landfill. The people of this suburb were primarily older residents plus a small but growing number of professionals. All told, the group had two or three hundred members of varied backgrounds. CCHW gave the group some basic advice: Organize. Put out a fact sheet. Go door to door to educate the public. Petition. Get people involved.

In the months that followed, the group called CCHW frequently for advice. Each time they were given the same advice: action. The group seemed to agree, yet took no action. At the outset they had hired a prominent lawyer from the area. He was well respected in the county and had numerous official contacts. The group relied on his suggestions and would not take any action that contradicted them. Effective methods like canvassing door to door, putting out flyers, and petitioning he considered "undignified." The group, he said, should not engage in any activity that might upset any court action.

Within a year, the ribbon-cutting ceremony was held for the unlined landfill the group had formed to oppose. Of the group's hundreds of members, ten or fifteen carried signs that day—their first public demonstration. Their fight had been lost by their lawyer. Anticipating a loss of the court fight, he had been calling for a lined landfill.

In the process the group accumulated legal fees amounting to nearly $300,000. The group's only courtroom victory came after they had lost their major fight. By dropping a subsequent suit against the county, they were able to recover $75,000 of their legal fees from the county.

Today the landfill is leaking and the group is now taking that issue to the streets with some success. At last, they are learning from their mistakes.

NOTES

1. This discussion of when to hire a lawyer draws much of its inspiration from articles by the Citizens Clearinghouse on Hazardous Waste.
2. Federal Rules of Civil Procedure, Rule 26(b)(1).
3. There is a trend in the courts to increase rather than decrease the range of agency actions viewed by the courts as "committed to agency discretion." See *Heckler v. Chaney*, 105 S. Ct. 1649 (1985).
4. A court may overturn agency actions "in excess of statutory authority or short of statutory right"; 5 USC sec. 706.
5. In *Citizens to Preserve Overton Park v. Volpe*, 401 U.S. 402 (1971), a community group sued the secretary of transportation to block the release of funds to build a federal highway through a park. Federal law prohibited highways from being built through parks if a feasible and prudent alternative existed. There had been no formal findings issued by the secretary of transportation prior to planning.

The Supreme Court returned the case to the lower court with instructions that that court could require agency officials to testify to explain their actions and could require the agency to make formal findings for the court.

6. See, for example, *Seacoast Anti-Pollution League v. Costle,* 572 F.2d 872, 876 (1st Cir. 1978), requiring a formal hearing to protect rights of citizens at a specific site when an agency's action might deplete shellfish, fish, and wildlife at the site.

7. For an analogous case where denial of life was a basis for finding a right to at least an informal hearing prior to a government decision, see *Goldberg v. Kelly,* 397 U.S. 254 (1970), in which a government decision to terminate welfare benefits was held to threaten the recipient's ability to live.

8. Telephone conversation with Rick Parrish, Environmental Task Force.

9. Attorney's fees are not generally recoverable in lawsuits to force agency action. The citizen suit provisions are an exception.

10. CERCLA sec. 113 (h)(4).

11. See EPA's *Community Relations in Superfund: A Handbook* (1983), chap. 6.

12. 50 Fed. Reg. 47914, 47933 (November 20, 1985).

13. CERCLA sec. 122. Alternatively, if an off-site RCRA disposal site is used for wastes from a facility or permanent destruction of materials at the facility is expected, then a full release from future liability to the United States must be granted in any agreement; sec. 122(f).

14. Federal Rules of Civil Procedure, Rule 24(a)(2).

15. In *Southeast Alaska Conservation Council, Inc. v. Watson,* 35 Fed. R. Serv. 2d 1255 (9th Cir. 1983), a fishermen's association was allowed to intervene because its economic interests might not be adequately represented by plaintiffs pursuing aesthetic and recreational goals.

16. *United States v. Stringfellow,* No. 84-5682 (9th Cir., February 18, 1986).

17. CERCLA sec. 113(i).

18. 28 CFR 50.7(c).

19. The action must be one that would lead to liability if the actor were a private party. See Federal Tort Claims Act, 28 USC secs. 1291, 1346(b)(c), 1402(b), 1504, 3110, 2401(b), 2402, 2411(b), 2412(c), 2671–2680.

20. 28 USCA <2680(a).

21. For instance, the Coast Guard was successfully sued when its failure to maintain a beacon caused a shipwreck; *Indian Towing Co. v. United States* 350 U.S. 611 (1955). The Forest Service was sued when its neglect in fighting a fire caused property damage; *Rayonier Inc. v. United States* 352 U.S. 315 (1957).

22. But *Butz v. Economou* 438 U.S. 478 (1978) afforded quasi-judicial action by agency officials even broader immunity.

23. For example, *Roughton v. Thiele Kaolin Co.* 209 Ga. 577, 74 S.E.2d 844 (1953); *Whalen v. Union Paper Bag Co.* 208 N.Y. 1, 101 N.E. 805 (1913).

24. *Environmental Defense Fund v. Lamphier* 714 F.2d 331, 13 ELR 21094 (4th Cir. 1983).

9

Local Campaigns and the Law

SANFORD LEWIS

Grassroots activists are transforming the way that government and industry handle toxic chemical problems. Your efforts on the local and state levels, and perhaps on the national level, can play a part in the movement toward truly effective controls over toxics. In the coming years, activists will need to focus their attention on two dramatic gaps in the system: enforcement and prevention.

While an impressive body of toxics laws are on the books, they are only as strong as their enforcement. Generally, the laws are scarcely being enforced. Citizens taking on a local problem for the first time are often surprised to discover that government seems to be playing ball with businesses that jeopardize the public's health. Government officials have no shortage of excuses for allowing pollution to continue. For instance:

- "We don't have the staff to think through all of the issues." There are no across-the-board emission standards for many toxics. Proceeding case by case is difficult, time consuming, and costly.
- "We don't have the inspection staff." Violators are not detected due to inadequate field inspections.
- "The company may have been a lawbreaker in the past, but now it has agreed to do all that it can." Violators are given extensions or waivers due to "extenuating" circumstances or "good faith" efforts.
- "We don't have the power or staff to punish all of the violators." The

legal authority and personnel are lacking to punish every violator that's detected.

Citizen activists are changing this picture by insisting that more resources go for enforcement, pushing laws to step up agency powers, conducting innovative enforcement projects, and generally refusing to accept the standard excuses for government inaction.

The only truly effective way to prevent toxic hazards is to reduce the use of the most dangerous chemicals. Not only is citizen pressure needed to increase law enforcement, but it also must convert nearsighted enforcement into preventive enforcement. Citizen pressure can move agencies to enforcement strategies that don't just shift toxic by-products from air to water to land like a toxic shell game but, rather, take toxics out of the environment once and for all by reducing and even eliminating their use.

The saga of Saco, Maine, is a vivid example of how citizens can win such a campaign. After many years of dumping its electroplating wastes into the river, in 1985 a local manufacturer was ordered by state officials to correct its illegal practices. The firm proposed piping the wastes across town to discharge further downstream, which would dilute its chromium to a legally tolerated level.

Local residents sought another solution. Instead of going along with this typical "nonsolution" to toxic pollution, they joined with the National Toxics Campaign (NTC) and the Maine People's Alliance (MPA) to ask the firm to reduce its chromium discharge at the source. NTC showed how similar companies had actually eliminated the need to use toxics. MPA showed the citizens how to get the word out and build their clout.

The "new pipe vs. toxics reduction" battle began to escalate. Soon it was the top story in local newspapers. Sportsmen and concerned citizens lined up on one side, the firm on the other. Eventually the controversy became an election issue. Five of the six candidates who supported toxics reduction won their races, creating a new majority on the city council. The toxics issue was clearly the deciding factor in turnover of council members. The new town council required the company to study toxics reduction and report back to them. In the meantime, the town withheld the permit needed to build the pipeline. In July 1986, the company's study showed that the wastes didn't have to be dumped into the river at all. Finally, the company agreed to eliminate its toxic river dumping.

You can win your local toxics fight by following Saco's example. Consider using every feasible opportunity—permits, technical information, inspections, policy debates, elections—to raise issues of toxics enforcement and prevention. Your local campaign may range from an all-out community organizing effort to a citizens' lawsuit to a series of press conferences. Your campaign can be carried out no matter how little money and people power you have. A campaign to get local businesses to reduce their production of hazardous wastes and use of toxics, for example, might take any of these approaches:

- The tin-plated approach: Send a letter to twelve local companies requesting them to allow you to review their in-plant toxic reduction efforts. Hold a press conference publicizing the results of your inquiries.
- The silver-plated approach: Send a small delegation of your organization's members to local plants with the same request. Arm your members with additional questions or requests of company officials.
- The gold-plated approach: Establish a new community group concerned with toxic enforcement and prevention. Do door-to-door canvassing to announce the group's formation. Bring in national experts. Formulate a detailed list of issues you want the target firm to address— a complete toxics prevention platform. Stage a major neighborhood meeting to deliver this platform to the target firm's executives.

PREPARING FOR YOUR LOCAL CAMPAIGN

Toxics issues are so complex that many a fight has been lost by bogging down in endless research. Minimize the amount of time you must spend in the library; maximize the time you spend on the politics of the issue. In this section we'll look at the key questions to ask during the first step of your campaign.

CLARIFY YOUR GOALS

At the outset, you'll need enough information to select the major focus of your local campaign—a company, a cluster of companies, or a government agency. If you already know who you'll target, you can start the information gathering. Don't wear yourself out doing detailed research on every possible target! Instead, clarify your goals. Pinpoint your key concerns first. For example:

- Hot issues
- Known problem sites

- Districts that are politically important
- Media interest and coverage
- Objectives of your group

GATHER TECHNICAL INFORMATION

After you've narrowed the possible targets to a few specific companies or agencies, begin your research. Using Freedom of Information Act (FOIA) and right-to-know requests, start gathering information.

Key questions in your research relate to the importance of toxics and to possible lawbreaking. Try to learn the types and locations of toxics. Consider the amount of toxics being dumped, emitted, or stored. Is anything known about human exposure via water, air, land, or food? What do scientists say about the health damage the substances may cause? Is the agency or company breaking the law? Find out if there are any known violations by target firms. Are federal or state officials aggressively prosecuting violations? Are some firms likely to be using toxics without being regulated?

Remember: You need not gather enough details to prosecute violations yourself. Just get enough information to state a clear public concern over problems at target firms or agencies. Later, though, you may want to expand your information. Here are a few examples of technical questions that can take longer to answer:

- How much of a toxic chemical is handled and emitted by a firm?
- What are the firm's safety practices?
- Are there EPA standards for this industry and these toxics?
- Are there ways of reducing the toxics used and disposed of in this industry?
- What legal loopholes may apply? Are they being abused here?

You may not want to wait for answers before launching your campaign.

ASSESS YOUR RESULTS AND DESIGNATE TARGETS

After you've got your information, assess it and select a target. One aspect of this targeting is judging how serious the toxics problem is at a given site, agency, or firm compared with other problems. You may want to select a group of companies or agencies you'll ultimately want to address and also a top-priority target on which to start. But you must also consider many other political and strategic questions:

- Is the proposed campaign winnable? How long is it likely to take to win?
- Will your campaign capture the public's and the media's attention? Are the local media receptive to covering toxics issues?
- Is the target industry or agency big enough or bad enough to give your campaign a "David and Goliath" or "Robin Hood" theme?
- Who runs the target firm or agency? Would they make an exciting focus?
- Is the community organized? If it is, would a campaign help to revitalize the organization? If it isn't, what are the indications that the community is a likely place to organize? Is there community interest? Is there a core group of people who'd be interested in creating an organization?
- Would working on the campaign help meet your organization's needs—say, building membership and bringing in new coalition partners? Would your campaign reach out to unions, seniors, or other constituencies?
- Would working on the campaign help to expand or strengthen your organization's leadership? Would your allies in high places support you?
- If you have a door-to-door canvass, how would it fit in this campaign?
- Would the campaign enhance your group's credibility with the media, opinion leaders, and other key institutions?
- How would the campaign relate to other work your group has done in the community?
- What level of staff, door-to-door canvass, and financial resources will your organization dedicate to this campaign?
- Do you have technical experts at your disposal for this effort? Can you get such support elsewhere (say, from NTC)?
- Could your campaign be made a crucial issue in an upcoming electoral fight? Will there be a key congressional race in your district? Will you create a strong constituency on toxics issues for a key congressional representative?

PLANNING YOUR CAMPAIGN

When you are about to enter a campaign against a polluter, it's important to design a campaign plan that makes best use of the legal handles available to you. Before launching a major effort, use the information in the following pages to help focus your campaign plan and map out the strategy that will bring you success.

PROFILE THE TARGETS AND LIST THE ISSUES

Prepare short "fact sheets" that convincingly document any violations, the extent of toxic dumping, or potential public health and environmental threats from the target firms or agencies. Try to dramatize the problem by estimating the amount of toxics going into the environment every day or every year. (For other strategies, see Chapter 2.)

Next list the concerns that will be the focus of your campaign, featured in letter writing, petitions, meetings, and other efforts. Here's a list of typical issues:

1. Enforce existing pollution control laws.
   - Ensure that all businesses are being regulated. Have they applied for the appropriate permits? Does the agency know of all toxics uses and discharges?
   - Ensure that the government strictly limits allowable pollution. Are agencies actually regulating the full range of toxics that are used or emitted? Are all restrictions applied to toxics as strict as they can be?
   - Ensure strong enforcement of government restrictions. Are industries largely allowed to monitor their own pollution? Are there frequent government inspections? Are lawbreakers promptly and properly penalized? Are lawbreakers promptly brought into compliance?

2. Establish preventive activities beyond the legal requirements.
   - Does the public take action on local toxic uses, emissions, and management?
   - Is there a toxics reduction program at each local firm?
   - Is there an accident prevention program at each local firm using highly toxic chemicals?
   - Are neighborhood inspections conducted?

3. Apply the "polluters must pay" principle.
   - Do major toxics users pay for enforcement by government and citizens?
   - Do major toxics users pay for independent public review of their toxics reduction and accident prevention programs?

• Do major toxics users pay for all environmental and human harm caused by pollution?

You can use this outline to draw up a list of issues that apply to *your* campaign.

CONSIDER ALL THE LEGAL HANDLES

Now that you know what you want, how are you going to make it happen? Your campaign strategy depends on your leverage, local politics, and your resources. Make a list of all the legal handles your group could conceivably use to press your target for action. If you're targeting a firm, consider whether any of following apply:

• Does the company have state or federal permits for air pollution, water pollution, or hazardous waste?
• Does the company have local permits for storage of flammables or toxics or the use of underground tanks?
• Are any of the state or local permits up for renewal, due soon, or subject to being "reopened"?
• Does the company lease property from the town?
• Does the company plan to make changes that will require zoning variances or other local permits?
• Does the company have special state financing? Does it need to apply for such financing?
• Are environmental actions being taken against the firm for past or current violations? Are there violations that could warrant such attention?
• Do banks, insurers, or stockholders have a special interest in the firm's toxics handling practices?
• Is the firm vulnerable to bad press?
• Are there incentives (such as financial or technical assistance) to move the firm to act?

Later in this chapter we'll discuss where you can find handles and how to make the most of them. Never start with the assumption that handles don't exist. You may be surprised to find little-known laws that can be of help. For example, the City of Cincinnati wanted to prevent the transportation of hazardous materials via an interstate highway that went through the city. Rather than passing a new local ordinance, they discovered a little-known federal regulation banning the transport of hazardous materials through cities. Local police simply began enforcing the law, giving $75 tickets to truckers of hazardous materials.[1] According to Dr. Fred Millar of the Environmental Policy Institute, this was actually the first time that citations had been issued under this long-standing federal rule!

CHOOSE YOUR STRATEGY

Your group must make a realistic assessment of its strengths, its resources, and how these strengths and resources can be improved. Can you enlist the help of actual or potential allies, such as other groups, the media, unions, and politicians? Finally, select the best strategies based on such considerations as:

- The most effective means of building your organization's power.
- Your target's weaknesses and your understanding of what's most important to the target.
- Time frames. (Will the water pollution permit be renewed in two years, or is a decision impending immediately?)
- Your organization's long-term goals.

Consider combining several strategies for maximum effectiveness. You might, for example, direct part of your strategy at state-level enforcement: publicizing a firm's pollution violations, asking the attorney general to seek stiff penalties, and asking that the state's schedule for correcting the violations include a toxics reduction plan. Simultaneously, at the local level you could organize opposition to the company's request for a zoning variance or building permit until it proposes an effective toxics reduction plan.

CAMPAIGNING TO WIN

No matter which legal handles you choose, adopt a winning strategy for your local campaign. Motivate the right person to make the right decision. Consider the motivating factors of key decision makers. Put yourself in their shoes. What would make it easy to decide in your favor? What would make it hard to decide against you? It might mean holding private meetings with these key figures or with people who influence them. It might mean organizing huge demonstrations showing overwhelming public sentiment.

It might mean bringing in experts to show that your solution is technically possible and credible.

Remember that hearings and legal angles alone are not nearly so useful if you don't also demonstrate public concern through a strong organizing effort. A great example of massive organizing to oppose facility licensing occurred in North Carolina, where a radioactive materials incinerator had been proposed by U.S. Ecology. Three or four thousand people organized by community, clergy, and civil rights groups appeared at hearings to oppose the license.

Shape the debate to *win*. What are the opposition's best arguments? Have you truly rebutted them? What questions still linger in decision makers' minds? Which members are having an attack of conscience? How can you help translate such attacks into votes in your favor? Some decision makers may ask themselves, "What's the worst that can happen if I decide against the citizens?" What *is* the worst that can happen? Could it cost politicians or others their jobs? Would anyone be embarrassed? Are you prepared to escalate your efforts? To do whatever it takes to win? How can you get the press coverage you need? Is your information condensed into simple quote-sized bites for the press?

Look for ways to force the issue. Is there a convenient link between your local economy and your toxics problem that will force people to stand up and take notice? In New Jersey, beaches were closed a record-breaking thirty-five times during the summer of 1986 due to detection of high coliform levels (an indicator of sewage contamination). The loss of business in resort communities, whose economy is based on the beaches, is beginning to move state, county, and local officials to strengthen enforcement of proper operation of sewage treatment plants.[2]

Take first things first. Decide what you hope to achieve during each phase of your campaign. (Sort out opponents and allies, raise public awareness, win intermediate victories, and so on.)

USING DIRECT NEGOTIATIONS

Simply pushing for more government action isn't always enough, however, for often the government's programs ensure only minimum protection. By dealing directly with the polluter you can often secure more reliable protection. What you can see for yourself—through direct inspections with your own expert—may be far more reliable than a government inspector's report about conditions in a plant. A firm's written agreement with your group may give your neighborhood far more protection than a government agency can provide. For one thing, you may want some guarantees that the government is unwilling or unable to provide. For example, without a direct agreement with the company (or the passage of new laws) you may be unable to obtain:

- A company toxics reduction plan
- Technical assistance funding to review the firm's activities
- The right to inspect the firm periodically
- Comprehensive safety protection at the facility
- The right to ongoing participation in the company's toxics handling decisions

While you don't ordinarily have a legal right of access to neighboring plants for inspection or negotiations, these rights can be won through strong organizing and the use of handles such as those described here. Working with Massachusetts Fair Share, for example, residents of numerous Massachusetts communities have fought for—and, in some cases, won—the right to inspect dangerous industrial facilities accompanied by their own safety experts. After the inspections revealed safety problems, citizens have won improvements in toxics handling through direct negotiations with companies. In another case, a transporter and recycler of hazardous wastes was inspected by local citizens five times. After the first inspection the group and their industrial hygienist scored numerous improvements. While these changes cost the company thousands of dollars initially, they paid for themselves within a year due to savings in materials and operational costs.

GUIDELINES FOR ACTION

If you're getting nowhere with action by the government or the company, you might want to explore direct negotiation. But before you enter any phase of negotiation you must be sure the conditions are right. Publicity, for example, might be undesirable to either side. You may want to be sure the company is prepared to negotiate in good faith before allowing them the good publicity that could arise from the image of hearty cooperation. You may want to precondition early conversations on absolute secrecy, so that no one outside of your group and company officials will be told of these exploratory talks.

If exploratory discussions do take place, you can use them to allow each player to define exactly what he means by "negotiation." Are there concerns that both sides are interested in discussing? Would the company be willing to reach a binding agreement enforceable by your group? Remind them that you've got an arsenal of tactics ready to use in the event that negotiations fail.

If your group decides that it's appropriate, enter formal negotiations with the firm's executives. At the end of this process, you'll want a written, verifiable agreement. Here are some ground rules to keep in mind.

Appoint a negotiating team for your group. If your group is large, chances are that not everyone will participate in discussions with the company. If a smaller group is delegated to meet with the firm, give this negotiating team explicit instructions about how far they can go in the session and what kinds of issues must be brought back for a group decision.

Negotiating requires listening. Companies need to listen to community residents. Community residents should also be prepared to listen to companies. Important information may be gained.

Do not surrender your power. You may want to keep up your pressure tactics throughout the negotiation—for instance, you can picket or sue the company and negotiate at the same time. In any event, don't give up your right to picket, to sue, to organize, or to do whatever else is needed, just because a company is willing to talk with you.

Plan your negotiating strategy carefully. Before entering negotiations with the firm, decide who from your group will chair the meeting and what will be said (and not be said) in the session. Be clear about what kinds of disclosures you want to make and avoid. It's generally inadvisable to disclose your "bottom line" in a negotiation, for instance, or to reveal the hidden weaknesses in your group's power or strategy.

Be prepared for give and take. Set your initial demands high enough that there's room to compromise on some points. Be clear about your most crucial interests, and be clear on the difference between your interests and your negotiating posture. You may be calling for the company to shut down, for example, but your real concern may be securing your neighborhood's health and safety. If the firm can guarantee your safety without closing, would you be willing to discuss that?

Decide whether, when, and why you want lawyers present at the bargaining table. If you're engaged in formal proceedings against the firm, both your lawyer and the firm's lawyers are likely to be precluded by legal ethics from talking with the opposition's client unless the opposing lawyer is present or has given permission to meet with his or her clients.[3] If the presence of lawyers is likely to impede your ability to speak for yourselves and listen to company executives, you may want to shut all lawyers out. But if you're negotiating the detailed terms of an agreement or other legal issues will be discussed, it may make sense to have lawyers present.

Be sure that you're talking to the right people. Verify that the people sent to negotiate by the company have the authority to make the decisions needed. If not, insist on meeting with those people.

Carefully consider the role of any outsiders in the negotiation process: politicians, environmental officials, reporters, and mediators. Before allowing any of these figures into the negotiation room, your group should consider the pros and cons of each. Some typical concerns are:

- With reporters present, neither side may be able to speak frankly. But you may want the media present to show the public how unreasonable the company is being.
- You may want politicians present who are strong allies and can exert pressure on the company if negotiations fail. But less strongly allied politicians can be a problem. They may participate in the process and then steal all the credit. Their presence might also force you to compromise more than you'd like, since they may press for what *they* consider to be a reasonable outcome. Politicians like to act as mediators. Sometimes this is okay, but beware of their pressure to settle for less.
- Environmental officials must be consulted on any aspects of your agreement that will have to be enforced by their agencies. They can also be a key source of technical information. But inviting them to all the meetings may focus the discussion on narrow technical issues.
- Mediators can help both sides set ground rules to make a negotiation work. They can help keep the discussion on track. They can even act as a go-between between your group and the company. But the costs of having a mediator can also be high. Not only must they be paid but, acting as a go-between, they may miscommunicate information for both sides. A poor mediator can distract from the heart of discussion and even make inappropriate comments that undermine your leverage or results. Remember: A mediator is not an ally of your group but a neutral party. If you do have a mediator, carefully work out the ground rules for his or her participation—such as the aspects of the negotiation they will be involved in and exactly what their role is. Be sure the members of your group understand that the mediator must be treated just as cautiously as the firm.

Try to have your speaker chair the meeting, following an agenda agreed upon with the firm. Begin with a short presentation: Why are you there and what are you asking for? Sum up the results at the end of the meeting. Such simple procedures can help keep the meeting on track and focused on your issues.

During your negotiation sessions, ask all the "what if" and "why not" questions. You can make major headway in negotiations by showing that a company is being unreasonable when they say "it would be impossible for us to . . ." You can ask them "why not?" and insist on proof.

Consider using some public record or forum to document whether the firm is being cooperative. A firm with permit applications pending before an agency, for example, may tell that agency they're negotiating with you to demonstrate their good faith. If they're cooperating, say so; if not, document this on the public record.

Caucus during and between negotiating sessions. If any member of your team is unsure what to say during a session, take a break out of earshot from the company officials and other outsiders to consider your strategy. Don't hesitate to walk out of the session if the firm is being uncooperative. In between negotiating sessions, you'll probably want to get together with other members of your group and discuss strategy, progress, and issues raised in your discussion. List all the issues on a flipchart and discuss them one by one during these group strategy sessions.

Get any agreement in writing. But before you do, think about what could go wrong. Are there any loopholes, intentional or unintentional, in your proposed agreement? Any agreement you reach should be put in writing so that you have a permanent record of what you've agreed to. Try to have the agreement written as a legally binding contract. Have a lawyer assist you in drawing one up. Here are some examples of the terms of such a contract:

- The creation of a fund, paid for by the company but managed by your group, that allows you to hire needed experts.
- Provisions allowing you to verify action by the firm consistent with your agreement—such as the issuance of a toxics reduction report by the company by a specific date or the right to a number of unannounced inspections by your group.
- A clause requiring company compliance with all environmental and health and safety laws and allowing your group to enforce these laws directly and penalize the firm for violations.
- Easy enforcement clauses—such as the right of your group to require binding arbitration if the firm appears to be violating the agreement; to have large stipulated fines prepaid in an escrow account or bonded and

paid to your group or a designated charity upon determination of a breach of the agreement; or to have your attorney fees paid by the firm in the event that you must sue to enforce the agreement.
- A clause stating that if a court voids any part of your agreement, the remaining provisions will remain in effect.

Be sure the agreement is signed by the right officials. Check your state's laws to ensure that the company officials who sign your agreement have the power to bind the corporation to comply.

USING THE LAW

The law offers plenty of strong handles for preventing toxic usage, incidents, and exposure. Local activists must understand, however, that often you may want a firm to do something the laws do not actually require. Obtaining this action may thus become a matter of using political and legal tools to your maximum advantage. The target firm may meet your demands because what you want is common sense or because it wants to end the uncertainty or costs you are imposing on it.

Local toxics reduction campaigns are a good example of how using an arsenal of agencies and laws can lead to winning your desired results. Although this discussion focuses on toxics reduction measures, it applies as well to other actions you may want a firm to undertake. As we will see, there are no current laws that order firms to reduce their usage of toxics. Yet there are many laws you can use to pressure a firm into reducing its toxics. Before we turn to environmental law, however, let's look at the basic elements you'd want a company to incorporate in its toxic reduction program—in other words, the things to ask for in your negotiations:

- A Plan: The company should develop a plan detailing its reduction of toxics usage and waste production.
- Toxics Inventory: The company should list quantities of chemicals entering, used, and leaving the plant via all routes, broken down process by process. This inventory, known as a *mass balance,* is the chemical equivalent of balancing a checkbook.
- Priority Framework: Based on the results of the inventory, the firm should set priorities. Chemicals receiving the most attention would be selected according to such factors as toxicity, volume, and cost of material losses.

- Process Changes: The firm should evaluate alternatives for reduction and develop a list of planned changes, alternatives evaluated, and toxics with no reduction alternatives.
- Schedules and Targets: The firm should prepare a timetable for implementing the reductions.
- Evaluation Plan: The firm should devise a plan for reviewing progress.
- Company Programs: The firm should name the highest-ranking official with direct responsibility and identify the programs aimed at waste reduction such as employee training or research and development.
- Broad Focus: The plan should cover hazardous wastes, water and air discharges, and risks of accidental releases.
- Preparation by Engineer: The plan should be prepared or reviewed by a licensed professional engineer prior to submission.
- Review Process: Members of the concerned public must have an opportunity to review the plan, along with their own experts, and to comment at a public forum regarding selection of alternatives under the plan. A government body should review the plan for completeness and require further work if the plan is incomplete. The public must have access to sufficient information about the facility and its production processes, including the toxics reduction plan in draft and final forms.

FEDERAL AND STATE LAWS

The RCRA Requirement

One federal environmental law, the Resource Conservation and Recovery Act (RCRA), directly encourages reduced toxics usage and waste production on a company-by-company basis. Every facility that generates more than 1,000 kilograms a month of hazardous waste is supposed to have "a program in place to reduce the volume or quantity and toxicity of such waste to the degree determined by the generator to be economically practicable." Generators sign a "boilerplate" clause asserting these facts on the form that accompanies each of their waste shipments. To document these assertions, they must submit, at least once every two years, a report "setting out the efforts undertaken during the year to reduce the volume and toxicity of waste generated, and [comparing] the changes in volume and toxicity actually achieved during the year in question . . . with previous years to the extent such information is available for years prior to [1984]."[4]

Legally, this requirement is so weak that it seems unlikely that EPA would actually use it to make a company reduce its wastes. In fact, the EPA has virtually stated that its enforcement efforts in this area will be limited to ensuring that a waste generator signs the waste minimization statement and submits the required reports. Other than that, EPA says that each generator should make a "good faith effort" to minimize waste.

Guidelines for Action

- Use the Freedom of Information Act to request the manifest forms of any local firms who ship hazardous wastes off-site (to see whether they've signed the statement that they are reducing their wastes) and biennial reports of all local hazardous waste generators (to review the extent of their waste minimization efforts). Generators were required to issue their first biennial waste reduction report in March 1987 and in March of each odd-numbered year thereafter.
- Request information directly from the firm beyond what you get through the Freedom of Information Act. Since there are no detailed EPA regulations governing the scope of a company's waste minimization reports, there is no assurance that these reports will do anything but skim the surface of what the firm has or hasn't done about reducing the use of toxics. Insist on detailed reports on in-plant toxics reduction with enough information for a plant's neighbors to judge for themselves whether a company has exercised "good faith" in its waste minimization efforts. (Compare the firm's efforts with the basic elements of a toxics reduction program described previously.)
- Pose questions to the target company and the EPA: Has the firm evaluated all available alternatives for reducing the major waste streams generated at the facility? Who did an evaluation? How thoroughly did they consider the economics and technology of toxic reduction? Does the firm plan to review every waste stream for its toxics reduction potential? How often will the firm conduct its toxics reduction study to consider new technologies and changing economics? When the firm makes in-plant changes, will they automatically consider the potential for toxics reduction? Has the firm evaluated the feasibility of elementary steps to toxics reduction—such as separating mixed waste streams (waste segregation)? Does the firm take a broad approach to toxics reduction—not only evaluating legally defined hazardous wastes but considering all waste streams and toxic hazards?

Your Right to Know Under Superfund

Amendments to the Superfund law enacted in 1986 established extensive right-to-know requirements, as well as state emergency response commissions and local emergency planning committees with responsibility for chemical accident preparedness. By August 13, 1987, each state had to designate members of the local emergency planning committees including environmental and community group members. By October 13, 1988, local committees had to complete their plans for local toxic emergencies.

Prevention, not evacuation, ought to be the first line of defense against local toxic hazards. Yet the emphasis under Superfund is on the aftermath of a toxic incident: how to give notice, evacuate the area, and clean up the mess. Ultimately, federal amendments will be needed to create a strong nationwide toxics prevention program. But in your local campaign you can reorient these local committees to meet your preventive agenda.

Guidelines for Action
- After you obtain information about a company's toxics usage or emissions, using your right to know, publicize the chemicals and their health effects. Call on the company to explain the need for these chemicals.
- Use the information gathered during the emergency planning process for details on toxics reduction. The local committee is specifically entitled by law to any information from facility owners and operators deemed "necessary for developing and implementing the emergency plan." The local committee can even bring a civil suit against a facility to obtain the information. You can urge the committee to request any relevant details of chemical usage, technologies, and alternatives needed to achieve toxics reduction at a target firm.
- When committee members are appointed under the Superfund law, issue a preventive challenge. Call on the industry appointees to set a good example for the rest of the industrial community by disclosing their own toxics reduction and chemical safety practices.

Other Federal/State Programs and Permits

The RCRA waste minimization provision does not call for reduction of toxic wastes and materials that are not technically designated as hazardous wastes. In fact, the government gives firms permission every day to dump toxic contaminants into our air and water without first reducing their toxics to the extent feasible. While probably more chemicals are spewed into the environment through smokestacks and drainpipes than via hazardous waste barrels, few "waste minimization" requirements exist for air and water toxics. And although the risks of a major chemical accident are pervasive, there are no rules requiring minimization of large-scale chemical storage.

Chapter 7 described the federal/state structure of environmental law. Any of the federal and state environmental laws may give you leverage for your toxics reduction demands.

Guidelines for Action

- Link toxics reduction to enforcement action by state or federal agencies and attorneys general. Call for violators to be required by consent decrees or compliance schedules to minimize use of their most toxic and most prevalent hazardous substances. They should be required to evaluate alternatives for toxics reduction, develop a timetable for implementing all feasible changes, and describe all alternatives evaluated. Public review of this plan should be allowed.
- Use the proposed renewal or issuance of a firm's environmental permits—on air pollution, water pollution, wetlands, or hazardous waste—as an opportunity to call for a complete company-wide program to reduce toxics usage. Oppose the permit on whatever grounds are valid within the agency's own regulations, laws, and guidelines. At the same time, even though the agency's regulations may not currently require it, insist that the firm be denied the permit until they prove a need to use and dispose of toxics through a complete company-wide toxics reduction plan. Couch your opposition in terms of a gradual phaseout of toxics. You could call for "zero discharge" of the most toxic substances to all environmental media within ten years, for example, unless the company proves that toxics reduction alternatives are infeasible.
- Link local dumpsite cleanup to the toxics reduction issue. Government negotiations with polluters at Superfund dumpsites do not often go beyond issues of site cleanup. Yet the same firms responsible for the dumps routinely produce hazardous wastes today, subjecting the public to continuing toxic risks even as they negotiate to minimize their cleanup responsibilities. Organize for a stronger role in the settlement process—both to gain a real role in cleanup bargaining and to press for

toxic use reduction by polluters as part of any settlement. Review their biannual RCRA waste reduction reports to the EPA.

LOCAL POWERS

In many instances you can combine local powers and laws as an arsenal of tools to press companies to reduce the amount of toxics they handle. Among the tools that may already be on the books in your area are health board powers, zoning and building codes, state EIR requirements, leases and property acquisition by local government, aquifer protection ordinances, local emergency planning committees, and eminent domain powers. Your pressure on local agencies to deny permits or take enforcement action can lead to the effective use of these powers for toxics reduction.

Health Boards

Local health boards typically have a broad mandate to address local public health matters. In Massachusetts, for example, the health boards have broad authority to "make reasonable health regulations."[5] These regulations may include requirements for local firms to obtain permits and pay fees. Health board orders to companies are enforceable in court. Most health boards also have the power to regulate and shut down "nuisances" that may damage the public health. Often states have given specific toxics duties to local health boards, such as the implementation of right-to-know laws and aspects of siting hazardous waste facilities.

Guideline for Action. Press for creative use of your local health board's powers. For instance, the County Health Department in Ventura, California, has issued a detailed survey to local firms asking them to submit waste reduction plans—including statements on what toxics reduction measures they have explored.

Variances, Permits, and Zoning

Local governments issue a wide range of permits for construction, digging, filling, and many other activities. Most companies need some form of local permit to operate. Virtually all construction requires a building permit. If a project doesn't meet local zoning criteria, a variance may be required after a full public hearing. Those who build in a floodplain or near a wetland or water supply generally need a permit from a local conservation commission. Firms storing flammable chemicals may need a permit from the local fire department. Find out what permits a target firm has and what permits are due for renewal. These handles may give you leverage in your local campaign. Consider not only what permits are being applied for but also whether any existing permits can be revoked.

Guidelines for Action

- Oppose zoning variances or any other local permits for firms that have failed to prepare complete toxics reduction plans.
- Oppose variances and all local permits for toxics users that should be located in industrial zones and away from residences.
- In opposing a variance or permit, raise as many objections as possible. One way to defeat a project is to bury it in conditions that the applicant won't be willing or economically able to meet. A zoning commission in Henderson, Kentucky, imposed twenty-six zoning permit conditions on Union Carbide when they proposed building a PCB facility there.[6] These conditions effectively stopped the plant from being built.
- Enact a local resolution making toxics reduction the top priority for solving local pollution problems. Use the resolution to argue that companies must demonstrate toxics reduction before applying for permits.

Sewage Authorities

The Clean Water Act requires local sewage agencies to establish a program requiring industries to "pretreat" the toxics they're dumping into the sewers. (See Chapter 7.)

Guideline for Action. Press local sewage authorities and state government for enforcement of pretreatment requirements. Push them to require the submission of toxics reduction plans by all local sewer dumpers.

Other Ideas

Local governments sometimes lease property to local businesses or help to finance them. In doing so, they may have the freedom to put whatever terms they wish into the contract. Local governments also have diverse powers related to local land use—such as the power to buy property for public use (eminent domain) and the power to buy or grant rights of way through property for such public uses as utilities, pipelines, and roadways.

Guidelines for Action

- Insist that local government include requirements for company toxics management and reduction planning in government contracts and financing.
- Block the granting of rights of way to firms that have not prepared toxics reduction plans. Remember: It was the threatened denial of a simple right of way that led to the pollution prevention victory in Saco, Maine, described earlier in this chapter.
- As a last resort, seek to have local government actually buy property or buy the right to use hazardous chemicals on the property from a landowner in order to block the usage of toxics.

LAWSUITS AGAINST THE TOXICS USER

Consider using your right to sue for damages or court orders as one way of gaining leverage over the target firm. The issue of toxics reduction could be brought up as part of settlement discussions. See Chapter 8 for more information on your recourse against polluters.

MAKING MONEY TALK

Often your strongest leverage may come from people, organizations, and laws that are far from what you might think of as "environmentally oriented." In the corporate world, money talks. The strongest leverage may come from other businesses and players a corporation relies on for its financial support—its own board of directors, shareholders, lenders, customers, suppliers, and insurers. The corporation may also be a subsidiary of a larger corporation. Through marketplace pressures and through direct interactions, each of these outside players may become sympathetic to your concerns and may even be enlisted to help. Even without direct public pressure, some financial institutions have begun to consider toxics issues in their transactions. Banks and insurance companies, for example, are beginning to review toxic hazards on-site prior to issuing loans or insurance coverage to toxics users.

As a concerned citizen, you can help to sharpen awareness and concern for toxics reduction. This in turn will increase your leverage to get a corporation to prepare a toxics reduction plan. Consider appealing to any of the individuals or institutions the firm does business with. By providing these figures with toxics information, you'll ensure they can take better account of the financial risks and moral implications of their dealings with the company. Moreover, many laws govern the relations between the corporation and these other parties. Here are some ideas on how you can use such laws as you interact with outside players in your campaign to improve a firm's toxics management.

The Board of Directors

The board of directors is elected by the shareholders to oversee the managers of a corporation. In the past, the directors were allowed and even encouraged by law to take a "do nothing" attitude, with no role in the day-to-day operations of the firm. Their role was virtually limited to hiring and firing of top executives. Now, however, some state courts require directors to use reasonable care that the corporation is properly managed and in compliance with applicable laws.[7] Unless directors can show they used "due diligence" in overseeing the corporation's activities, they might even face personal liability for corporate mismanagement or lawbreaking.[8]

Guidelines for Action
- Meet with prominent members of the board of the target corporation. Urge them to press for an audit of the company's compliance with state and federal environmental requirements and to use every opportunity to reduce toxics usage. You might also have a lawyer inform board members about their legal obligation to monitor compliance with toxics laws. Supporting your program might help them meet any such diligence requirements.
- If board members take no action, you can threaten to inform insurers who cover company directors and officers. If they aren't monitoring the company's compliance with "due diligence," substantial insurer payouts could result. This point might also help you to enlist the insurer in your preventive efforts.
- In some cases, you might consider acquiring shares of the company's stock and filing a "shareholder's derivative suit" against the heads of the corporation. These are suits brought by shareholders in the name of

the corporation that target company managers and directors. For instance, you might bring a shareholder's suit to hold a manager personally liable for penalties imposed on the corporation for violating an environmental law. But be sure to obtain a lawyer's advice before seriously considering such action, since state laws strictly limit these suits. For more information, see Chapter 3 on corporate campaigns.

Shareholders

The law does not demand much involvement of shareholders in corporate affairs. They simply invest their money and then, if they're lucky, reap the benefits. But federal rules do give shareholders *rights*—to obtain information and to vote on major policy issues.

The Securities and Exchange Commission (SEC) prescribes rights of shareholders of "public-issue" corporations—that is, corporations registered with the SEC. SEC tries to ensure that investors have the information they need to make intelligent investment decisions. This information—on environmental penalties, suits, and expenditures needed for legal compliance—is presented in the corporation's annual report to shareholders.

Specifically, the SEC requires public-issue corporations to disclose lawsuits or agency proceedings that might require significant spending. Environmental proceedings must be reported if it's obvious that the typical investor would want to know of them or if the resulting cost could be more than 10 percent of the firm's assets (or more than $100,000 if the government is party to the case).[9] Aside from lawsuits and government agency actions, corporations must also report any changes in financial condition of which an "average prudent investor ought to be reasonably informed."[10]

The SEC also allows shareholders to vote on social and political questions relevant to the corporation. Any holder of voting stock can pose the questions for all shareholders to vote on.[11] Thus activists can use shareholder meetings to raise issues and place pressure on corporate officials to change the company's policies.

Guidelines for Action
- After buying shares of the corporation's stock, formulate a proposal for action by shareholders. Your proposal should recommend action by the firm's management or suggest an amendment of the corporate

by-laws. It should relate to overall company policy rather than day-to-day decisions—for example, you can have the shareholders vote to request that the company's executives prepare a report on what the firm is doing to reduce its toxics usage and prevent chemical accidents.

• Often companies have two different stories about toxics cleanup and prevention costs. They tell their shareholders in their annual report that they expect no major losses; at the same time, they tell government agencies that cleanup or pollution controls would be so expensive it could put them out of business. To enlist shareholders and directors in your local toxics campaign, inform them of such discrepancies and emphasize the enormous losses that could result from continued toxic abuses.

• Begin a divestment campaign against a toxics-abusing firm. Encourage shareholders—institutions, unions, and public leaders—to sell their stock and reinvest in "clean" stocks and money market funds. Two socially responsible funds that reportedly invest only in nonpolluting businesses are the Working Assets Money Fund (230 California St., San Francisco, CA 94111) and the Calvert Group (1700 Pennsylvania Ave. NW, Washington, DC 20006). These funds generally pay interest comparable to other money market funds. Write them for information.

Industrial Financing Authorities

State and local governments often finance the construction or expansion of local industries by issuing bonds or providing other financing. To obtain this financing, a company is usually required to demonstrate that a public benefit will be provided through the funding—such as creating jobs and restoring depressed neighborhoods.[12] Although waste disposal and resource recovery facilities may be construed to fulfill this requirement, activists may argue that an applicant with a poor toxics management record does not provide a public benefit because it actually operates against the public's best interests.

Guidelines for Action. If a target firm plans to build a new plant or expand an existing one, find out if it's applying for financial assistance. Pressure the firm to meet your toxics reduction demands by threatening to oppose public financing. If this approach doesn't yield the desired results, you can oppose the financing by taking the following actions:

- Request to make a counterpresentation as a community representative at the financing authority's meeting in which the applicant presents its proposal.
- Make community presentations at the public hearing on the proposal and submit other comments in writing.
- Usually the city council or mayor must approve a government-financed project. If so, request a full investigation by that official of the company's toxics practices prior to any approval. Organize to win disapproval of the project if your concerns are not addressed.

Banks

Your local banker may seem an unlikely ally in environmental and community issues. Yet banks have a unique sensitivity to money matters and may become reluctant allies in your fight to clean up a toxic hazard.

Banks may risk serious financial losses if property on which they have issued loans becomes contaminated. In some states, contamination can actually cost banks their collateral (the property on which they hold rights while a loan is outstanding). In these states with "superlien" laws, the state environmental agency can conduct a cleanup and then foreclose and auction the property to recover the state's costs. Sometimes a bank may even face liability to pay for the cleanup.

Banks guard their public image. While it's important to keep a steady flow of banking customers, the bank's larger concern may be the potential impact on its federal and state licensing. Banks insured by the Federal Deposit Insurance Corporation (FDIC) or chartered by the federal government are subject to federal Community Reinvestment Act (CRA) regulations. (Most financial institutions are covered by one of these two categories. Exceptions are credit unions, mortgage bankers, and mortgage brokers.) These requirements become crucial when a bank changes its business by establishing or relocating a branch, merging with other banks, or acquiring assets.[13] For permission to take such action, the bank must apply to one of four federal agencies and submit to public comments.[14]

A challenge to a bank's proposal to take such action could be very costly to the bank—indeed, these transactions often involve billions of dollars. If a public challenge drags on for months, the uncertainty caused by the delay in obtaining a final decision can itself be very costly to the bank.

This is why you may find your local bank willing to go out on a limb to help you resolve a toxics issue. The bank might even provide the money for cleanup or the funding needed for a citizen group to obtain technical assistance.

Guidelines for Action

- Contact a bank that holds collateral in a site where toxics are mismanaged. Remind bank officials of the possible loss of collateral that may result from toxic releases and exposure. Ask for their help in cleaning up the firm's mismanagement practices.
- If you know that the target firm is a mess, invite its banker to join you in a tour of the facility. By demonstrating the hazardous conditions there, you might just make progress on your local problems based on good relations with the bank.
- If your state environmental agency has power to impose toxics liability on the bank or a superlien on the bank's collateral, you can use these powers to press for bank action. If the bank is uncooperative, inform them that you'll lobby the state to use its powers unless they work with you to restore the environment and implement toxics reduction.
- If the lender is insured by the FDIC or chartered by the federal government, you can file a complaint in the bank's Community Reinvestment Act (CRA) file and threaten to challenge every action of the bank that falls under the act. The most effective campaigns using the CRA are multiple-issue campaigns calling for the bank to improve its lending practices in a number of areas. To use the CRA effectively, your group must assess the community's credit needs, evaluate the lender's performance in regard to those needs, and then use the CRA as leverage to get the bank to address your demands. While a loan recipient's toxics may be your group's key concern and a top negotiating issue with the bank, you must also document the bank's failures in regard to the factors assessed under CRA regulations:[15]

1. Failure to ascertain the community's credit needs and to communicate with community members regarding the availability of credit.
2. Failure to publicize its credit services. (Check with real estate brokers on the extent to which they've received letters describing the bank's services.)

3. Failure to offer credit applications equitably (such as the un-availability of application forms at certain branches and the terms of loans compared with other banks).
4. Failure to treat women, minorities, the elderly, or the handicapped equitably.
5. Failure to participate in local community redevelopment programs.

You can file a CRA complaint at any time by submitting comments at either the bank's head office or the relevant branch. Comments must relate to the bank's performance in helping to meet the community's credit needs; you must not include any comments that "reflect adversely upon the good name or reputation of any person other than the bank."[16] This means you need to steer a fine course between describing the bank's tendency to expose the community to toxic hazards—which would be an acceptable comment—and complaining about a specific company. Ignoring this rule might allow the bank to exclude your comments from the file.

When a bank covered by the CRA requests the government's permission to change its structure or acquire assets, this is a specific opportunity for public comment. Although public comments are usually submitted to the government in writing, you may file a written request for a formal or informal hearing—which could lead to substantial delays for the bank.[17]

For more information on CRA strategies, obtain *The Community Reinvestment Act: A Citizen's Action Guide,* available from the Center for Community Change, 1000 Wisconsin Ave. NW, Washington DC 20007.

Insurance Companies

Companies that store and use toxics have traditionally been insured under their general liability policies to cover the cost of lawsuits for bodily injuries and property damages arising from sudden chemical accidents (such as fires and spills). But owners and operators of certain hazardous waste facilities are legally required to insure against both sudden and nonsudden occurrences.

Insurance to cover a business's pollution liabilities has become increasingly expensive and hard to obtain since the mid-1980s. In fact, many hazardous waste facilities were shut down at that time due to the unavailability of insurance. Other toxics-using firms were operating without insurance for toxic pollution liabilities—opening the possibility that an incident at their facility would leave them bankrupted with no one but the victims to bear the resulting losses. The federal government and most states currently provide no backup compensation schemes for such incidents.

The key questions for a local toxics campaign are typically:

- Does the target firm have pollution insurance?
- If it doesn't, will the firm itself be able to pay the cost of any property damages and personal injuries that could result from an incident at the site? Or would residents of the neighborhood be forced to bear the losses themselves?
- If the firm does have pollution insurance, is it adequate to protect the public? (See Chapter 7 for the major shortcomings in hazardous waste insurance and some ideas on how to plug these loopholes.)
- If the firm has pollution insurance, can its insurer be enlisted to pressure the company to meet your concerns?

Guidelines for Action
- Find out whether the targeted toxics user has pollution liability insurance. Request a copy of the insurance policy from the firm, and work with groups like NTC to review its adequacy.
- If the firm is uninsured or the insurance policy is inadequate, raise this concern during any state or local permit hearing involving the toxics user. Insist that the firm obtain adequate insurance or shut down. If no insurance company finds the risks at the facility to be acceptable, why should you and your neighbors underwrite the dangers?
- Insurers may be recruited to support better toxics management. Pollution insurers generally want to know when there are unnecessary toxic risks at an insured site, since they might ultimately have to pay the costs. They may even screen the pollution risks themselves to help them set rates and decide who to insure. Since such reviews generally occur only at the time insurance is issued (or renewed), insurers may welcome your report of goings-on at the site in the interim. Notify the insurer if you have reason to believe that the insured firm is creating unnecessary hazards for which the insurer may be held liable. Encourage the insurer to pressure the firm to change its toxics management practices under the threat of increased rates or even loss of insurance coverage.
- If the insurer is uncooperative in moving the firm toward better toxics management, consider getting tough by setting in motion the state monitoring that applies to insurance companies. Insurers are licensed and regulated by the state. If an insurance company is unable to pay

potential liabilities, its license could be suspended or revoked.[18] To use this approach, estimate the insurer's potential liability given the amount of toxics on the site and the extent of people and property in the vicinity. Work with a friendly insurance expert to compare this figure with the insurer's available capital and other liabilities. If your analysis indicates that the insurer may be undercapitalized, ask stockholders, creditors, or policyholders to call for a state investigation of the insurer's financial strength. If this action moves toward possible delicensing of the insurer, you could attempt to take part in the proceedings as a member of the affected public.

Buyers and Sellers

Aside from these diverse legal tactics, remember that the power of the marketplace may itself be the strongest source of leverage over your target. Enlist buyers and sellers in your local campaign. In one local campaign in Massachusetts, a firm that sold specialized products to a limited number of buyers (five other firms) found that at least one of its buyers began to seek alternative sources of the materials when it became public that the neighbors were intending to shut the firm down. The buyer's business relied on a steady flow of supplies. Given the threat of a stoppage in production, they hedged their bets by seeking other suppliers. Sometimes a pragmatic appeal to buyers and sellers carries just as much weight as a moral appeal.

CREATING A CITIZENS' TOXICS BOARD

Your local agencies may not be getting the job done. Your local health board, for example, probably has broad powers covering everything from inspecting food establishments to inspecting septic tanks. They may have little time to attend to toxic chemical issues that involve intensive effort. Your health board may even be a stagnant bureaucracy, harder to change than to replace with another agency. Your concerns may need a stronger vehicle for expression. Maybe you need a citizens' toxic board. A new institution can bring fresh energy and ideas to solving the toxics problem.

A citizens' toxics board can take various forms—from an official body created by local ordinance and elected by the community to a self-appointed citizen group that begins to work *around* the local bureaucracy. A citizens' toxics board can initially focus on a local firm. Citizens might form the

"Ajax Citizens' Toxics Board," for example, which would begin scrutiny of that local firm's handling of toxics. Regardless of the circumstance, a citizens' toxics board would ask tough questions and demand answers, inspect facilities, oversee cleanup of toxic messes, and so forth. This board could oversee other agencies and have the power to override their bad decisions.[19] It could also serve as a sounding board for citizens regarding careless health board decisions. Finally, the toxics board could be a better-integrated substitute for the health board, fire department, or other local agencies charged with monitoring toxics.

Your proposal to create a local toxics agency may improve local toxics management regardless of whether the proposed board is actually created. By suggesting that existing agencies are not doing their job, you may force them to stay on their toes. A campaign for a local toxics board might be combined with specific demands on these agencies, so that they may view the new board as a worse option than responding to your current needs.

If you do create a new board, public access should be ensured. Strong public involvement should be built in. Consider the following issues:

- Relation to other agencies? How will the new board relate to other community agencies, such as the local emergency planning committee and the health board?
- Elected or appointed members? An appointed membership could mean that the same officials who appointed your current "do-nothing" officials will now appoint the toxics board members. To avoid making the board "window dressing," require separate elections of members.
- Labor representation? Representation of workers in the target plants could be especially important to understanding and solving toxics problems.
- Staffing? The new board should be run by a trusted person, not an industry yes-man. Consider how this person will be hired.
- Public notice of meetings? How far in advance will the public be notified?
- Funding of board experts and staff? Will local toxics users be required to pay for the board's operation? Since their practices have created the need for the board, this seems to make sense.
- Continuing role of local activist groups? A local toxics board is no substitute for organized local citizens. Unless there is strong and unified public activism outside of government, there may be little a government agency can do to solve local toxics problems. Both strong activism and responsive agencies are needed. Will you continue to

build grassroots activism in the community with the new board in place? Unless there are enough trustworthy players for both "insider" and "outsider" roles, it may be better for you and your group to remain outsiders than to create this new institution.

PASSING NEW LAWS

Oddly, it may be easier to pass a new law than to get a firm to manage its toxics safely. If you're getting nowhere with the existing laws, you may want to press for a new local law that requires the target firm and all similar firms to handle their toxics as you deem appropriate. Concern over "supertoxic" nerve gas materials at one firm led the health commissioner of Cambridge, Massachusetts, to enact a regulation banning the storage, testing, and transportation of nerve gas within the city limits. Several California communities have enacted regulations requiring firms to file toxics reduction plans with the local government.

Of course, you may meet local resistance to your proposed new toxics law. Your proposal could easily become the crux of a local political fight. Just as hazardous waste cleanup became the leading issue for the 1989 New Jersey gubernatorial race, toxics prevention could become the big issue in your local electoral campaigns. Candidates for mayor or town council could be asked whether they'd support using new or existing local laws to require local businesses to reduce their usage of toxics.

Whether or not a new law is needed to win your local toxics fight, your group is unlikely to ensure sound toxics management throughout the community or the state without new legal enactments. Any victory over the negligent use of toxics is cause for celebration. But you'll need new legislation or across-the-board policies to make preventive habits routine for every toxics user.

NOTES

1. 49 CFR 397.9.
2. *New Jersey Hazardous Waste News,* September 1986.
3. Model Code of Professional Responsibility, DR 7-104.
4. Hazardous and Solid Waste Amendments of 1984, sec. 224, amending secs. 3002, 3005, and 8002 of RCRA.
5. Mass. Gen. Laws, chap. 111, sec. 31.

6. *Action Bulletin,* Citizens Clearinghouse on Hazardous Waste, September 1986.
7. A. Emerson, "The Director as Corporate Legal Monitor: Environmental Legislation and Pandora's Box," *Seton Hall Law Revew* 15 (1985):593.
8. *Ibid.,* pp. 609 and 595.
9. 17 CFR 229.103, Instruction 5. Similar government actions are allowed to be grouped in the company's report, which reduces the usefulness of these materials in toxics activists' research.
10. 17 CFR 229.303(b)(1) requires reporting of material changes in financial condition; 17 CFR 210.1-02(n) defines "material."
11. Rule 14a-8, 17 CFR 240, 14a-8 (1979); L. S. Black, Jr., and A. G. Sparks, "SEC Rule 14a-8: Some Changes in the Way the SEC Staff Interprets the Rule," *Toledo Law Review* 11 (1980):957.
12. See, for example, *Boston Industrial Development Bond Program,* Boston Industrial Development Financing Authority (1985), p. 8.
13. 12 CFR 262.3(a), (b).
14. 12 CFR 262.3(b).
15. See, for example, 12 CFR 228.7.
16. See, for example, 12 CFR sec. 25.5 (a)(1).
17. See, for example, 12 CFR 262.3 (e). A request for a hearing on any changes in the bank's status should identify the protester, state the basis for objection to approval of the bank's proposed action, provide written evidence to support the objection, and, if a meeting or hearing is requested, state that members of the public wish to be heard. The objection must relate to factors that the government is entitled to consider: the financial and managerial resources of the institution, the effects on competition, and, most important to toxics activists, the convenience and needs of the communities to be served; 12 CFR 262.25(d)(1)(ii). See also the Community Reinvestment Act, 30 USC, sec. 2901(a)(3). ("The Congress finds that . . . regulated financial institutions have a continuing and affirmative obligation to help meet the credit needs of the local communities in which they are chartered.")

   After a decision is made by the governing agency, you may request, within fifteen days, a reconsideration of the agency's decision; 12 CFR 262.25(d)(4), 262.3. If a decision has been delegated by the board to its staff, however, review of the staff decision can be obtained by filing a petition with a board member within five days of the delegated decision requesting review of the decision as an adversely affected party; 12 CFR 262.25(d), 265.3.
18. See, for example, 211 Code of Massachusetts Regulations 4.01(2)(i).
19. This model has worked effectively at the state level in Michigan's Toxic Substances Control Commission. In the event of a toxic emergency, that independent commission can override health and environmental agency decision making.

PART III

The Ultimate Solution

10

Preventing Pollution

DAVID ALLEN

Environmental laws and programs established in the United States during the past twenty years have not proved all that effective in protecting human health and the environment from industrial toxins. Current environmental programs are largely designed to control industrial wastes, emissions, discharges, and pollutants at the end of the pipe and only after critical decisions have already been made to use toxic materials. While this strategy has merits, there are limits to the amount of environmental protection that can be achieved within the pollution control framework.

One possible reaction is to do nothing—to accept as inevitable the limits of pollution control or even to weaken existing programs. This has been the direction of the 1980s. Another response is to focus solely on broadening and strengthening existing pollution control programs. Using this approach, the government would put all of its resources into the expansion of traditional programs, systems, and activities for controlling pollutants.

These two options are not the only ones, however. There is a superior approach that is open to the United States. The nation could begin to take advantage of opportunities for preventing pollution.

In fact, there is a critical choice to be made. Are we to continue to rely almost exclusively on traditional pollution control programs, or are we to shift at least some of our resources, money, and commitment toward the goal of pollution prevention?

Preventing pollution requires that the nation make a major commitment to reducing the use of toxic materials in production and commerce. In addition, a related goal is to reduce the generation of wastes and pollutants

269

in all environmental media (air, water, and land). Considerable evidence indicates that companies can readily change the technology of production to reduce the toxics they use and the wastes and pollutants they generate.

A strategic shift toward pollution prevention is not only superior environmentally. It could help to revitalize the U.S. economy by stimulating technological innovation, by creating long-term business investment patterns, by renovating and changing production processes, by introducing new and environmentally benign products and services to the market, by demonstrating a new commitment to developing the skills of American workers, and by making a major national commitment to tailoring U.S. technologies and products to the environmental situation of the twenty-first century.

Citizen concern about hazardous substances and industrial waste has been the driving force behind environmental protection legislation in the United States since 1970. Public awareness that the air and water were seriously polluted by industrial emissions and discharges led to the passage of the Clean Air Act (CAA) and the Clean Water Act (CWA). Similarly, citizen fears and concerns about toxic and hazardous waste led to the passage of the Resource Conservation and Recovery Act (RCRA) and the Comprehensive Environmental Response, Compensation and Liability Act (CERCLA), or Superfund.

Despite these laws and programs, as the United States enters the twenty-first century it continues to face major environmental problems. Hazardous waste disposal sites still abound, billions of pounds of toxic air pollutants are routinely emitted from industrial facilities across the nation, public drinking water supplies have been contaminated, and toxic materials steadily make their way into the foodchain. The nation's bays and estuaries are contaminated, acid rain is destroying many of the nation's forests and lakes, and the specter of global environmental catastrophe haunts the public.

At the root of many of our most pressing environmental problems are the technologies and materials of modern production. Many people argue, for example, that the greatly increased production of synthetic organic chemicals and petrochemicals, especially halogenated organics, has wrought major changes in the technical organization of the nation's production system, with very serious environmental and public health effects following in its wake. In 1940, roughly 2 billion pounds of synthetic organic chemicals and petrochemicals were produced in the United States; by 1988, some 214 billion pounds of such chemicals were being produced.[1] The figure is much higher if nonsynthetic chemical production is added to the total. Not all of these materials are toxic, but many of them are. Some of these chemicals are known or believed to cause or contribute to cancer, birth defects, neurological and behavioral disorders, immunological deficiencies, and ecological disruption.

Modern production technologies and materials are a root cause of the hazardous waste generation and environmental pollution that now proceeds at an alarming pace. The government estimates that 569 million metric tons of RCRA hazardous wastes were generated by U.S. industry in 1985, reflecting a per capita waste generation rate of approximately 2 tons per American each year.[2] This may be an underestimate. The true figure of annual hazardous waste generation may well be closer to 1 billion metric tons, exclusive of hazardous pollutants released to the nation's air and water. Figures such as these point to the potential for a public health and environmental crisis of major proportions and raise serious questions regarding the overall effectiveness of the nation's environmental protection strategy.

THE INSTITUTION OF POLLUTION CONTROL

Initial attempts to deal with environmental problems have focused on controlling pollution after it already exists. In essence, we do little more than physically manage the wastes, discharges, emissions, and pollutants that are generated. Surface impoundments, hazardous waste incinerators, wastewater treatment units, slurry walls, waste recycling units, deep-well injection operations, air pollution control filters, leachate collection systems, monitoring wells, and similar technological fixes have been installed or used at the end of the pipe to deal with environmental wastes and pollutants.

After twenty years of environmental progress the nation has succeeded in creating a huge and politically influential pollution control and waste management industry, much of it structured like a public works program. As this industry has developed, the various technologies and strategies that have been designed and put into place to physically manage wastes and pollutants have met with little outstanding success.

How do we, as a nation, attempt to manage the hundreds of millions of tons of hazardous industrial wastes and pollutants that are created each year? To answer this question we must ask how technology is used to deal with problems created by technology. To begin with: The control of pollution can only take place at some physical point after wastes and pollutants have been created. Once pollution exists, there are three broad strategies for physically controlling it. All three strategies are unavoidably risky, costly, and liable to technological failure:

- Recycling: Wastes and pollutants are recycled in the environment. While recycling may appear relatively sound for certain wastes—such as relatively nonhazardous municipal solid waste (MSW)—it is usually quite problematic where toxic and hazardous waste is concerned. Recyclable hazardous wastes and pollutants are burned in industrial furnaces, boilers, and cement kilns, applied to the land, handled, stored, and recycled at off-site locations, and incorporated into construction materials such as road asphalt and cement blocks. Recycling of hazardous industrial waste is often poorly regulated and in many cases exempted from regulation.
- Treatment: Wastes and pollutants are treated through chemical, biological, or mechanical means to minimize their toxic and hazardous characteristics. Sometimes treatment is little more than a euphemism for dispersing wastes to the environment. One treatment method, for example, involves evaporating volatile fractions of hazardous waste in surface impoundments to prepare the solid fraction of the waste for land disposal.
- Disposal: Wastes and pollutants are disposed of in or on the land or are dispersed to air, surface water, groundwater, and marine environments.

Some people argue that at least some progress has been made under the pollution control system, and it is difficult to argue with them. In fact, pollution control works for conventional pollutants or nontoxic materials such as sewage, nonchemical agricultural runoff, and other biodegradable nontoxic wastes. But evidence now suggests there are limits to the amount of environmental and public health protection that can be achieved using only pollution control. The point is that the pollution control approach is not all that effective in dealing with the many toxic wastes of industry. It is necessary but not a sufficient environmental protection strategy. Consider the following facts:

- Nationally, there are now 1,219 sites on the federal Superfund list alone, with many other state Superfund sites not included on the federal list. New sites are proposed annually, and there is limited progress in cleanups as the number of sites rapidly continues to increase. The federal Superfund program alone will cost the government more than $100 billion over some decades—exclusive of the cost of cleaning up military sites and exclusive of costs to industry and society.[3]
- Concern about groundwater and public drinking water supplies is

growing. About 50 percent of the nation depends on groundwater as a source of drinking water.[4] The Center for the Study of Responsive Law reports that 19 percent of the public water systems tested in the nation show toxic contamination.[5]

• Toxic air pollution is a major national problem. Toxic chemical release data submitted by only the largest producers and users of toxic chemicals as defined under Section 313 of the Federal Emergency Planning and Right-to-Know Act indicate that more than 2.7 billion pounds of toxic chemicals were released to the atmosphere by major manufacturing facilities in 1988 alone.[6] Emission standards have been developed by EPA that address only seven of potentially hundreds of toxic air emissions.[7]

• Toxic air emissions are not the only problem. In general, releases of toxic chemicals to air, water, and land are substantial. EPA's toxic release data for 1988 indicate that roughly 20 billion pounds of toxic chemicals were released to the environment in 1988 by industry. Actual environmental releases may be greater by a factor of twenty. One federal agency, in recent testimony before the U.S. Senate, stated that as many as 400 billion pounds of toxic chemicals are emitted, discharged, or released as wastes and pollutants each year.[8]

• In 1986, there were 12,282 reported incidents involving major releases of toxic and hazardous substances—through accidents and spills.[9]

• Toxic compounds can be readily identified in the body tissue of most if not all Americans. A recent EPA analysis of human fatty tissue found several compounds—including styrene, xylene isomers, 1,4-dichlorobenzene, and ethylphenol—in all samples tested.[10] A government review of relevant literature readily identified more than 200 industrial chemicals and pesticides in human body tissue.[11]

Something is wrong with our environmental programs. There are alarming inadequacies that cannot simply be explained away by pointing to slashed environmental budgets and inadequate enforcement of laws. What twenty years of national experience shows is that when used in the absence of stategies that reduce pollution, the pollution control system in and of itself is not an effective or reliable a way to deal with the many environmental problems that stem from the use of toxic materials.

Meanwhile, few adherents to the doctrine of pollution controls seriously question whether pollution and the materials that contribute to it could be avoided, reduced, or eliminated *before* wastes and pollutants must be controlled. Instead, waste and pollution are increasingly taken for granted.

In fact, pollution control has become a national institution, tenaciously sustained by entrenched bureaucracies in government, industry, and the environmental movement.

Nontheless, American communities where pollution control is practiced know firsthand of the inferiority of this approach. And general criticism of the pollution control approach is also beginning to be heard. A recent study by the Office of Technology Assessment (OTA), an analytical arm of the U.S. Congress established in 1972 to address problems associated with technology and society, questions whether pollution control alone is sufficient.[12] The president's Council on Environmental Quality (CEQ) echoes such sentiments. According to the CEQ:

> In recent years progress under [pollution control] has become . . . slow and uncertain. . . . It is not just that [the pollution control approach] is difficult to implement and often overly expensive in terms of benefit achieved. It is that the scale of the problem—the number of pollutants, the number of diverse sources, and so on—militate against [the pollution control] system having a substantial effect . . . in any but the very longest run. . . . What we are doing now . . . is not working at all well. The . . . system is marked by substantial noncompliance, delay, consent decrees, and . . . legalistic combat, rather than by steady reduction of toxics.[13]

Dr. Barry Commoner, a noted environmentalist, in a review of national environmental progress that has occurred since the first "enthusiastic outburst of Earth Day in April of 1970" provides the following critical assessment:

> The regulations mandated by the Clean Water Act, and more than a hundred billion dollars spent to meet them, have failed to improve water quality in most rivers. . . . The occurrence of three serious pollutants—nitrate, arsenic, and cadmium—has increased considerably. . . . The once valuable catch of herring and whitefish dropped off sharply after 1950 [and has] not recovered between 1960 and 1980. . . . A national survey of changes in water quality between 1972 and 1982 showed almost no progress in lakes. . . . In the past twenty-five years [groundwater has] become increasingly polluted by nitrates and toxic chemicals. . . .
>
> Since 1950 the roster of serious chemical pollutants has seriously expanded. . . . For the first time in the three-and-a-half-billion-year history of life on this planet, living things are burdened with a host of man-made poisonous substances. . . . Members of the general American population now carry several dozen man-made chemicals, many of them carcinogenic, in their body fat (and generally in the fat of mother's milk as well). Toxic chemicals now seriously

pollute important segments of the foodchain. . . . Tumors are found on fish with increasing frequency. . . .

There are two general ways in which a pollutant may be prevented from entering the environment: either the pollutant is eliminated from the activity that generates it, or a control device is added to trap or destroy the pollutant before it enters the environment. . . . The few real improvements have been achieved not by adding control devices or concealing pollutants (as by pumping hazardous chemical wastes into deep water-bearing strata) but simply by eliminating the pollutants. . . . This [insight] directs our attention to the technology of production—the vast and varied machinery of industry, agriculture, and transportation. . . . The effort to deal with environmental pollution has been trivialized. A greal deal of attention has been paid to designing—and enforcing the use of—control devices that can reduce hazardous emissions only moderately. Much less attention has been given to the more difficult but rewarding task of changing the basic technologies that produce the pollutants.[14]

SIX UNAVOIDABLE PROBLEMS WITH POLLUTION CONTROL

National commitment to the institution of pollution control has remained fundamental, deep-seated, almost devotional, despite the fact that many pollution control strategies have proved notoriously ineffective. In essence, despite the fallibility of pollution control doctrine, institutional commitment to pollution control has proved exceedingly difficult to overcome. There is, however, potential for change. New instrumentation, analytical techniques, and information increasingly throw light on the high rate of failure of pollution control techniques. The general public is becoming more aware of—and vocal about—environmental problems that are not being solved. Our national infatuation with pollution control has enough of a history to allow us to begin to evaluate it critically.

Common sense alone should tell us that something is wrong with this environmental option. Local incidents involving community and workplace exposures, chemical contamination of public drinking water supplies, waste management facility upsets, industrial accidents, and other local disasters are now routinely reported in the press with alarming monotony. And even these stories are overshadowed by evidence that pollution control is not reliably dealing with broader national and international environmental problems. During the late 1980s an emerging consensus seems to be crystallizing around the view that pollution problems are worsening, even in the face of major efforts to control pollution.

There are at least six basic flaws in the pollution control approach that help to explain its relative ineffectiveness:

1. End-of-pipe focus
2. Cross-media waste shifting
3. Environmental transport of pollutants and wastes
4. Sanctioned release
5. Failure to regulate many toxic materials
6. Economic inefficiency

END-OF-PIPE FOCUS

Pollution control focuses on the end of the pipe where wastes and pollutants exit from stacks, discharge pipes, and processes. An end-of-pipe emphasis contributes to widespread public and community concern about the environment. This is because workers and communities are affected by wastes and pollutants managed in their midst. A misplaced focus at the end of the pipe also fails to address the *cause* of pollution problems, which resides in the technology, operations, and materials of production.

CROSS-MEDIA WASTE SHIFTING

Pollution control allows the shifting of wastes and pollutants between different environmental media. Evaporation techniques shift hazardous waste from land to air. Leachate collection systems shift hazardous wastes from landfills to publicly owned treatment works and surface water. Scrubbers installed in smokestacks to control air emissions transfer pollutants from air to groundwater.[15]

Lee M. Thomas, a former administrator of the EPA, described how it is possible for industry to engage in waste-shifting practices under the pollution control regime. As Thomas points out: "It is entirely possible . . . that somewhere in the country toxic metals are being removed from the air, transferred to a wastewater stream, removed again by water pollution controls, converted to a sludge, shipped to an incinerator, and returned to the air."[16]

ENVIRONMENTAL TRANSPORT OF POLLUTANTS AND WASTES

Wastes and pollutants released within one environmental medium are transported to distant locations where they cause problems. The pesticide Silvex, applied to crops in the southwestern United States, is transported in the atmosphere to the Great Lakes where it contaminates the aquatic foodchain. Tall smokestacks built in the Midwest, required under air regulations to disperse emissions, are now implicated in acid rain that deposits chemical pollutants hundreds of miles from the source of pollution in forest topsoil and lakes.[17]

SANCTIONED RELEASE

Pollution control sanctions the release of wastes and pollutants at rates that might be considered reasonable on a case-by-case basis, but these releases accumulate and contribute to unacceptable levels of pollution. For example, permits administered under the Clean Water Act are required before pollutants can be legally released to surface water. They are based not on health or environmental standards but on what is technologically feasible for the company applying for the permit. Once the permits are authorized, the permitted activities are not adequately reviewed by government officials. In addition, many known toxins are not regulated in the permits.

Hence toxic discharges are released to surface waters to build up to unacceptable levels in the environment. One case in point is Chesapeake Bay. EPA estimates that more than 3,000 tons of toxic metal wastes are entering Chesapeake Bay each year from companies in Maryland and Virginia. A recent OTA study discusses this problem: "Many believe that cumulative discharges of hazardous waste have played a role in the declining marine life of the bay. (For example, even while environmental regulations have escalated, commercial catches of striped bass fell from 6 million pounds in 1970 to 600,000 pounds in 1983. Oyster harvests have dropped by two-thirds in the last 20 years.)"[18] The decline of the Chesapeake Bay ecosystem is not an isolated case. In general, it is believed that "estuaries and coastal waters are in deep trouble around the nation."[19]

FAILURE TO REGULATE MANY TOXIC MATERIALS

Pollution control programs fail to regulate a sufficient number of toxins. For example, the federal government identified 145 cancer-causing chemicals in its Fourth Annual Report on Carcinogens. Yet many of these materials, which can only be listed in the annual report if significant numbers of the U.S. population are exposed, "have not been acted on by [federal] agencies and programs."[20]

ECONOMIC INEFFICIENCY

Economic issues are of great concern to the majority of Americans. Plant closings throughout the rust belt, a troubling trade imbalance with foreign nations, and other pervasive economic problems linked to declining innovative dynamism in the U.S. economic and social system are real concerns. Complying with government pollution control regulations is a social responsibility of industry. Nonetheless, economic decline raises big questions about the extent to which even an environmentally alert and activist government would be politically able to impose only additional pollution control requirements on U.S. industry in the long term.

Pollution control calls for end-of-pipe "add-ons" such as air pollution filters, equalizing tanks, and wastewater treatment units. In the broadest sense, it also involves site remediation strategies that contain, shift, transport, or destroy wastes and pollutants in the environment. However necessary they may be, these pollution control expenditures are nonproductive, providing only limited technological and economic advantages for U.S. industry.

The fundamental problem is that environmental strategies designed to control pollution at the end of the pipe fail to renovate manufacturing technology, do not constructively deal with the declining performance of U.S. industry, fail to systematically develop the skills of workers, and do not promote beneficial technological innovation and management reorganization within American industry. However necessary it might be, pollution control is without doubt an inferior economic option.[21]

PREVENTION VS. POLLUTION

Recognizing the inferiority of the pollution control approach, the question arises: Is it time to break with tradition by advancing a more reliable and effective option for environmental protection? The question only makes sense if a better alternative exists.

In fact, a superior alternative does exist. This better alternative—one that involves the systematic reduction of toxic chemicals, wastes, and pollutants before they are created—is known as pollution prevention. The nation can seriously assist industry to escape the regulatory burdens, uncertainties, and economic costs of pollution control, not by helping industry to avoid pollution control responsibilities but by helping to reduce, avoid, or eliminate the pollution that needs to be controlled. The aim is not to weaken pollution control programs but to provide the technical, economic, and institutional basis for industry to produce less of the toxic materials, wastes, and pollutants that must be managed in the first place.

Preventing pollution is not some abstract goal in the distant future. With today's technology, it is possible to make major strides in reducing, avoiding, or eliminating the use of toxins and the generation of hazardous waste and pollution at the point of production itself. Indeed, pollution prevention provides the most reliable and effective environmental protection while promoting industrial innovation and industrial competitiveness.

Those who might counter that preventive environmentalism is too radical an option should be reminded that pollution prevention has historical roots extending into the 1970s. We have known for at least a decade that the principles of prevention could be pragmatically applied to environmental protection—as was done when EPA reduced exposures to certain air toxics by phasing down the use of lead in gasoline or when it required low-solvent coating operations in certain industries. Thus the Toxic Substances Strategy Committee convened by the president's Council on Environmental Quality spoke with the authority of practical experience, and not just theory, when it said that "prevention is the key to controlling many diseases and environmental problems caused by toxic chemicals."[22]

Pollution prevention is not yet widely practiced, however, and it has yet to be elevated to its rightful place among environmental options. Although there are many opportunities for practicing pollution prevention, opposition to this superior strategy persists. Veiled opposition has been particularly strong at EPA in recent years despite recent talk to the contrary,[23] and industry has not been at all supportive.[24] Without an organized advocacy and widespread public knowledge about the unique benefits of preventing pollution, it is likely that pollution prevention will remain underutilized, buried within the dominant tradition of pollution control, its progress blocked by stubborn institutional, behavioral, and cultural obstacles.

REDUCING INDUSTRY'S USE OF TOXIC CHEMICALS

The most effective, reliable, and simple strategy for reducing some of the worst forms of pollution involves reduction of the use of toxic materials.[25] (Unless otherwise stated, the words *toxic* and *hazardous* are not intended to be scientifically precise terms, nor are they used here in their statutory or regulatory sense, but simply to refer to materials that, when exposed to people in sufficient amounts, are harmful.) Reducing the use of toxic synthetic organic chemicals and other industrial toxic materials—a relatively new environmental approach that cuts against the grain of current environmental and industrial practice—is readily achievable by changing the basic technology, operations, and materials of modern production.[26]

True toxics use reduction can only be achieved by altering production technology, operations, and materials. Actions that do not modify the production process but deal with wastes after they already exist—recycling spent solvents at hazardous waste management facilities, for example, or reclaiming lead from used batteries—are not true use reduction strategies. They are pollution control approaches with all the unavoidable problems, risks, liabilities, and costs of pollution control.

Toxics use reduction goes directly to the center of many of our environmental problems. In essence, it is based on the recognition that industrial production is the root factor that determines society's overall rate of exposure to toxic substances. Industrial production as it is now organized demands the extraction of massive amounts of toxic materials from the earth, necessitates the release of vast quantities of toxic materials to our air, water, and land, damages the health of American workers, and systematically incorporates toxic materials into products and building materials. Thus by the simple expedient of changing the technology, operations, and materials of production we can effectively take advantage of diverse opportunities to avoid, reduce, or eliminate all facets of society's exposure to industrial toxics. The reduction and elimination of toxic materials is achievable using a variety of technical approaches that often overlap.

Chemical Pathway Redesign: Companies can change the series of chemical reactions and steps required to produce an end product—thus avoiding certain highly toxic intermediate processes that generate by-products, waste, and pollution. ARCO Chemical produces propylene oxide through a synthetic chemical pathway that does not use a chlorohydrin intermediate. Propylene oxide is used in the production of antifreeze. Previously propylene oxide manufacturers had to use chlorinated alcohol intermediates. ARCO eliminated these materials—and their many hazardous by-products—by designing a new synthetic route to propylene oxide. ARCO still produces propylene oxide, but employs a fundamentally different chemistry. In essence, an alternative chemical production pathway was developed. The production of propylene oxide via the ARCO method is cheaper and less polluting than production using the chlorohydrin. In fact, the ARCO process is beginning to dominate propylene oxide production.[27]

Input Substitution: Companies can change the raw materials they use, substituting nontoxic or less toxic materials for hazardous chemicals. Cryodynamics Inc. produces refrigeration units and cooling systems for application to military, aerospace, and industrial high-performance requirements. Refrigerators and cooling systems typically require the use of trichlorofluoromethane (CFC-11), which with halons and certain chlorinated solvents contributes to the destruction of the ozone layer. As ozone is destroyed, more harmful ultraviolet radiation penetrates to the earth's surface with potentially disastrous public health and environmental effects.

Cryodynamics employed an alternative equipment design concept that allowed it to substitute helium for CFC-11 in its production. Helium, which is used by Cryodynamics as a cryogenic cooler rather than a refrigerant, has no adverse effects on the ozone layer. Refrigeration units and cooling systems manufactured by Cryodynamics using the CFC-free technology are more energy efficient, reliable, and effective than those using CFCs. They are lighter, contain no valves, and require less lubrication. Cryodynamics has produced cooling systems for NASA and is under contract to design a prototype air conditioning system for use in buses manufactured in Winnipeg, Canada. Moreover, the firm has been contacted by European auto manufacturers expressing an interest in its patented technology and has signed a memorandum of understanding with the Chinese government to help produce 1 million home refrigeration units for the Chinese.[28]

Cleo Wrap, a relatively large company and the world's largest producer of Christmas gift-wrapping paper, converted from organic solvent-based inks to water-based inks in its printing operations. By shifting from chemical to water-based technology Cleo Wrap eliminated the need for storing, handling, and transporting toxic solvents, reduced fire hazards, was able to apply for lower fire insurance premiums, eliminated waste storage capacity, and eliminated hazardous waste disposal costs. The company cut the costs of toxic material management, reduced workers' exposure to solvents, and eliminated atmospheric emissions of solvent vapors.[29]

End-Product Reformulation: Companies can change the design, composition, or specifications of end products to reduce, avoid, or eliminate the use of toxics. Polaroid, through its innovative Toxics Use Reduction and Waste Reduction Program, eliminated the use of mercury by redesigning the batteries used to power its cameras. This product reformulation was in part a response to regulations in Switzerland that imposed limits on the allowable level of mercury in carbon/zinc batteries. The conversion to mercury-free batteries resulted in a simplified manufacturing process, eliminated material costs for mercury, and reduced costs of complying with industrial hygiene and occupational safety regulations. The company also eliminated mercury from environmental wastes at its battery production facility.[30]

Equipment Modification: Companies can change the technology of production by means of equipment redesign, equipment renovation, or plant modernization with the goal of reducing the use of toxic materials. Microfinish—a small electroplating company—provides an example of how changes in the basic technology and equipment of production, including modernization and renovation, can result in the reduced use of toxic materials. Microfinish accomplished this by installing a cyanide-free plating system. This modification of the technology of production slashed pollution control costs and eliminated cyanide from the workplace. The system offered advantages not only in occupational hygiene and environmental protection but in efficiency and energy conservation as well.

The manufacturer and supplier of the cyanide-free system used by Microfinish compared the costs of technological options for different plating systems. The comparison assumed a waste effluent generation rate of 16 barrels per hour, at 250 days per year, totaling 16,000 barrels per year. Annual pollution control or waste treatment costs for a cyanide-intensive plating system would be $8,700; for the cyanide-free system, however, pollution control costs are reduced to $100 per year.[31]

Improved Plant Operations: Companies can better oversee plant operations and systems through routine equipment maintenance, expert handling of toxic materials, increased training of shop floor personnel, expert monitoring of process equipment, and more attention to planning. This approach results in more efficient use of toxic materials, reduction of workplace emissions, decreased generation of environmental wastes and pollutants, reduced demand for toxic materials from industrial suppliers, and safer operations with a reduced likelihood of Bhopal-type accidents.

Exxon Chemical America installed floating roofs over its tanks of volatile solvents, thereby cutting emissions of volatile organic compounds (VOCs). This operational improvement is reported to have greatly reduced VOC emissions, cut materials costs, and allowed the company to reduce its purchases of chemicals from industrial suppliers.[32]

Dow Chemical reduced its chemical input requirements for a crude-product drying system by installing a computer and on-stream analyzer to adjust the amount of chemical drying agent needed in the operation. Material requirements for the drying agent dropped by more than a third, and waste generation was similarly reduced.[33]

Recycling as Part of a Production Process: Companies can return potential wastes and potential environmental pollutants to production operations within the parameters of production itself to reduce the volume or amount of virgin toxic materials that are used.

Daly-Herring Company modified a dust collection operation so that manufacturing wastes from a variety of processes and operations could be reintroduced into the processes that generated them. The company cut materials and disposal costs and reduced waste storage and transport.[34]

GTE Sylvania installed an electrolytic metal recovery cell to recover copper wastes from rinsewater. The process change allows for recirculation of rinsewater, the sale of recovered copper, and reduced disposal costs for copper sludge wastes.[35]

An expanding list of case studies in the technical literature describes how reducing the use of toxics has been both practical and economically sound in company after company, both in the United States and in foreign nations. It is important to distinguish, however, between two different types of reduction: toxicity reduction and toxic material loss reduction.

The most desirable environmental strategy involves toxicity reduction of processes and products—whether this involves reducing the toxicity of chemical production processes, the toxicity of operations for manufacturing paper, or the toxicity of end products such as furniture polish and batteries. Reducing the toxic material content or toxic property of a process, by-product, or product is known as *toxicity reduction*.

The second reduction strategy, which is less desirable, does not alter the toxicity of the process or product but uses toxics in the production process more efficiently, usually through operational improvement or through the use of closed-loop systems. A given product—for example, a computer, an automobile part, or a machine tool—is made with the same materials, but the technology of production is tightened up so that fewer environmental toxics are released during production. This is known as *toxic material loss reduction*.

REDUCING INDUSTRY'S HAZARDOUS WASTES

Reducing the use of toxic materials is unexcelled as a strategy for dealing with the entire spectrum of risks, costs, problems, liabilities, and concerns posed by toxic materials, by-products, wastes, pollutants, and products. It is not, however, the only effective option for achieving pollution prevention. A related option is industrial hazardous waste reduction as defined by the congressional Office of Technology Assessment. The importance of industrial hazardous waste reduction should not be underestimated.[36]

Industrial hazardous waste reduction has much in common with use reduction of toxic materials. First, waste reduction changes the technology and materials of production. Second, it cannot be achieved through traditional pollution control strategies that focus on controlling wastes and pollutants at the end of the pipe. Third, waste reduction is an economically sound response to many of the problems posed by environmental waste and pollution.

Nonetheless, these two reduction strategies have slightly different goals. This difference could have major environmental implications if one approach is adopted to the exclusion of the other. For example, waste reduction often deals with potentially hazardous materials and pollutants that may not be regulated as toxic but nevertheless may cause environmental harm. Certain industrial materials such as ignitable, reactive, and corrosive materials and wastes may or may not be considered toxic but are amenable to waste reduction. In addition, in cases of scientific and regulatory uncertainty about toxicity, it may be possible to make a stronger case for waste reduction than for toxics reduction.

Waste reduction is not necessarily an effective means for achieving toxicity reduction of certain processes and products, however. For example, there is no clear evidence in the pollution prevention literature that waste reduction has resulted in a major shift to chemical pathway redesign. Moreover, waste reduction seldom results in input substitution and end-product reformulation—which is where the most significant toxicity reduction gains can often be achieved.[37] In fact, waste reduction might stimulate engineering strategies that incorporate toxic materials in the products themselves in order to reduce the toxicity and quantity of hazardous wastes generated by a company. To illustrate, Monsanto eliminated a waste stream by reformulating an adhesive so that hazardous constituents remained in the product, rather than the waste stream.[38]

One weakness of waste reduction becomes clear when one reviews the indoor air pollution problem. EPA has recently cited indoor air pollution as a major health risk for Americans. While indoor air pollution does not yet rank high in the public's view of environmental problems, EPA believes that it might prove to be one of the major environmental problems of the 1990s.[39] A recent study by the Massachusetts Special Legislative Commission on Indoor Air Pollution states that perhaps as much as 50 percent of all illnesses are caused by indoor air pollution.[40]

Volatile organic compounds are a major contributor to toxic indoor air pollution. Hundreds of VOCs released from products, consumer items, and building materials are easily identified in the indoor environment. Many VOCs are known or suspected irritants, neurotoxicants, and carcinogens.[41]

While waste reduction tends to encourage the most efficient industrial production technologies and strategies—thereby reducing the generation of both regulated and nonregulated environmental waste and pollution at manufacturing plants—it does not *frontally* address the composition, specification, and design of products, building materials, and consumer items. Hence waste reduction does not always foster a clear-cut strategy to reduce, avoid, or eliminate toxic materials in products. This shortcoming is of particular concern not only for indoor air pollution. It is also relevant for household hazardous waste, municipal solid waste, and occupational exposure problems.

POLLUTION PREVENTION: AN ECONOMIC ENVIRONMENTALISM

Whatever their relative merits, toxics use reduction and waste reduction are two interrelated facets of pollution prevention. Pollution prevention, in turn, is an economically sound environmental strategy. By promoting changes in the technology and materials of production, in industrial processes and operations, and in attitudes, pollution prevention can contribute to structural improvements in the U.S. economy. In fact, reduction policies for pollution prevention should be seen as a means for jointly achieving environmental and economic goals. For the first time there is an effective environmental option capable of being linked to policies of economic transition, economic restructuring, industrial innovation, and long-term industrial development in the United States.

It is instructive to compare strategies for revitalizing the U.S. economy with those for preventing pollution. A recent study, conducted by the MIT Commission on Industrial Productivity,[42] cites six interrelated patterns of industrial behavior that can be held to account for the steady decline of U.S. manufacturing:

- Outdated production strategies
- Short-term rather than long-term planning and investment
- Weaknesses in research and production
- Consistent failure to develop human resources

- Failure to develop cooperative relationships within companies, between companies, and between companies and other societal institutions
- Cross-purpose action between government and industry[43]

Note that in every one of these cases, policy options for pollution prevention can be made to dovetail neatly with actions that could help revitalize the U.S. economic system.[44]

There is little doubt that the pollution prevention approach can promote innovative production strategies that contribute to the competitiveness of U.S. industry. Pollution prevention stimulates long-term, rather than short-term, planning and investment patterns. It strengthens industry and government research programs and contributes to scrutiny of and investment in production processes. Pollution prevention also develops the skills of workers, requires a higher level of technological literacy throughout company and government operations, calls for a higher order of cooperation within and between companies, requires cooperation between industry and other social institutions, and, finally, reduces cross-purpose action between industry, government, labor, and environmental interests.

In short: Pollution prevention is eminently suited to be linked to economic policies that could increase the productive performance of American industry and open up new markets for U.S. producers through the development of safer technologies, materials, and products. To continue to overemphasize end-of-pipe pollution control options (recycling, treatment, and disposal) at the expense of a strong, long-term commitment to pollution prevention could be a serious economic mistake.

Other nations may already have a head start. Various foreign countries (France, West Germany, Sweden, Norway, Denmark, The Netherlands, Austria) are already taking steps toward pollution prevention.[45] Coupled with the well-documented decline in U.S. manufacturing, our failure to exploit the economic and environmental benefits of pollution prevention could be a major strategic error on the part of American government and industry.

THE UNIQUE BENEFITS OF PREVENTING POLLUTION

In the final analysis, the benefits of an environmental option serve as the rationale for its adoption and consequent placement in a hierarchy of priorities for environmental protection. The benefits of preventing pollution are unequaled among environmental options, and these unique benefits call for its rapid and systematic adoption as the strategy of choice—over and above strategies for controlling pollution.

It should be borne in mind that preventing pollution has great logical and practical appeal on a number of fronts. As an environmental option, pollution prevention is unequaled in:

- Providing the most certain means for ensuring environmental, public health, and worker protection
- Reducing production, regulatory compliance, liability, and insurance costs for industry
- Contributing to industrial innovation and industrial competitiveness by systematically changing the technology, operations, and materials of production
- Increasing public confidence in government activities, operations, and programs for environmental protection
- Lessening long-term governmental responsibilities, costs, and uncertainties associated with the environment
- Providing moral and political authority to U.S. policymakers as they address issues relating to international and global environmental security

RESISTANCE AT EPA

Despite its unique benefits, however, true pollution prevention is not being seriously promoted by the government and has found no credible advocates at EPA. There is no significant authority to promote preventive changes across the total array of environmental problems in the nation. In the case of toxic materials, the Toxic Substances Control Act (TSCA), originally intended to address chemical risks at the point of production, manufacture, or use, has not brought about *broad-based* reductions in toxic material usage and was never intended to do so. Many people question the effectiveness of TSCA even in testing new and existing chemicals.

Although the EPA in the 1980s has slowly lumbered toward the implementation of pollution prevention by creating a small Pollution Prevention Office within EPA's Office of Policy, Planning, and Evaluation, this development is largely the result of pressure from outside the agency. In addition, a close analysis of the EPA effort shows that it promotes waste minimization, not pollution prevention.[46] Whatever the motivation, EPA's current effort could not have been better designed to obscure important policy distinctions while undercutting true pollution prevention. Agency efforts are not only ill defined, underfunded, and poorly coordinated, but they have limited institutional visibility in the total context of EPA activities, operations, and programs, despite all recent attempts to demonstrate otherwise.[47]

EPA is apparently more committed to the unavoidably risky pollution control strategy of recycling wastes and pollutants in the environment than it is to achieving true pollution prevention.[48] In 1988, EPA testified against pollution prevention legislation being considered by Congress that would have established an effective pollution prevention program.[49] In 1989, EPA designed its own legislation despite the fact that well-designed pollution prevention legislation was already being considered by Congress.[50] In general, it is difficult to imagine EPA policies and actions that would more effectively undermine prospects for toxics use reduction and industrial waste reduction than those that have thus far been considered, designed, and promoted.

CONCLUSION

Pollution control has not met with outstanding success over a twenty-year span. Nonetheless, there is a superior environmental protection strategy based on principles of preventing pollution. And there are mutually complementary incentives, options, and enhancements available to us to advance pollution prevention. (See Appendixes A and B, below.)

Preventing pollution—with all of its unique benefits—does not have to remain, as it has thus far been, a theoretical goal in the distant future in relation to which there is much idle talk but no real action. With today's technology, major progress can be made. Many of the available industrial, governmental, and public options for preventing pollution are beginning to be seriously discussed and debated in a variety of contexts. Some promising activities in industry, government, and public life are beginning. But this is no more than a beginning. The fundamental and system-changing shift toward pollution prevention has not yet taken place.

Clearly, pollution prevention is an aspect of sound industrial practice. It could provide unique environmental, economic, and political benefits as we enter the twenty-first century. Yet only a handful of exceptional American companies are committed to it. Long committed to the inferior strategy of pollution control, weakened from a decade of negligence, and suffering recent cuts in critical areas of environmental spending, the EPA, the nation's top environmental agency and perhaps the most significant such agency worldwide, has thus far failed to provide leadership.

To gain the full advantages of pollution prevention will require a major shift in environmental protection values—a return to the common sense and clear thinking that were present when the modern environmental ethic made itself felt in the "enthusiastic outburst of Earth Day" nearly twenty years ago. To embrace preventive values means going beyond the limiting language of pollution control, the prevailing language in the world of slowly declining American industries and entrenched governmental and environmental bureaucracies. An Archimedean lever will have to be located in the public world of environmental politics and environmental activism—a lever that can be used to shift environmental protection priorities not from the center of political power but from its periphery. For those who would commit themselves to this task—within industry, government, and the environmental movement—the minimum requirement may first be that they recognize the environmental reality of our time.[51]

The question then becomes: Can support for serious pollution prevention be mobilized in the environmental movement? If it can, and if pollution prevention achieves primacy over pollution control, there are many untapped opportunities to improve our environmental and economic security as America enters the twenty-first century.

APPENDIX A: GOVERNMENT OPTIONS FOR PREVENTING POLLUTION

What we need is a practical reform of the hierarchy of priorities that have thus far guided the environmental movement, the government, and industrial decision making. The major thrust of environmental activism and government activity must be altered to provide serious support for pollution prevention. Here, in summary form, is a series of practical actions—some already implemented, some still being debated in legislative, administrative, and public contexts—that can be considered as part of an overall structural framework for bringing about pollution prevention in the United States. These actions need not all be implemented. Yet in principle they could be readily used or may well be used at some point in the future. It is important to see them as ideal components of a total *system* of pollution prevention options. They are presented here to bring conceptual clarity to the discussion of options for preventing pollution.

NEW LAWS AND PROGRAMS

New environmental laws are required that are specifically designed to bring about pollution prevention. It is not possible to establish effective pollution prevention programs in the absence of new legal authority and new government policies that give primacy to the pollution prevention option.[52]

Moreover, new government programs must be established at EPA and in other federal and state agencies.[53] Some basic program options include:

- Establishing an administratively autonomous Office of Pollution Prevention—an all-agency office, with high visibility and strong institutional position, headed by an assistant administrator at EPA—to focus specifically on preventing pollution[54]
- Coordinating actions of the EPA Office of Pollution Prevention with other federal and state government agencies[55]

Following these minimum requirements for pollution prevention, there are a number of interrelated actions that could be used to achieve rapid and reliable progress.

SIX TYPES OF ACTION TO ACHIEVE PROGRESS

Six broad areas of government activity should be considered when designing pollution prevention programs.[56] By taking into account the widest array of factors and policy instruments for promoting preventive environmental protection, the government will be in the best possible position both to spur pollution prevention and to avoid unintended consequences that sometimes result when different factors are excluded from program analysis and program design. If the government does not use certain options available to it, a rationale should at least be provided as to why the program option was not adopted.

Information Collection and Management

All government programs require data for their organization and administration. In the area of pollution prevention policy, the need for information is particularly acute.

Chemical Usage and Waste Generation Inventories: Comprehensive information is required about hazardous material inputs, industry-specific and company-specific patterns of chemical use, and waste outputs to air, water, and land. This information would include a mass-balance calculation of chemicals brought on-site, chemicals that are created on-site, and chemicals that are either managed on-site or leave in the form of pollutants or product.

General Industry Information: Information is required concerning types, characteristics, and numbers of companies that are to be included in a government pollution prevention effort. Such information is needed for designing, targeting, and assessing government programs.

Assessment Activities

Rational allocation of government resources is an important goal, particularly where the government has multiple responsibilities and cannot address every problem. As a basis for rational use of limited government resources, and in order to track the efforts and progress of specific industries and companies, it is necessary to undertake a number of different types of assessment.

Toxics Use Reduction and Waste Reduction Measurement: Measurement of actual progress in preventing pollution is an important responsibility of industry and government.

Analysis of Alternative Preventive Technologies and Strategies: Assessment of available and emerging pollution prevention technologies and methods is another important responsibility.

Toxicity and Hazard Assessment: Toxicity evaluations and identification of high-hazard materials and process technologies is a related responsibility.

An important question is whether assessments should be undertaken on an ad hoc or periodic basis. Ideally, assessments should be carried out periodically to identify changes in industrial practice and in technical and scientific knowledge. In the case of pollution prevention measurement, periodic assessment is needed to identify trends in hazardous material usage and waste generation.

Education, Training, and Assistance

Education programs and technical assistance are almost universally regarded as important for the success of pollution prevention. Education, training, and assistance efforts inform industry about the availability and cost effectiveness of pollution prevention opportunities.

Industrial Assistance: A program to assist trade associations, business organizations, educational institutions, labor groups, and public interest organizations can be established. Such assistance programs can be implemented by state pollution prevention boards.

University-based Activities: University programs can be created to educate and train engineers, environmental planners, and other pollution prevention specialists. Such programs can also be designed to develop knowledge about techniques for preventing pollution and to provide on-site managerial and technical assistance to industry. One way of ensuring proper training and education is through the creation of a Pollution Prevention Institute in the university system.

Company Planning Requirements: Government can require that companies draw up pollution prevention plans. This quasi-educational approach has a great deal of intrinsic merit. An important function of required plans is that they initiate a "self-educating" function in industry. They contribute to beneficial changes in the strategic focus, competitive emphasis, innovative capacity, and materials management focus of industry with a minimum of intrusive government involvement. Plans also assist the government in identifying industries and companies that operate inefficiently or suboptimally and therefore require special government services.

Economic Activities

In the final analysis, economic factors play a critical role in industry decision making and in government program administration. Two basic questions involve the raising of revenue for a government program and the design of economic incentive systems to spur pollution prevention by industry.

Government Revenue: Revenue-generating mechanisms are an important aspect of every government effort. One option, particularly useful for pollution prevention, is to impose a charge at the point of production, sale, or purchase of toxic and hazardous industrial materials.

Input Charges: A front-end tax or charge on hazardous and toxic materials raises revenue for government programs and, in addition, operates psychologically to shift the materials management focus of companies away from an end-of-pipe to a front-end environmental protection emphasis. The aim is to focus industrial attention at the juncture where the initial decision to produce, use, or purchase dangerous materials occurs. Input taxes are already assessed in a number of states in order to generate revenue for state Superfund programs.

Financial Assistance: A different economic issue involves the development of financial assistance mechanisms for industry. Financial assistance can be selectively used to develop different networks and types of knowledge for pollution prevention in industry, educational institutions, labor groups, consumer groups, and environmental groups. There are two basic types of potentially useful financial instruments: *Grant programs* can be established primarily for building institutional networks, knowledge, and expertise; *loan programs* can be established to directly assist firms operating under capital formation constraints.

Full Cost Accounting: Companies can be required, as an aspect of pollution prevention planning, to fully assess the costs and expenditures associated with hazardous and toxic material production, use, storage, management, and pollution. This can have a significant impact on company decision making where hazardous materials are concerned.

Regulatory Activities

Regulatory programs for control and management of toxic materials and wastes may be made more effective in promoting pollution prevention by raising the industrial costs associated with regulatory compliance. Existing laws and programs, however, were not purposely designed to promote pollution prevention. They fail to provide the necessary technical assistance, information, and direct economic incentives. As pollution prevention incentives, therefore, they are not purposeful.

Nonetheless, although existing regulatory programs do not constitute direct means for achieving pollution prevention, they could be made to function more effectively as indirect promoters of pollution prevention.

After adjustment, regulatory programs could be made to promote pollution prevention, particularly if used in conjunction with information, technical assistance, and economic enhancements. The options for indirect regulation include the following possibilities.

Regulatory Expansion and Coordination: Existing regulatory programs that monitor and control environmental wastes and pollutants released to air, water, and land could be coordinated with the primary aim of promoting pollution prevention. One aspect of this strategy involves broadening regulatory coverage of hazardous and toxic chemicals and pollutants under Clean Air, Clean Water, Hazardous Waste, Safe Drinking Water, and Occupational Safety and Health programs.

Enhanced and Coordinated Enforcement: Enhanced enforcement and coenforcement of existing pollution control programs and regulations is another option. Enhanced enforcement involves the establishment of a stronger enforcement presence by government agencies. It may also involve mechanisms for community initiation of government enforcement actions. Coenforcement involves the coordinated and simultaneous enforcement of all pollution control laws at a given facility, which can reduce government enforcement costs.

Integrated Inspection: Inspections typically deal with land, air, or water pollution. Single-media inspections do not provide for a comprehensive multiple-media review of all chemicals released as waste, however, and may not identify cross-media shifting of pollutants. But integrated inspections— in which releases to air, water, and land are simultaneously reviewed— could provide a more comprehensive understanding of pollution at specific companies and might result in fewer opportunities for shifting pollutants from one medium to another. By limiting opportunities for cross-media pollutant shifting, industry could be motivated to reduce pollution.

Regulatory Flexibility: The government could administer a program of temporary compliance extensions or regulatory waivers that would be selectively issued to promote pollution prevention. These have been variously described as "innovation waivers" or "regulatory concessions." Regulatory flexibility can provide companies with the opportunity to reduce toxics use and to reduce waste in the face of impending regulatory requirements that might otherwise force them to overinvest in pollution control.

Regulatory Review: Systematic review of existing regulations and programs can be undertaken for purposes of regulatory adjustment. The intent would be to determine the effect of government regulations on industrial practice and to adjust regulations in ways that directly promote pollution prevention, rather than additional pollution control.

In addition to indirect regulatory options, there are direct regulatory options for preventing pollution. These options directly address production.

Performance Standards: Some might advocate enforceable waste reduction standards. Waste reduction standards might take the form of efficiency requirements imposed on industries or companies generating waste. This is perhaps the most problematic option available.

First, waste reduction standards would be exceedingly difficult to administer, creating an administrative nightmare for government and industry. The amount of data and information required to enforce a system of waste reduction standards might rapidly overwhelm government's data management capabilities. Furthermore, standards could serve as a powerful incentive for illegal disposal and could contribute to systematic underreporting of waste generation by industry in order to avoid penalties associated with not meeting the requirements. In addition, in some cases standards could keep many companies from accomplishing even more waste reduction than the standards would require, and in this way a system of standards might inhibit innovations for waste reduction. But most important, many companies might be motivated to turn hazardous waste into product as a means of coming into compliance with the standard. Instead, a more appropriate strategy might involve the limited application of efficiency requirements or performance standards on toxic chemical usage.

Phaseouts and Bans: Phaseouts and bans of toxic chemicals constitute a direct regulatory means for bringing about pollution prevention. In cases where use of a specific material poses unacceptable health and environmental risks or significant economic costs, it is appropriate to phase out, restrict, or ban its use. Such actions do not in principle adversely affect economic activity since industry can typically innovate or diversify to remain competitive and viable—as in the case of DDT, PCBs, asbestos, and CFCs.

Phaseouts and bans of the most toxic and hazardous materials need not be economically disruptive. To illustrate, consider the policy option of eliminating lead in gasoline—an approach that even President Reagan's Council on Environmental Quality termed "sensible . . . from both a public health and an economic perspective." In some instances, it is more disruptive to the economic and social system to continue usage than it is to phase out such usage, as in the case of CFCs and other ozone depleters.

However, while phaseouts and bans are a direct and effective means for reducing toxic chemical use, they in no way eliminate the need for other pollution prevention options. Even if the range of banned chemicals were to increase markedly, a phaseout system would still fail to address the great majority of chemicals that are toxic but nevertheless unlikely ever to be banned.

Overall Program Coordination

Coordination of governmental and nongovernmental activities, operations, and programs is a crucial goal. One important means of organizing various activities is to develop and periodically update a government-wide pollution prevention report and plan. Another means of achieving the same end is to establish operational compatibility among various government agencies with responsibilities for pollution prevention, pollution control, waste management, public health protection, and economic development and to adjust them to promote pollution prevention. Government and industry programs that are not internally coordinated cannot be expected to establish clear government-wide and company-wide priorities and guidelines for pollution prevention.

Comprehensive Government Planning and Reporting: A comprehensive government plan and report on pollution prevention can be required. This formalizes program design, sets a public schedule for program evaluations and government actions, and provides for public accountability and legislative review.

General Coordination: Consistent with government-wide planning and administrative activities is the establishment of the organizational means for coordination and operational compatibility of relevant government and industry activities and operations.

None of the actions summarized above is as effective in isolation as it is when integrated into an overall system of activities. And the system as a whole is more effective when the public is involved.

APPENDIX B: CITIZEN INVOLVEMENT

The general public—not only government and industry—has a major role to play in preserving the environment and protecting human health. One responsibility involves changing consumption practices in order to reduce demand for products containing toxic materials. This measure can accelerate changes in industry and in government policy.

In fact, pollution prevention more readily involves citizens in preserving our environment than does pollution control. The public is better able to practice pollution prevention at the point of consumption than it is to engage in pollution control. For public and community pollution prevention strategies to succeed, however, more information must be made available to citizens about toxic materials in products, probably through national product labeling requirements. Other avenues of public and community activity are also open, however. History shows that community and political activism is often a potent factor in promoting organized changes in government policy and industrial practice.[57]

In addition, from the point of view of government policy it makes sense to instill public confidence by providing meaningful opportunities for public input. This democratic principle and social value is well established in U.S. environmental policy. In addressing the question of using democratic institutions and processes to manage and reduce environmental risk, for example, William Ruckelshaus, a former EPA administrator, stated that the point

> is not to say whether the sharing of the power to make risk management decisions is right or wrong: it is simply to state that it is a fact of life in the United States. We have decided, in an unprecedented way, that the decision-making responsibility involving risk issues must be shared with the American people, and we are very unlikely to back away from that decision. So the question before us is not whether there is going to be a sharing, whether we will have participatory democracy with regard to the management [or reduction] of risk, but how.[58]

The critical question is not whether public involvement in environmental decision making is acceptable, but how it is to be achieved.

There are six broad areas of public and community involvement:

- Information: The public could be given access to relevant information used for government decision making relating to pollution prevention. This right-to-know principle is already firmly established under certain major programs, such as the federal Community Right-to-Know program established in Title III of the Superfund Amendment and Reauthorization Act of 1986.
- Assessment Activities: The public could be provided with opportunities to have meaningful involvement in the interpretation of environmental information. This could be facilitated by establishing state

Pollution Prevention Boards with broad public, government, and industry representation.

• Education and Technical Assistance: The public could be provided with the means to hire and consult with technical experts who could articulate the public interest in public forums. This option has already been exercised under the federal Superfund program.

• Economic Assistance: Funding could be provided to enable more effective public and community participation, just as it is offered to sustain industry interest in pollution prevention.

• Regulatory Review: Opportunities could be provided for public and community review of regulatory actions, as in decisions involving the administration of pollution prevention innovation waivers or regulatory concessions to industry.

• Overall Coordination: Public review and comment could be solicited on government reports and plans, and public representatives could be included on any Pollution Prevention Board or other body required for the development of government plans.

NOTES

1. *Chemical Engineering News,* May 1989.
2. U.S. Congress, Office of Technology Assessment, *From Pollution to Prevention: A Progress Report on Waste Reduction—Special Report,* OTA-ITE-347 (Washington, D.C.: U.S. Government Printing Office, June 1987), p. 13. These figures are even more significant in light of the fact that EPA has made only limited progress in determining wastes that should be regulated. See U.S. Congress, General Accounting Office, *Hazardous Waste: EPA Has Made Limited Progress in Determining the Wastes to Be Regulated,* GAO/RCED-87-27 (Gaithersburg, Md.: U.S. General Accounting Office, December 1986). According to this GAO report: "The first step to successful nationwide regulation . . . of hazardous wastes is identifying which wastes present a clear threat to human health and the environment. Despite the importance of this, however, EPA has made limited progress in identifying hazardous wastes. EPA does not know whether it is controlling 90 percent of existing hazardous wastes—or 10 percent; likewise, it does not know if it is controlling the wastes that are most hazardous. At present, the disposal of dangerous wastes, such as certain pesticides and known carcinogens, is not being regulated by EPA."
3. U.S. Congress, Office of Technology Assessment, *Superfund Strategy,* OTA-ITE-252 (Washington, D.C.: U.S. Government Printing Office, April 1985).
4. U.S. Congress, Office of Technology Assessment, *Protecting the Nation's*

Groundwater from Contamination, OTA-O-233 (Washington, D.C.: U.S. Government Printing Office, October 1984).

5. *Troubled Water on Tap* (Washington, D.C.: Center for the Study of Responsive Law, January 1988), p. i.

6. U.S. Environmental Protection Agency, *Environmental News: EPA Releases Toxic Inventory Data,* April 12, 1989.

7. Council on Environmental Quality, *Environmental Quality 1984, 15th Annual Report* (Washington, D.C.: U.S. Government Printing Office, 1984), pp. 53–55.

8. *Statement of Office of Technology Assessment Before the Subcommittee on Environment and Public Works,* U.S. Senate, May 10, 1989.

9. Personal communication with Deborah Sheiman, Natural Resources Defense Council, December 1987.

10. U.S. Environmental Protection Agency, *Broad Scan Analysis of the FY82 National Human Adipose Tissue Survey Specimens,* vol. 1—Executive Summary, EPA-560/5-86-035, December 1986.

11. U.S. Environmental Protection Agency, National Institutes of Health, Department of Energy (Interagency Collaborative Group on Environmental Carcinogens), *Chemicals Identified in Human Biological Media: A Data Base,* March 1980.

12. U.S. Congress, Office of Technology Assessment, *Serious Reduction of Hazardous Waste: For Pollution Prevention and Industrial Efficiency,* OTA-ITE-317 (Washington, D.C.: U.S. Government Printing Office, September 1986); U.S. Congress, Office of Technology Assessment, *From Pollution to Prevention.*

13. *Environmental Quality 1985: The Sixteenth Annual Report of the Council on Environmental Quality—1987,* pp. 18–23; cited in Joel S. Hirschhorn, "Congressional Opportunities to Support Waste Reduction," *Fourth Annual Massachusetts Hazardous Waste Source Reduction Conference Proceedings,* Department of Environmental Management, Office of Safe Waste Management, October 1987.

14. Barry Commoner, "A Reporter at Large: The Environment," *New Yorker,* June 15, 1987.

15. See U.S. Congress, Office of Technology Assessment, *Serious Reduction of Hazardous Waste,* pp. 147–148. See also Conservation Foundation, *Examples of Cross-Media Pollution Problems and Control Approaches in North America,* prepared for the Environment Directorate, Organization for Economic Cooperation and Development, Paris, May 7, 1986. The fact that cross-media pollutant shifts are not effectively addressed by the pollution control system has been a major concern for some time. See, for example, U.S. Congress, General Accounting Office, *Environmental Protection: Agenda for the 1980's,* GAO/CED-82-73 (Gaithersburg, Md.: U.S. General Accounting Office, May 1982), chap. 8: "Most legislation is enacted along separate pollution lines—such as

air, water, hazardous wastes, and toxic substances—which do not address the multimedia pollution problem" (p. 30).

16. Lee M. Thomas, quoted in *The New York Times,* "Week in Review" section, May 11, 1986.

17. Conservation Foundation, *Examples of Cross-Media Pollution Problems and Control Approaches in North America.*

18. U.S. Congress, Office of Technology Assessment, *Serious Reduction of Hazardous Waste,* p. 18. See also *Washington Post,* "The Poisoning of Chesapeake Bay," June 1, 1986, p. 1.

19. U.S. Congress, Office of Technology Assessment, *Wastes in Marine Environments,* OTA-O-334 (Washington, D.C.: U.S. Government Printing Office, April 1987), p. 47.

20. U.S. Congress, Office of Technology Assessment, *Identifying and Regulating Carcinogens,* OTA-BP-H-42 (Washington, D.C.: U.S. Government Printing Office, November 1987), p. 21.

21. Current figures and estimates offered by the Commerce Department suggest a national cost of over $80 billion for pollution control each year. The congressional Office of Technology Assessment suggests that the true cost may be much higher, perhaps more than $100 billion annually. America spends a larger percentage of its GNP on pollution control than any other nation. See *Statement of Office of Technology Assessment Before the Subcommittee on Environment and Public Works,* U.S. Senate, May 10, 1989. It should be noted, however, that these figures do not reflect missed economic opportunities associated with failing to invest in the production system of U.S. industry. Opportunity costs of not engaging in pollution prevention may be considerably higher than the simple costs of administering and complying with pollution control. By focusing on the end of the pipe, the United States is missing economic opportunities for industrial innovation, industrial restructuring, product and technology development, and renovation of process equipment and operations.

22. Council on Environmental Quality, *Toxic Chemicals and Public Protection: A Report to the President by the Toxic Substances Strategy Committee* (Washington, D.C.: U.S. Government Printing Office, May 1980), p. 21.

23. For an analysis of problems in EPA's pollution prevention policy that is as relevant today as it was when it was first published, see U.S. Congress, Office of Technology Assessment, *From Pollution to Prevention.* EPA has recently been less than forthright in responding to weaknesses in its public policy. For a general review of this problem, see "Dead Fish and Red Herrings: How the EPA Pollutes the News," *Columbia Journalism Review,* November/December 1988.

24. For example, several members of the Subcommittee on Pollution Prevention of the EPA Science Advisory Board noted that, with respect to pollution prevention, industry is opposed to letting EPA "in the door under any circumstances"; see *Environment Reporter,* March 1989, p. 2465.

25. The policy option of "toxics use reduction" is a cognate concept to OTA's industrial hazardous waste reduction. Toxics use reduction, as the term is specifically employed here, was first conceived of and developed as a policy instrument sharing many features of OTA's waste reduction. The term, and the policy consonant with it, refer to actions and goals, however, that shift attention from simple reduction of environmental wastes and pollutants to reduction in the *use* of toxics in the U.S. production system. For an early work that helped set the stage for the idea in 1985, see Richard C. Bird, *Promoting Improved Toxic Chemical Management and Source Reduction,* Massachusetts Department of Environmental Quality Engineering, Bureau of Solid Waste Disposal, April 1985. See also David W. Allen and John T. O'Connor, *Review of Source Reduction Policy and Program Development—A Background Report,* Massachusetts Department of Environmental Quality Engineering, June 1985. A variant of the term is "hazardous substance use reduction," as the term is employed in the New Jersey Pollution Prevention and Hazardous Substance Reduction bill of 1989.

26. Toxics use reduction involves "changes in production materials, technologies, processes, operations, or products that reduce, avoid, or eliminate the use of toxic materials so as to reduce health and environmental risks." See David W. Allen, "Toxics Use Reduction: For Pollution Prevention and Other Benefits," unpublished paper prepared for the National Toxics Campaign and PIRG Toxics Action, December 1987. It is important to note that this definition excludes the redistribution of risk, as in cases where risk is shifted from wastes to products, or from general to occupational environments, or from one environmental medium to another. Likewise, toxics use reduction does not involve conventional recycling of already created wastes and pollutants, as at solvent recycling operations. Conventional recycling is a pollution control strategy with unavoidable risks, costs, and liabilities. For example, 10 percent of the federal Superfund sites in 1986 were previously recycling and treatment facilities for already-generated wastes.

27. Personal communication with Marco Kaltofen, chemical engineer, National Toxics Prevention Fund, April 1989. See also *Chemical Business,* March 1988, and Philip J. Chenier, *Survey of Industrial Chemistry* (New York: Wiley, 1986).

28. Personal communication with Marc Goldberg, Cryodynamics, May 1989. See also *A Consumer's Guide to Protecting the Ozone* (Boston: National Toxics Campaign, 1989).

29. U.S. Congress, Office of Technology Assessment, *Serious Reduction of Hazardous Waste,* p. 82.

30. Personal communication with Harry Fatkin, Polaroid, April 1989. See also *A Report on the Environment* (Cambridge, Mass.: Polaroid Corporation, May 1989). Polaroid's innovation also had a positive impact on the municipal solid waste stream. Previous to the elimination of mercury, Polaroid's batteries were contributing to mercury contamination of municipal garbage. In fact, nine

times the actual physical quantity of mercury was being disposed of by consumers of Polaroid's camera products in the form of municipal solid waste as was being disposed of by Polaroid at its manufacturing operations.

31. United Nations Environment Program, Office of Industry and the Environment, *Low- or Non-Pollution Technology Through Pollution Prevention*, prepared by 3M Company, p. 27.

32. U.S. Congress, Office of Technology Assessment, *Serious Reduction of Hazardous Waste*, p. 81.

33. Ibid., p. 80.

34. Donald Huisingh et al., *Proven Profit from Pollution Prevention* (Washington, D.C.: Institute for Local Self-Reliance, 1985), pp. 79–80.

35. Ibid., p. 118.

36. U.S. Congress, Office of Technology Assessment, *Serious Reduction of Hazardous Waste;* see also U.S. Congress, Office of Technology Assessment, *From Pollution to Prevention*. These pioneering studies on waste reduction (or "source reduction") remain unequaled in their scope and significance.

37. U.S. Congress, Office of Technology Assessment, *Serious Reduction of Hazardous Waste*. One indication that there is lack of attention to toxicity reduction when waste reduction alone is pursued can be found in this OTA report. OTA assessed the relative frequency of different waste reduction techniques reported in the literature. Of 258 case study examples of waste reduction in the literature in 1986, only 22, or less than 10 percent, involved either input substitution or end-product reformulation.

38. David Sarokin et al., *Cutting Chemical Wastes* (New York: INFORM, 1985), p. 89. This practice is not so unusual as some may claim: 3M and Dow have boasted of similar waste reduction accomplishments. And it is quite common in chemical production that hazardous by-products are used in a secondary process to produce a marketable product.

39. U.S. Environmental Protection Agency, Office of Health and Environmental Assessment, EPA Indoor Air Quality Implementation Plan, EPA-600/8-87/014 (Washington, D.C.: U.S. Government Printing Office, June 1987).

40. Commonwealth of Massachusetts, Special Legislative Commission on Indoor Air Pollution, *Indoor Air Pollution in Massachusetts: Final Report*, April 1989. Health costs in the United States, not necessarily related to indoor air quality, are $100 billion per year. According to an EPA study cited by the commission, "organic contaminants can occur indoors at up to 10 times the outdoor levels found in either industrial or rural areas" (p. 14).

41. In *Indoor Air Pollution in Massachusetts*, the commission states that "careful selection of building materials, furnishings and household cleaning products would drastically reduce indoor air levels of VOCs . . . [but] additional characterization of . . . indoor products is needed to make these product selection determinations" (p. 190). Even more effective yet would be reduction of the

use of toxic VOCs by industry in its production of consumer items, furnishings, and building materials—an option that the commission's study does not consider.

42. Michael L. Dertouzos, Richard K. Lester, Robert M. Solow, and the MIT Commission on Industrial Productivity, *Made in America: Regaining the Productive Edge* (Cambridge, Mass.: MIT Press, 1989). See also Suzanne Berger et al., "Toward a New Industrial America," *Scientific American,* June 1989, pp. 39–47.

43. Berger, "Toward a New Industrial America," pp. 39–47. In relation to these six problems, Berger, a member of the MIT Commission on Industrial Productivity, states: "Although an increasing number of American companies are recognizing what it takes to be the best in the world, many U.S. firms have not yet realized that they will have to make far-reaching changes in the way they do business. They will need to adopt new ways of thinking about human resources, new ways of organizing their systems of production and new approaches to the management of technology."

44. See, for example, U.S. Congress, Office of Technology Assessment, *Serious Reduction of Hazardous Waste;* see also U.S. Congress, Office of Technology Assessment, *From Pollution to Prevention.*

45. U.S. Congress, Office of Technology Assessment, *Serious Reduction of Hazardous Waste,* pp. 19–20. According to this OTA report: "Many Western European governments have actively encouraged waste reduction for many years. To the extent that their 10-year lead in waste reduction results in more efficient processes and increased productivity among European industries, U.S. firms in similar industrial sectors may be placed in an inferior economic position."

46. For an analysis of the faulty logic, inherent ambiguity, lack of clear commitment, and failure of leadership embodied in EPA's pollution prevention policy, see U.S. Congress, Office of Technology Assessment, *From Pollution to Prevention.* EPA initially used the term *waste minimization* as opposed to waste reduction. Waste minimization is, however, a greatly inferior option. A much criticized environmental strategy, waste minimization promotes pollution control actions such as conventional recycling of already existing wastes and pollutants. Recently, EPA has adopted the term *pollution prevention,* which overlays, like veneer, its original waste minimization policy.

47. In the *Statement of Office of Technology Assessment Before the Subcommittee on Environment and Public Works* (May 10, 1989), p. 8, we find:
EPA's efforts remain several levels below the Administrator in the organization and are underfunded.

EPA's continuing attempt at establishing a pollution prevention policy has not been able to resolve a basic definitional issue: Should pollution prevention remain faithful to the goal of reducing waste generation at its source? If so, then it should not include conventional recycling efforts; recycling may be the best form of waste management, but that is not the same thing as not producing waste to begin with.

EPA has not made much progress in using its current information collection systems to measure national waste reduction.

State programs lack significant funding and are often misdirected to assisting companies with regulatory compliance [for pollution control].

48. See, for example, Public Comment on EPA's Proposed Pollution Prevention Policy Statement (in response to *Federal Register*, Notice, January 26, 1989, pp. 3845–3847), David Allen, National Toxics Campaign, April 15, 1989, RCRA Docket Number F-88-SRRP-FFFFF, available from the National Toxics Campaign. See also David Allen, "Recycling?", paper presented at the Fifth Annual Woods Hole Waste Reduction Conference, June 21–23, 1989, Woods Hole, Mass.

49. According to the *Hazardous Materials Intelligence Report* (Cambridge, Mass.: World Information Systems, 1988): "A bill that Representative Howard Wolpe (Democrat–Michigan) has introduced to encourage hazardous waste generators to reduce their waste production would unnecessarily duplicate the U.S. Environmental Protection Agency's (EPA's) efforts . . . according to EPA Assistant Administrator James Barnes testifying before the U.S. House of Representatives' Energy and Commerce Committee's Transportation, Tourism, and Hazardous Materials Subcommittee. . . . A separate waste [reduction] office within EPA would 'serve to diffuse the [agency's] effort, not intensify it,' Barnes told the subcommittee." In fact, EPA was doing virtually nothing to seriously promote waste reduction as defined in the Wolpe bill.

50. Testimony of William K. Reilly, administrator, Environmental Protection Agency, before the Subcommittee on Transportation and Hazardous Materials, Committee on Energy and Commerce, U.S. House of Representatives, May 25, 1989, "Consideration of H.R. 1457, 'The Waste Reduction Act.' "

51. Kurt H. Wolff, *Surrender and Catch: Experience and Inquiry Today* (Dordrecht: D. Reidel, 1976).

52. See "Is There a Need for Legislative Action?" in U.S. Congress, Office of Technology Assessment, *From Pollution to Prevention*. See also the statement of Dr. Joel S. Hirschhorn, senior associate, Office of Technology Assessment, before the Subcommittee on Transportation and Hazardous Materials, Committee on Energy and Commerce, U.S. House of Representatives, May 25, 1989, "Consideration of H.R. 1457, 'The Waste Reduction Act'": "A *legal* definition of what our nation sees as the most important way to prevent and solve environmental problems is critical. . . . Legislation, after all, is our democratic way to institutionalize the national will and implement a social value. . . . If we want waste producers to change their processes, products, operation and management systems, and attitudes, then public policy as

embodied in statute needs to make the new rules and objectives crystal clear."

53. An organizational focal point must be established to promote pollution in a way that is consistent with the recognized superiority of this option. See U.S. Congress, Office of Technology Assessment, *Serious Reduction of Hazardous Waste;* U.S. Congress, Office of Technology Assessment, *From Pollution to Prevention.*

54. Current EPA efforts in this regard have been insufficient. See the statement of Office of Technology Assessment before the Subcommittee on Superfund, Ocean and Water Protection, Committee on Environment and Public Works, U.S. Senate, May 10, 1989.

55. Administrative options for state-level programs involve the creation of state pollution prevention boards, offices, divisions, and interagency councils. See, for example, "The Toxics Use Reduction and Waste Reduction Act," state legislation suggested by the National Toxics Campaign (1987); the Massachusetts Toxics Use Reduction bill (1985, 1987), prepared by MassPIRG in association with the National Toxics Campaign; the Indiana Preventive Environmental Protection and Waste Reduction Assistance bill (1988), prepared by the National Toxics Campaign Fund in association with Indiana Citizens Action Coalition; the Texas Pollution Prevention and Waste Reduction Assistance bill (1989), prepared by the National Toxics Campaign Fund in association with Texans United. See also David Allen, *State Programs in Waste Reduction,* May 1986, pp. 1–180; David Allen, *State Policy and Program Options for Reduction of Hazardous Waste,* South Carolina Hazardous Waste Task Force, Subcommittee on Waste Reduction, January 25, 1988, pp. 1–154; David Allen, *Policy and Program Options for Reduction of Hazardous Waste in Texas,* prepared for the Texas Task Force on Waste Management Policy by Texans United and the National Toxics Prevention Fund, July 16, 1988, pp. 1–89.

56. This is a comprehensive system-structural model. The initial attempt to develop a comprehensive approach can be directly traced to early work in Massachusetts by staff and former staff of the National Toxics Campaign. See Richard C. Bird, *Promoting Improved Toxic Chemical Policy and Source Reduction,* April 1985; see also David Allen and John T. O'Connor, *Review of Source Reduction Policy and Program Development,* June 1985.

For the formalization of this approach using a specific six-sided model, see David W. Allen, "A Systems Framework for Presenting Waste Reduction Program Elements of the States," in *State Programs in Waste Reduction,* U.S. Congress, Office of Technology Assessment, Background Contractor's Report, December 1985–May 1986, pp. 1–180. The model is subsequently applied in David Allen, *State Policy and Program Options for Reduction of Hazardous Waste;* see also David Allen, *Policy and Program Options for Reduction of Hazardous Waste in Texas,* pp. 1–89. This comprehensive, six-sided model and its conceptual basis were originated by David B. Zilberman for application to special problems in systems theory and model building; see papers and publications on modal methodology, Zilberman Archive, Boston University. A "comprehensive-systemic" approach has since been adopted by others; see, for example, Warren Muir and Joanna Underwood, *Promoting Hazardous Waste Reduction: Six Steps States Can Take* (New York: INFORM, September 1987).

57. See, for example, Chapter 2 of this book in which a community environmental rights model—the Three Rights Model—is presented. The model provides for serious community and public participation in environmental decision making. Chapter 2 also discusses the role of the public in affecting political campaigns so that elected officials are more responsive to the public's desire for effective environmental protection.

58. William D. Ruckelshaus, "Overview of the Problem: Communicating About Risk," in J. Clarence Davies, Vincent T. Covello, and Frederick W. Allen (eds.), *Risk Communication: Proceedings of the National Conference on Risk Communication, Washington, D.C., January 29–31, 1986* (Washington, D.C.: Conservation Foundation, 1987).

Resources

GENERAL READING

Berman, Daniel M. *Death on the Job: Occupational Health and Safety Struggles in the United States.* New York: Monthly Review Press, 1978. Also available in Spanish.

Berman, Daniel M., and Vicente Navarro (eds.). *Health and Work Under Capitalism: An International Perspective.* Farmingdale, N.Y.: Baywood Publishers, 1983.

Brown, Michael. *The Toxic Cloud: The Poisoning of America's Air.* New York: Harper & Row, 1987.

Carson, Rachel. *Silent Spring.* Boston: Houghton Mifflin, 1962.

Castleman, Barry. *Asbestos: Medical and Legal Aspects.* New York: Harcourt Brace Jovanovich, 1984.

Chavkin, Wendy (ed.). *Double Exposure: Women's Health Hazards on the Job and at Home.* New York: Monthly Review Press, 1984.

Commoner, Barry. *The Closing Circle.* New York: Bantam, 1971.

Davis, Lee Niedringhaus. *The Corporate Alchemists—Profit Takers and Profit Makers in the Chemical Industry.* New York: Morrow, 1984.

Davis, Mike. *Prisoners of the American Dream: Politics and Economy in the History of the U.S. Working Class.* London: Verson, 1986.

Epstein, Samuel S. *The Politics of Cancer.* Garden City: Anchor/Doubleday, 1979.

Freudenberg, Nicholas. *Not in Our Backyards! Community Action for Health and Environment.* New York: Monthly Review Press, 1984.

Gorz, Andre. *Ecology as Politics.* Boston: South End Press, 1980.

————. *Paths to Paradise: On the Liberation from Work.* Boston: South End Press, 1985.

Illich, Ivan. *Energy and Equity.* New York: Harper & Row, 1974.

Ives, Jane H. *The Export of Hazard: Transnational Corporations and Environmental Control Issues.* Boston: Routledge & Kegan Paul, 1985.

Kazis, Richard, and Richard Grossman. *Fear at Work.* New York: Pilgrim Press, 1982.

Mott, Lawrie, and Karen Snyder. *Pesticide Alert: A Guide to Pesticides in Fruits and Vegetables.* San Francisco: Sierra Club Books, 1987.

Rosner, David, and Gerald Markowitz (eds.). *Dying for Work: Workers' Safety and Health in Twentieth Century America.* Bloomington: Indiana University Press, 1987.

Stellman, Jeanne. *Women's Work, Women's Health.* New York: Pantheon, 1977.

————. *Work Is Dangerous to Your Health.* New York: Vintage, 1973. Also available in Spanish, Portuguese, and Italian.

Trost, Cathy. *Elements of Risk: The Chemical Industry and Its Threat to America.* New York: New York Times Books, 1984.

Van Strom, Carol. *A Bitter Fog.* San Francisco: Sierra Club Books, 1983.

Vyner, Henry. *Invisible Trauma: The Psychological Effects of the Invisible Environmental Contaminants.* Lexington, Mass.: Lexington Books, 1988.

Wegman, David H., and Barry S. Levy. *Occupational Health—Recognizing and Preventing Work-Related Disease.* Boston: Little, Brown, 1983.

Weir, David. *The Bhopal Syndrome.* San Francisco: Sierra Club Books, 1987.

Weir, David, and Mark Schapiro. *Circle of Poison: Pesticides and People in a Hungry World.* San Francisco: Center for Investigative Reporting, 1984. Available in many languages.

Wirka, Jeanne. *Wrapped in Plastic: The Environmental Case for Reducing Plastic Packaging.* Washington, D.C.: Environmental Action Foundation, 1988.

SELECTED RESOURCES

Chapter 2: Organizing to Win

Alinsky, Saul D. *Rules for Radicals.* New York: Vintage Books, 1972.

Kahn, Si. *Organizing: A Guide to Grassroots Leaders.* New York: McGraw-Hill, 1982.

Staples, Lee. *Roots to Power: A Manual for Grassroots Organizing.* New York: Praeger, 1984.

Chapter 3: Corporate Campaigns

How to Find Information About Companies. This and several other guides to corporate research, though pricy, are available from Washington Researchers, Washington, D.C.

Manual of Corporate Investigation. A superb, comprehensive manual available from the Food and Beverage Trades Department, AFL-CIO.

Raising Hell: A Citizen's Guide to the Fine Art of Investigation. Available from *Mother Jones* magazine in San Francisco.

Chapter 4: Getting Information

Finding Out What a Company Produces

- *Industrial Directory.* To find out what a suspected polluter produces, first check the *Industrial Directory* for your state. Published by the Chamber of Commerce or a private publisher, the directory (sometimes called the "Manufacturing Directory") classifies firms according to the Standard Industrial Classification (SIC) code. SIC codes categorize businesses according to the goods and services they provide. The federal government's *Standard Industrial Classification Manual,* a fixture in most libraries' reference section, defines industry-by-industry classification codes. Two-digit industrial codes are general; four-digit codes are more specific.
- *Thomas' Register.* This supplement to the *Industrial Directory* is a good source for the details of a product. It offers photos of products in the Products and Services section.

Other Library Sources

- *Encyclopedia of Occupational Health and Safety,* 3rd rev. ed. (New York: International Labor Organization, 1983). Two-volume set. Provides a good overview of common production processes, materials used, and occupational hazards. Available from Unipub, 205 East 42nd Street, New York, NY 10017. ($155.00)
- William A. Burgess, *Recognition of Health Hazards in Industry: A Review of Materials and Processes* (New York: Wiley, 1981). ($36.00)
- Lester V. Cralley and Luther Cralley, *Industrial Hygiene Aspects of Plant Operations* (New York: Macmillan, 1982). ($130.00 for two-volume set)
- Marshall Sittig (ed.), *Pesticide Manufacturing and Toxic Materials Control Encyclopedia* (Park Ridge, N.J.: Noyes Data Corp., 1980). ($96.00)
- *Encyclopedia of Chemical Technology,* 3rd ed. ($5,000 for 24-volume set)
- J. Stellman and S. Daum, "Occupational Index" in *Work Is Dangerous to Your Health* (New York: Vintage Books, 1973). ($2.95)
- "Development Document for Effluent Limitations Guidelines, New Source Performance Standards and Pretreatment Standards for [Name of Industry]," Point Sources Category, EPA, Office of Water, Effluent Guidelines Division, EPA Publication Division. This series of documents shows the concentrations of specific chemicals expected in industrial wastewater streams using various control technologies.
- *Treatability Manual,* EPA, Office of Research and Development, July 1980 Two-volume set. Volume 2 is especially helpful because it contains descrip-

tions of major industrial processes and concentrations of chemicals expected in wastewater.

- *Publications Catalog,* National Institute of Occupational Safety and Health, 6th ed., August 1984. This catalog contains numerous contract reports and hazard assessments of specific industrial sectors. For example: "Hazard Assessment of the Electronic Component Manufacturing Industry," NIOSH Contract 210-80-0058, February 1985, NIOSH Publication 85-100.
- *Industrial Process Profiles for Environmental Use.* For example: Chapter 9, The Synthetic Rubber Industry, February 1977, PB 281-480. Prepared for the Industrial Environmental Research Laboratory, Cincinnati, by Radian Corporation. Overview and description of processes used in industry. Includes list of companies, their locations, and products (though somewhat outdated). Includes process flow diagrams and estimated waste loads for certain kinds of plants. About thirty industrial processes have been profiled in this series.
- *Locating and Estimating Emissions from Sources of* [for example] *Acrylonitrile.* Prepared for the Office of Air Quality Planning and Standards by Radian Corporation, EPA 450/4-84-007a, PB 84-200609, March 1984. For processes that produce or use the subject chemical, each document in this series gives an overview of processes, emissions, and source test results. Chloroform, carbon tetrachloride, formaldehyde, nickel, and ethylene dichloride have also been covered in these reports.
- Donald Huisingh, Larry Martin, Helen Hilger, and Neil Seldman, *Proven Profit from Pollution Prevention: Case Studies in Resource Conservation and Waste Reduction* (Washington, D.C.: Institute of Local Self-Reliance, 1986). ($26.00)

Tips on Targeting Federal Offices

- *Federal Activities in Toxic Substances* (EPA.560/TIIS-83-007). Part of the EPA's Toxic Integration Information Series. Although it costs $30.00 and was written in 1983, it is the only comprehensive, accessible guide to "who does what" to control toxics in the federal government.
- Washington Monitor's *Federal Yellow Book.* This is essentially a phone book to federal departments and agencies. The Yellow Book allows you to find the "information specialists" who manage information for the regulators.
- *Using the Freedom of Information Act: A Step-by-Step Guide.* A concise "roadmap through the bureaucratic thicket" for lay people. Available from: Center for National Security Studies, 122 Maryland Avenue NE, Washington, DC 20002. ($3.00)

Information on Worker Health Records

- *Occupational Safety and Health Cases.* Companies may appeal OSHA citations and penalties to the OSHA Review Commission, an independent three-member panel. This resource publishes the commission's decisions. (Try a law library to find this publication.) You can find an index to employers in the back of each volume.

- To get information on the company you are dealing with, submit a FOIA request to: Freedom of Information Officer, Executive Secretary's Office, OSHA Review Commission, 1825 K Street NW, Washington, DC 20006.

Other Resources

- National Institute for Occupational Safety and Health (NIOSH) Health Hazard Evaluations. NIOSH performs occasional workplace inspections called Health Hazard Evaluations (HHEs). To find out whether a HHE has been published since 1981 on the plant you are interested in, contact the NIOSH Division of Technical Services at 513-841-4287.
- A report summarizing the 1980 attempt of the U.S. Department of Transportation (DOT) to develop comprehensive hazardous materials management plans (then called the State Hazardous Materials Development program) is available from Valerie Sandstrom (202-366-4439).
- The Environmental Policy Institute. A good source of information on the development of model legislation for local governments attempting to regulate hazardous materials transportation. Emphasis on information gathering. Contact Fred Millar, 218 D Street SE, Washington, DC 20003 (202-547-5330).
- *The Emergency Response Handbook.* Information on how to find out what hazardous materials are being transported through your community by deciphering the chemical codes on the back of trucks and railroad cars. Available at no cost from Research and Special Programs, DHM-51, U.S. DOT, 400 Seventh Street, Washington, DC 20590 (202-426-2301).
- Public Data Access, a database research company, offers several databases useful to citizens researching toxic waste problems. Contact Public Data Access, 30 Irving Place, New York, NY 10003 (212-529-0890).
- National Conference of State Legislatures, "State Hazardous Materials Policy: Issues Raised by the Bhopal Incident," State Legislative Report, vol. 10, no. 1, January 1985.
- The federal *Equal Employment Opportunity Commission* covers the entire country. File an FOIA request with the nearest district and regional offices. You can get the address by calling 1-800-USA-EEOC.

Useful Mailing Lists

- National Institute for Occupational Safety and Health (NIOSH), Publications Dissemination, 4676 Columbia Parkway, Cincinnati, OH 45226. (513) 684-8235. Quarterly announcements of publications, many of them free.
- National Air Toxics Information Clearinghouse (NATICH), Pollutant Assessment Branch, Office of Air Quality Planning and Standards, EPA, Research

Triangle Park, NC 27711. (919) 541–5519. Attention: Nancy Riley. Bimonthly newsletter.
• Office of Toxic Substances, TSCA Assistance Office (TS-799), EPA, 401 M Street SW, Washington, DC 20460. (202) 554–1406. "Chemicals in Progress" bulletin.

Toll-Free Telephone Numbers

• EPA RCRA/Superfund Hotline: 1-800-424-9346
• EPA TSCA Assistance Office: 1-800-424-9065
• EPA Chemical Emergency Preparedness Program: 1-800-535-0202
• National Pesticide Information Clearinghouse: 1-800-858-7378

Chapter 5: The Neighborhood Inspection

Useful Reading

Burgess, William A. *Recognition of Health Hazards in Industry.* New York: Wiley, 1981. Excellent general reference on workplace hazards.

Clayton, George D., and Florence E. Clayton (eds.). *Patty's Industrial Hygiene and Toxicology.* 3rd rev. ed., vol. 2B. New York: Interscience, 1981.

Cralley, L. V., and L. J. Cralley. *Industrial Hygiene Aspects of Plant Operation.* Vol. I: Process Flows; Vol. II: Unit Operations and Product Fabrication. New York: Macmillan, 1982–1984. A review of the hazards and controls of specific industries and production processes.

Cullen, Mark R. (ed.). *Workers with Multiple Chemical Sensitivities in Occupational Medicine: State of the Art Reviews.* Philadelphia: Hanely & Belfus, 1987. This may be the best single guide on processes, chemical hazards, and the like; international in scope.

DOT. *1987 Emergency Response Guidebook.* DOT P5800.4. Milwaukee: J. J. Kelley and Associates. A pocket-sized guide for emergency response to spills and fire associated with specific materials.

Levy, Barry, and David Wegman. *Occupational Health: Recognizing and Preventing Work Related Disease.* 2nd ed. Boston: Little, Brown, 1988. A little technical (it's meant for MDs) but an excellent reference.

National Safety Council. *Accident Prevention Manual for Industrial Operations.* 8th ed. Chicago: National Safety Council, 1980. Another good reference for specific industrial processes.

NIOSH. *Pocket Guide to Chemical Hazards.* DHEW (NIOSH) Publication 78-210, Government Printing Office Stock No. 017-033-00342-4, 5th printing, September 1985. A pocket-sized publication with a wealth of technical information. It's all here (for the listed chemicals) but a little hard to read.

Office of Technology Assessment. *Preventing Illness and Injury in the Workplace.* OTA-H-256. Washington, D.C.: Government Printing Office, April 1985. Excellent source of discussion and statistics on various subjects written as findings and recommendations to Congress.

Safety and Health Guide for the Chemical Industry. USDOL-OSHA Publication 3091, 1986. An excellent, in-depth, easy to understand guide for plant operation and emergency response. The question format is particularly useful for the community.

Sax, Irving N. *Cancer Causing Chemicals.* New York: Van Nostrand, 1981. A brief description of the positive evidence that various materials cause cancer.

Sax, Irving N., and Richard J. Lewis. *Hawley's Condensed Chemical Dictionary.* 11th ed. New York: Van Nostrand Reinhold, 1987. Good information on many chemicals and other issues in a dictionary format.

Health and Safety

Contact specific unions directly if they are known or call Peg Seminario at the AFL-CIO to find out who to speak to.

Peg Seminario
Department of Health, Safety, and Social Security
AFL-CIO
815 Sixteenth St. NW
Washington, DC 20006
(202) 637-5366

Freedom of Information Officer (FOIA)
Executive Secretaries Office
OSHA Review Commission
1825 K St. NW
Washington, DC 20006

- File FOIA requests with the nearest district and regional office. You can get the address by calling 1-800-USA-EEOU.
- For more information on whether HHEs have been published on the plant you're interested in, contact: NIOSH, Division of Technical Services (513) 841-4287.
- *Occupational Safety and Health Cases,* published annually by the Bureau of National Affairs, records the OSHA Review Commissions' citations and penalties.

COSH Groups

Alaska Health Project
417 West 7th Avenue, Suite 101
Anchorage, AL 99501
(907) 276-2864

ALCOSH [Allegheny Council on Occupational Safety and Health]
210 West 5th Street
Jamestown, NY 14701
(716) 488-0720

Alice Hamilton Occupational Health Center
410 Seventh Street, SE
Washington, DC 20003
(202) 543–0005

CACOSH [Chicago COSH]
33 East Congress Expressway, Suite 723
Chicago, IL 60605
(312) 939-2104

ConnectiCOSH [Connecticut COSH]
130 Huyope Street
Hartford, CT 06106
(203) 549-1877

CYNCOSH [Central New York COSH]
615 West Genessee Street
Syracuse, NY 13204
(315) 437-9401

LACOSH [Los Angeles COSH]
2501 South Hill Street
Los Angeles, CA 90007
(213) 749-6161

Maine Labor Group on Health, Inc.
Box V
Augusta, ME 04330
(207) 289-2770

MassCOSH [Massachusetts COSH]
241 St. Botolph Street, Room 227
Boston, MA 02115
(617) 247-3456

NCOSH [North Carolina OSH Project]
P.O. Box 2514
Durham, NC 27705
(919) 286-9249

NYCOSH [New York COSH]
275 Seventh Avenue, 25th Floor
New York, NY 10001
(212) 627-3900

ORVCOSH [Ohio River Valley COSH]
35 East 7th Street, Suite 200
Cincinnati, OH 45202
(513) 421-1849

PHILAPOSH [Philadelphia Project OSH]
511 North Broad Street, Suite 900
Philadelphia, PA 19123
(215) 386-7000

RICOSH [Rhode Island COSH]
340 Lockwood Street
Providence, RI 02907
(401) 751-2015

ROCOSH [Rochester COSH]
502 Lyell Avenue, Suite 1
Rochester, NY 14606
(716) 458-8553

Sacramento COSH
c/o Fire Fighters Local 522
3101 Stockton Boulevard
Sacramento, CA 95820
(916) 444-8134

SCCOSH [Santa Clara Center for OSH]
760 North 1st Street
San Jose, CA 95110
(408) 998-4050

SEMCOSH [Southeast Michigan COSH]
1550 Howard Street
Detroit, MI 48216
(313) 961-3345

TNCOSH [Tennessee COSH]
1515 East Magnolia, Suite 406
Knoxville, TN 37917
(615) 525-3147 or (615) 525-5090

WISCOSH [Wisconsin COSH]
1334 South 11th Street
Milwaukee, WI 53204
(414) 643-0928

WYNCOSH [Western New York COSH]
450 Grider Street
Buffalo, NY 14215
(716) 897-2110

Environmental Education

- "Air Pollution and Weather: Activities and Demonstrations for Science Classes," by Henry S. Cole. *The Science Teacher,* vol. 40, no. 9, December 1973. Copyright 1972 by the National Science Teachers Association, 1201 Sixteenth Street NW, Washington, D.C.
- "Household Toxics," a curriculum for fourth, fifth, and sixth graders available from Environmental Health Coalition, 1844 Third Avenue, San Diego, CA 92101.
- "Investigations: Toxic Waste," published by Educators for Social Responsibility, 11 Garden Street, Cambridge, MA 02138.

Chapter 7: Federal Statutes

Right to Know

- Chess, C., B. J. Hance, and P. M. Sandman. *Improving Dialogue with Communities: A Short Guide for Government Risk Communication.* New Brunswick, N.J.: Environmental Communication Research Program, New Jersey Agricultural Experiment Station, Cook College, 1988. An excellent guide to information resources. This report accompanies two related volumes: "Improving Dialogue with Communities: A Risk Communication Manual for Government" and "Encouraging Effective Risk Communication in Government: Suggestions for Agency Management."
- "Are We Cleaning Up?", a study of EPA activities conducted by the Office of Technology Assessment, 1988. To ask EPA questions about cleanup issues, call the EPA-CERCLA hotline: 1-800-424-9346.
- Walk or boat down local streams to find out which businesses discharge pollutants into local waters without federal or state permits. To obtain a guide to this process of "streamwalking" contact: NJPIRG at 609-393-7474 or MASSPIRG at 617-292-4800.

Pesticides and Herbicides

- *Pesticides: A Community Action Guide,* available for $3.00 from Concern, Inc., 1974 Columbia Road NW, Washington, DC 20009.
- "Shadow on the Land," a report on America's hazardous harvest, National Toxics Campaign, Boston, 1988.
- For pesticide strategies and up-to-date information on pesticides, contact the National Coalition Against the Misuse of Pesticides at 202-543-5450.

General Toxic Substance Controls

- To ask EPA questions about TSCA, call the EPA-TSCA hotline at 1-800-202-554-1404.

Consumer Goods

- Haas. "An Assessment of FDA's Track Record on Issues of Consumer Protection." *Food, Drug, and Cosmetic Law Journal* 253 (1985):40.
- Klayman. "Standard Setting Under the Consumer Product Safety Amendments of 1981—A Shift in Regulatory Philosophy." *George Washington Law Review* 96 (1982):51.
- Worobec, Mary Devine. *Toxic Substances Control Primer.* Washington, D.C.: Bureau of National Affairs, 1986.
- To complain to the Consumer Products Commission (CPSC) about products that are hazardous due to composition, inadequate labeling, or packing, call the toll-free hotine at 1-800-638-2772.

Chapter 8: Your Legal Recourse

National groups that may provide consultations or help you to find a lawyer include:

- National Toxics Campaign
  617-482-1477
- Citizens Clearinghouse on Hazardous Waste
  703-276-7070
- Environmental Defense Fund
  202-387-3500
- Environmental Action
  202-745-4879
- Natural Resources Defense Council
  212-949-0049

Chapter 9: Local Campaigns and the Law

Useful Sources

L. S. Black, Jr., and A. G. Sparks. "SEC Rule 14a-8: Some Changes in the Way the SEC Interprets the Rule." *Toledo Law Review* 11 (1980):957.

Boston Industrial Development Bond Program, Boston Industrial Development Financing Authority (1985).

The Community Reinvestment Act: A Citizen's Action Guide. Available from the Center for Community Change, 1000 Wisconsin Ave. NW, Washington, DC 20007. ($3.00)

A. Emerson. "The Director as Corporate Legal Monitor: Environmental Legislation and Pandora's Box." *Seton Hall Law Review* 15 (1985):593.

Preventing Another Bhopal

"Bhopal, the Continuing Story." *Chemical and Engineering News,* February 11, 1986 (entire issue).

"The Case Against Corporate Crime." *Multinational Monitor,* May 4, 1987.

Dembo, D., et al. (eds.). *Nothing to Lose But Our Lives: Empowerment to Oppose Industrial Hazards in a Transitional World.* Hong Kong and New York: ARENA Press/New Horizons Press, 1988. Available for $13.50 from BARC (Bhopal Action Resource Center, Suite 9A, 777 United Nations Plaza, New York, NY 10017).

Engler, Robert. "Many Bhopals: Technology Out of Control." *The Nation,* April 27, 1985.

Everest, Larry. *Behind the Poison Cloud: Union Carbide's Bhopal Massacre.* Chicago: Banner Press, 1986.

Galanter, Marc. "Legal Torpor: Why So Little Has Happened in India After the Bhopal Tragedy." *Texas International Law Journal,* vol. 20, no. 2, Spring 1985.

International Confederation of Free Trade Unions and International Federation of Chemical Energy and General Workers' Unions. The Trade Union Report on Bhopal. July 1985.

Lepkowski, Will, "Methyl Isocyanate: Studies Point to Systemic Effects." *Chemical and Engineering News,* June 13, 1988.

Morehouse, Ward, and Arum Subramaniam. *The Bhopal Tragedy: What Really Happened and What It Means for American Workers and Communities at Risk.* New York: Council on International and Public Affairs, 1986. Available from BARC for $13.50.

Perrow, Charles. *Normal Accidents: Living with High-Risk Technologies.* New York: Basic Books, 1984.

————. "Risky Systems: The Habit of Courting Disaster." *The Nation,* October 11, 1986.

Subramaniam, Arum, and B. Bhushan. "Bhopal: What Really Happened?" *Business India,* February 25–March 10, 1985.

Upendra Baxi and Clarence Dias. "Shiram Judgement: Companies 'Absolutely Liable' for Industrial Hazards." *Business India,* January 2–15, 1987.

Weir, David. *The Bhopal Syndrome: Pesticide Manufacturing and the Third World.* Penang: IOCU, 1986.

Chapter 10: Preventing Pollution

Useful Reading

Allen, David W. *State Programs in Industrial Waste Reduction.* Background report prepared for the congressional Office of Technology Assessment, OTA-ITE-317. Washington, D.C.: U.S. Government Printing Office, September 1986.

Allen, David W., and John T. O'Connor. *Review of Source Reduction Policy and Program Development: A Background Report.* Section VIII, "Planning and Source Reduction." Prepared for the Massachusetts Department of Environmental Quality Engineering, Bureau of Solid Waste Disposal, June 1985.

Bird, Richard C., Jr. *Promoting Improved Toxic Chemical Management and Source Reduction.* Massachusetts Department of Environmental Quality Engineering, Bureau of Solid Waste Disposal, April 7, 1985.

Campbell, Monica, and William Glenn. "Profit from Pollution Prevention." Toronto: Pollution Probe Foundation, 1982.

Geiser, Ken. "Critical Elements of a Waste Reduction Plan." Paper presented at Government Institutes Conference on Hazardous and Solid Waste Minimization, May 8–9, 1986.

Huisingh, Donald, et al. *Proven Profit from Pollution Prevention.* Washington, D.C.: Institute for Local Self-Reliance, 1985.

Sarokin, David, et al. *Cutting Chemical Wastes.* New York: INFORM, 1985.

Sittig, Marshall. *Handbook of Toxic and Hazardous Chemicals and Carcinogens.* 2nd ed. Park Ridge, N.J.: Noyes Publications, 1985.

Toxics Prevention Act: Model State Legislation. Prepared by the National Toxics Campaign, January 21, 1987. See especially Chapter 1, "Toxics Use Reduction and Waste Reduction Act," secs. 5 and 10.

U.S. Congress, Office of Technology Assessment. *Serious Reduction of Hazardous Waste: For Pollution Prevention and Industrial Efficiency.* OTA-ITE-317. Washington, D.C.: U.S. Government Printing Office, September 1986.

U.S. EPA. *Assessment of Industrial Hazardous Waste Practices in the Leather Tanning and Fishing Industry.* Reston, Va.: SCS Engineers, 1976.

Effects of Toxic Chemicals

Chemical Emergency Preparedness Program, Interim Guidance and *Chemical Profiles.* Washington, D.C.: EPA, 1985. Contains information on acute toxicity of nearly 400 acutely toxic chemicals.

Chemical Hazards Information Profiles (CHIPS). EPA 560111-80-011. Washington, D.C.: Environmental Protection Agency, Office of Pesticides and Toxic Substances, April 1980. This edition was updated on November 25, 1986. For a copy, contact EPA's Technical Assistance Office (202-554-1404).

Chemical Hazards to Human Reproduction. Council on Environmental Quality. Washington, D.C.: U.S. Government Printing Office, 1981. For a copy, contact CEQ Publications Office (202-395-5750) or NTIS at (703-487-4650).

Dangerous Properties of Industrial Materials. 5th ed. New York: Van Nostrand Reinhold, 1979.

Fourth Annual Report on Carcinogens—Summary. Research Triangle, N.C.: National Toxicology Program, 1985. For a copy, write Public Information Office, National Toxicology Program, P.O. Box 12233, Research Triangle Park, NC 27709.

The Health Detective's Handbook. Baltimore: Johns Hopkins, 1985.

IARC Monographs on the Evaluation of the Carcinogenic Risk of Chemicals to Humans. Lyon, France: International Agency for Responsible Research on Cancer, February 1983.

Mutagenicity and Carcinogenicity Assessment of [name of chemical]. Washington, D.C.: Environmental Protection Agency, Office of Health and Environmental Assessment, 1985. For a copy, contact Office of Health and Environmental Assessment (202-382-7326).

The Registry of Toxic Effects of Chemical Substances (R-TECS). Washington, D.C.: U.S. Government Printing Office, 1979. This book is particularly useful for getting the most recent information on chemical hazards. Try finding this resource in a technical library first. Copies are expensive. For a copy, contact National Technical Information Service, Springfield, Virginia (703-487-4650).

FEDERAL DATABASES

SARA Title III Section 313 Reports
Description: Tier I information lists chemical emissions by category and amount into air, water, and land by major chemical users and producers. Tier II breaks down information by chemical name and identifies treatment or disposal means for each waste stream. Critical information for any local toxics organizing effort. Available on database; some information accessible through home computer.
Agency and Office: EPA; state Emergency Planning Commissions; local Emergency Planning Committees. EPA's Title III information number: (800) 535-0202
Mailing Address: Title III Reporting Center
P.O. Box 70266
Washington, DC 20024-0266
(202) 488-1501

Hazardous Waste Data Management Systems
Description: Lists 90,000 generators, transporters, treatment, storage, and disposal facilities that have notified EPA of their activities. About 75,000 of these are regulated under RCRA. Segments of the system provide the following kinds of information:
- Waste types handled by waste codes as defined in 40 CFR 261.
- Status of permit development—plant capacity, facility management plan, exposure information, permit modifications, public notice, monitoring program, corrective measures
- Inspections of RCRA facilities—date, type, status
- Enforcement actions taken against RCRA facilities—violation type and penalties
- Major facility status sheets—outline adequacy of insurance and groundwater monitoring programs for about 10,000 major facilities

Data are collected by state or federal officials. Most states send their data to the EPA region to be entered into the system. Seven states enter data directly into the system. Data are also available from Public Data Access, Inc., 30 Irving Place, New York, NY 10003-9990 (212-529-0890).

Agency and Office: EPA, Office of Waste Programs Enforcement, Compliance and Implementation Branch

Mailing Address: FOIA Officer
U.S. EPA
A-101
401 M Street SW
Washington, DC 20460
(202) 382-4048

Biennial Reports

Description: By September 30, 1986, states authorized to enforce RCRA were required to provide EPA with summary information on active treatment, storage, and disposal facilities. The summaries merely list unit processes (landfill and surface impoundment, for example) used at a particular site. The kinds of waste and the quantities handled are submitted in aggregate form for the entire state, not site by site. Site-by-site information remains in the sole possession of state RCRA programs. Where EPA has not authorized a state program (ID, MT, WY, IA, AK) the regional EPA office has site-by-site data.

Agency and Office: U.S. EPA, Solid Waste and Emergency Response, Office of Solid Waste

Mailing Address: FOIA Officer
U.S. EPA
A-101
401 M Street SW
Washington, DC 20460
(202) 382-4048

Federal Underground Injection Control Database

Description: Inventory and classification of injection wells in the U.S. Includes facilities handling hazardous as well as nonhazardous wastes (oil brines and mining operations, for example). Each record merely lists the location of the well, name of owner, and a legal contact.

Agency and Office: EPA, Office of Drinking Water, Information Systems

Mailing Address: FOIA Officer (see above)

Hazardous Waste Injection Database

Description: For each underground injection well where hazardous wastes are disposed of, this database contains a full record detailing its location, amount handled, geological formation, confining zones, types of pipes used, presence of packers and fluid seals. Does not include facilities that handled only brines or other wastes defined as nonhazardous under RCRA.

Agency and Office: EPA, Office of Drinking Water, Underground Injection Control Branch
Mailing Address: FOIA Officer (see above)

Delisting Petition Tracking System
Description: Tracks industry petitions for delisting of hazardous wastes. Information is retrievable by waste code, facility/company address, and company name. Petitions are not included in the system; they are available from the RCRA Docket Office (202-382-4646).
Agency and Office: EPA, Solid Waste and Emergency Response, Office of Solid Waste
Mailing Address: Office of Solid Waste
                      U.S. EPA
                      401 M Street SW
                      WH-562B
                      Washington, DC 20460
                      (202) 382-4788

Incineration at Sea, Applications for Permits File
Description: Keeps track of incoming applications for incineration at sea, "research burns," and facilities.
Agency and Office: EPA Administrator for Water, Marine, and Estuarine Management
Mailing Address: FOIA Officer (see above)

Off-Site Waste Management Database
Description: Not an EPA Database. In researching the book *Hazardous Waste Management: Reducing the Risk* (Washington, D.C.: Island Press, 1986), the Council on Economic Priorities compiled a massive amount of data on the hazardous waste management industry. The book presents mostly aggregate statistics; the raw, site-specific data are contained in this computerized database accessible through Chemical Information Systems. Cost is $95 per hour in addition to $300 annual charge for using CIS.
Mailing Address: Chemical Information Systems
                      Fein-Marquart Associates
                      7215 York Road
                      Baltimore, MD 21212
                      (301) 321-8440

Surface Impoundment Assessment
Description: 1980 EPA-funded state survey of 160,000 pits, ponds, and lagoons. "Section One" describes the facility, location, ownership, SIC code, and NPDES permit number (if any). "Section Two," available for most industrial sites, assesses

the degree of hazard, proximity to drinking water sources, and hydrogeological characteristics.
Agency and Office: EPA, Office of Drinking Water, Information Systems
Mailing Address: FOIA Officer (see above)

Open Dump Inventory
Description: In 1979 EPA gave grants to states to evaluate "sanitary landfills" according to the federal criteria contained in 40 CFR 257. Landfills failing one or more federal criteria were termed "open dumps" and added to EPA's inventory. About 1,600 sites made the initial list. Over the years federal grant money has dried up and only a few states continue to evaluate sanitary landfills and file reports with EPA. The first three years were done on computer; since then the list has been maintained manually. The list was last updated in June 1985; whether additional updates will occur is uncertain due to a transfer of authority within EPA for sanitary landfills.
Agency and Office: EPA, Solid Waste and Emergency Response; Office of Solid Waste, state programs
Mailing Address: FOIA Officer (see above)

Comprehensive Environmental Response, Compensation, and Liability Information System (CERCLIS)
Description: EPA's ongoing inventory and tracking system for assessment, spending, and cleanup activities at sites identified on the now defunct ERRIS system and at Superfund sites. Supplants the now-defunct Project Tracking System.
Agency and Office: EPA, Office of Emergency and Remedial Response
Mailing Address: FOIA Officer (see above)
Public Data Access (see above)

Emergency and Remedial Response Information System (ERRIS)
Description: Until recently, ERRIS was EPA's comprehensive inventory of approximately 27,000 alleged and actual hazardous waste sites in the U.S. In 1985, however, EPA merged ERRIS into the CERCLIS database.
Agency and Office: EPA, Office of Emergency and Remedial Response
Mailing Address: Public Data Access (see above)

Superfund Enforcement Tracking System (SETS)
Description: Lists all companies suspected of having owned, operated, shipped, carried, generated, or treated wastes disposed of at all Superfund sites. Data can be retrieved site by site. The computer system is being revised to retrieve by company name, not just site.
Agency and Office: EPA, Waste Programs Enforcement
Mailing Address: FOIA Officer (see above)

Hazardous Site Control Division
Description: This office compiles information on Superfund spending and obliga-
tions for remedial actions (not removals) at all sites on the National Priorities List.
On a regular basis they produce two comprehensive documents: Site-Specific
Remedial Funding, a compilation of remedial action by site; and the Superfund
Comprehensive Accomplishments Plan (SCAP) showing actual and planned Super-
fund obligations reported by regional offices.
Agency and Office: EPA, Office of Emergency and Remedial Response
Mailing Address: FOIA Officer (see above)

Cost Documentation Management System
Description: Highly detailed system for tracking documentation of costs at
CERCLA sites (canceled checks, receipts, vouchers). Used to develop CERCLA
107 cost-recovery legal actions. Does not contain information on every single site,
only those where EPA is attempting to recover costs.
Agency and Office: EPA, Solid Waste and Emergency Response, Office of Waste
Programs Enforcement
Mailing Address: FOIA Officer (see above)

Technical Database (NPL)
Description: Values assigned to rating factors for each site ranked by the Hazard
Ranking System; the final site score for each site; and various technical data
supporting the determination of the HRS scores. Also contains specific substances
found at NPL facilities.
Agency and Office: EPA, Office of Emergency and Remedial Response, Discovery
and Investigation Branch
Mailing Address: FOIA Officer (see above)

National Emissions Data System (NEDS)
Description: Annual emissions of criteria pollutants from 100,000 plants nation-
wide. All states are required to submit these data annually to the regional offices.
The data are then transmitted to the National Air Data Center of OAQPS in North
Carolina.
Agency and Office: EPA, Research Triangle Park, National Air Data Branch
Mailing Address: FOIA Officer
                   Mail Drop
                   Research Triangle Park, NC 27711
                   (919) 541-5619

Compliance Data System
Description: List of approximately 26,000 stationary air pollution sources and
their compliance status. Approximately 1,000 of these are covered by NESHAP's
regulations for five toxic air pollutants.
Agency and Office: EPA, Stationary Source Compliance

National Air Toxics Information Clearinghouse (NATICH)
Description: Centralized computer database of information voluntarily submitted by state governments. Includes results of source testing, permit information, health-based standards, and risk calculations pertaining to air toxics. Degree of detail varies widely depending on the state agency. At a minimum NATICH has contacts in state agencies who have dealt with specific factory processes. NATICH may even include results of testing, including names of facilities, but its primary mission is to share toxics air data among state officials; citizen access is not one of its explicit goals. Use of FOIA may prove necessary. EPA's contractor (Radion Corporation) plans to print periodic summaries of all the data contained in NATICH. They have also prepared a number of useful bibliographies on air toxics.
Agency and Office: EPA, Office of Air Quality Planning and Standards

Air Toxics Monitoring Database
Description: Ambient air monitoring data covering 132 toxic chemicals obtained from more than 200 research reports and investigations appearing in the open literature from 1970 to 1980. Published in NTIS microfiche; computer tape also available.
Agency and Office: EPA, Office of Air Quality Planning and Standards

Toxics Air Monitoring System (TAMS)
Description: National network of state and local air pollution agencies that monitor for toxic air pollutants. So far includes six monitoring stations in three cities: Houston, Chicago, and Boston. Data gathering began in 1985. Information is now stored in an "interim air toxics database." When the conversion of SAROAD to AIRS is complete, TAMS will be added to AIRS.
Agency and Office: EPA, OAQPS, Monitoring Reports Branch, Data Analysis Section

Hazardous and Trace Emissions System (HATREMS)
Description: Similar to NEDS, but only for lead. Since 1978 only two states have submitted lead source testing data despite the lead reporting requirement. Ambient lead monitoring data are contained in SAROAD.
Agency and Office: EPA, Research Triangle Park, National Air Data Branch

National Air Audit System
Description: EPA periodically audits the air pollution permits that states and localities grant to industries. This database contains the results of EPA's audits and is used to determine whether to continue to authorize state and local programs under the Clean Air Act. Includes data on state and local enforcement performance.
Agency and Office: EPA, Office of Air Quality Planning and Standards

Environmental Radiation Ambient Monitoring System
Description: Ambient levels of radiation in air, milk, and water. For each medium (air, drinking water, surface water, milk) there are about sixty monitoring stations across the country. Common fission products and actinides are included. A quarterly report entitled "Environmental Radiation Data" is issued. The database also contains data from surveys and studies conducted by this lab.
Agency and Office: Eastern Environmental Radiation Facility
Mailing Address: Eastern Environmental Radiation Facility
1890 Federal Drive
Montgomery, AL 36109

STORET
Description: EPA's main repository of ambient water quality monitoring data. Contains analyses collected by local, state, and federal agencies at more than 600,000 sites in the U.S. Includes sewage treatment plants, industrial effluent pipes, and drinking water wells.
Agency and Office: EPA, Water Quality Analysis Branch
Mailing Address: FOIA Officer
U.S. EPA
A-101
401 M Street SW
Washington, DC 20460
(202) 382-4048

Permit Compliance System
Description: Computerized system for tracking permit, compliance, and enforcement status for the NPDES program under the Clean Water Act. Contains information on the more than 65,000 active water discharge permits issued to facilities throughout the nation, including monthly averages of effluent discharges that exceed permitted levels; data from "discharge monitoring reports" that NPDES permit holders are required to file with EPA; compliance deadlines and information from EPA inspections, evidentiary hearings, and other enforcement actions.
Agency and Office: EPA, Water Enforcement Permits
Mailing Address: FOIA Officer
Office of Water Enforcement and Permits
EN-338
401 M Street SW
Washington, DC 20460
(202) 475-8557

Federal Reporting Data System (Public DW System)
Description: Owners and managers of drinking water supply systems are required to submit annual and triannual monitoring reports to state and local government

agencies. Violations reported to EPA by state and local agencies are cataloged in this database along with enforcement information and data describing the community served by a particular drinking water supply.

Agency and Office: EPA, Office of Drinking Water, Office of Program Development and Evaluation

Application Tracking System (POTWs)

Description: Under Section 301(h) of the Clean Water Act, publicly owned treatment works (POTWs) may apply to EPA for a variance from secondary treatment requirements for a discharge into marine waters (oceans and estuaries). This database keeps track of waivers granted by state programs and EPA regional offices.

Agency and Office: EPA, Office of Water, Marine, and Estuarine Management

Mailing Address: FOIA Officer
U.S. EPA
A-101
401 M Street SW
Washington, DC 20460
(202) 382-4048

Ocean Data Evacuation System

Description: Only covers EPA's program under Section 301(h) of the Clean Water Act, which allows dischargers to win modifications to their ocean discharge permits. Database contains monitoring data that dischargers are required to submit to demonstrate compliance with the law.

Agency and Office: EPA, Office of Water, Marine, and Estuarine Management

Mailing Address: FOIA Officer (see above)

FIFRA and TSCA Enforcement System (FATES)

Description: Database contains (1) record of FIFRA and TSCA inspections and enforcement proceedings; (2) registration data for pesticide-producing establishments and annual pesticide production reports; (3) state grant-in-aid program and accomplishment data; and (4) program and financial status of TSCA inspection contracts. If you're interested in a particular facility, your search will be greatly expedited if you provide EPA with the plant's Dun and Bradstreet's number. Production volumes contained in part (2) above are considered confidential business information. Chemicals are identified by "Shaughnessy codes," an internal EPA coding system.

Agency and Office: EPA, Office of Pesticides and Toxic Substances, Enforcement

Mailing Address: FOIA Officer (see above)

Pesticide Incident Monitoring System

Description: Hospitalizations and emergency room data involving pesticide poisonings by EPA region.

Agency and Office: EPA, Office of Pesticide Programs, Exposure Assessment
Branch
Mailing Address: Office of Pesticide Programs
U.S. EPA
TS-769C
1921 Jefferson Davis Hwy.
Arlington, VA 22202
(202) 557-0320

Notice of Arrival of Pesticides and Devices
Description: EPA requires importers of pesticides and related devices to notify the
agency before the shipment arrives in the U.S. EPA uses this form in conjunction
with Customs to regulate these imports. Not a computerized system but a collection
of forms.
Agency and Office: EPA, Office of Pesticides and Toxic Substances
Mailing Address: FOIA Officer
U.S. EPA
401 M Street SW
A-101
Washington, DC 20460
(202) 382-4048

Pesticide Product Information System
Description: Consists of three files: product labeling file (toxicity, ingredient,
brand name, registrant information); site pest file (pests for which chemicals are
used and sites where they're used); and "24(c)" file ("special local needs" exemptions granted under FIFRA). Information is gained more rapidly (for a fee) from the
National Pesticide Information Retrieval System, Etymology Hall, Purdue University, West Lafayette, IN 47907 (317-494-6614).
Agency and Office: EPA, Office of Pesticide Programs

Criminal Docket System
Description: Comprehensive national automated system for tracking criminal en-
forcement from initial stages of investigation through conclusion under all environ-
mental statutes.
Agency and Office: EPA, National Enforcement Investigation Center
Mailing Address: FOIA Officer
National Enforcement Investigation Center
Building 53, Box 25227
Denver Federal Center
Denver, CO 80225

Judicial Case Officer Tracking System
Description: Tracks the status of administrative appeal cases handled by the judicial officer. In addition to tracking case information, used for maintaining a mailing list of participants in each case. Information is retrievable by company name.
Agency and Office: EPA, Administrative Staff Offices
Mailing Address: FOIA Officer
　　　　　　　　U.S. EPA
　　　　　　　　401 M Street SW
　　　　　　　　A-101
　　　　　　　　Washington, DC 20460
　　　　　　　　(202) 382-4048

High-Risk Workplaces
Description: List of factories where NIOSH suspects that workers are at high risk from occupationally related cancer.
Agency and Office: Health Research Group

Consent Decree System
Description: Computerized inventory of consent decrees to which EPA is a party. Summaries are on computer. Hardcopy library of full texts of consent decrees also operated and maintained at NEIC. Some date back to 1976, but most are 1980 or later.
Agency and Office: EPA, National Enforcement Investigations Center
Mailing Address: FOIA Officer
　　　　　　　　National Enforcement Investigations Center
　　　　　　　　Box 25227
　　　　　　　　Denver, CO 80225
　　　　　　　　(303) 236-5100

Facilities Index System
Description: Master index to 250,000 facilities in U.S. and the EPA programs that regulate them. Information retrievable by company name, location, and NPDES number.
Agency and Office: EPA, Management and Information Services Division
Mailing Address: FOIA Officer
　　　　　　　　U.S. EPA
　　　　　　　　A-101
　　　　　　　　401 M Street SW
　　　　　　　　Washington, DC 20460
　　　　　　　　(202) 328-4048

Enforcement Docket System
Description: Tracks all civil and criminal enforcement actions taken by EPA or designated states under all major environmental statutes.
Agency and Office: EPA, Enforcement and Compliance
Mailing Address: FOIA Officer (see above)

Federal Facilities Information System
Description: Tracks 3,000 federal facilities' compliance with environmental regulations.
Agency and Office: EPA, Office of Legal and Enforcement Counsel
Mailing Address: FOIA Officer (see above)

Dioxin Tracking System
Description: Over the last three years EPA regional offices have collected samples at dozens of dioxin sites around the country.
Agency and Office: EPA, Solid Waste and Emergency Response, Waste Programs Enforcement

National Human Adipose Tissue Data
Description: Database of levels measured in human adipose tissue. Consists of approximately 22,000 samples covering twenty chemicals. Data are usually retrieved only by EPA region or U.S. Census Division (nine nationwide); may also be retrieved state by state. Database covers years 1970–1983; now trying to expand survey.
Agency and Office: EPA, Office of Toxic Substances, Exposure Evaluation Division
Mailing Address: Chief Field Studies Branch
U.S. EPA
Office of Toxic Substances
TS-798
401 M Street SW
Washington, DC 20460
(202) 382-3570

Asbestos Information System
Description: Data collected under Section 8(a) of the Toxic Substances Control Act (40 CFR 763, Subpart D) for development of proposed rules on asbestos. Details users of asbestos—amounts, locations, processes, and so on. Large portions of this database are considered confidential business information. Although EPA will discourage you from requesting *any* information, you're entitled to non-CBI under the Freedom of Information Act.
Agency and Office: EPA, Office of Toxic Substances, Information Management Division

Mailing Address: FOIA Officer
U.S. EPA
A-101
401 M Street SW
Washington, DC 20460
(202) 328-4048

Environmental Impact Statement Review Tracking System
Description: Index system to environmental impact statements that federal agencies are required to file in advance of major construction and other projects (according to the National Environmental Policy Act of 1970). Early years are sketchy, but data are reliable from about 1979 to the present. Citations to EIS reports can be retrieved by state and county, approximate date of filing, and federal agency. Copies of the reports themselves are not available from EPA.
Agency and Office: EPA, External Affairs, Office of Federal Activities
Mailing Address: Office of External Affairs
U.S. EPA
401 M Street SW
A-104
Washington, DC 20460
(202) 382-5074

Asbestos in Schools Hazard Abatement System
Description: Contains asbestos abatement applications from "local education agencies." Supports the grant award decision-making process and is used to draw up grant award documents. Does not track progress of work under the grant.
Agency and Office: EPA, Administration and Resources Management, Office of Information Resources Management
Mailing Address: FOIA Officer
U.S. EPA
A-101
401 M Street SW
Washington, DC 20460
(202) 328-4048

National Response Center
Description: Accidental releases of oil and CERCLA hazardous chemicals.
Agency and Office: U.S. Coast Guard
Mailing Address: FOIA Officer
U.S. Coast Guard
Management Analysis Division
G-CMA
2100 Second Street SW
Washington, DC 20593
(202) 267-2324

Hazardous Materials Information System
Description: Central computer system for hazardous materials transportation spill data since 1971. Includes telephone reports to National Response Center (see above) as well as written reports that carriers must file and other interested parties may file (49 CFR 171). Contains approximately 135,000 records.
Agency and Office: Department of Transportation, Research and Special Programs
Mailing Address: Office of Hazardous Materials Transportation
Policy and Development and Information Systems Division
U.S. Dept. of Transportation
400 Seventh Street SW
DHM-63, Room 8112
Washington, DC 20590
(202) 472-0534

Truck Accident File (TAF)
Description: Motor carrier accidents since 1973 involving fatality or injury or at least $4,200 in property damage. Includes carrier identification, description of cargo, and certain accident characteristics, so you may be able to retrieve some hazardous materials incidents from it.
Agency and Office: Department of Transportation, Bureau of Motor Carrier Safety, Federal Highway Administration
Mailing Address: FOIA Officer
Bureau of Motor Carrier Safety
400 Seventh Street SW
Room 4428
Washington, DC 20590
(202) 366-0534

Railroad Accident/Incident Reporting System
Description: More than 80,000 railroad accidents/incidents, approximately 1,000 involving hazardous materials. Must be a collision or derailment involving at least $4,900 in damage to rails or equipment. Can tell you how many cars in the train carried hazardous materials; whether any derailed or were damaged; how many released hazardous materials; and how many people were evacuated.
Agency and Office: Department of Transportation, Federal Railroad Administration, Office of Safety
Mailing Address: FOIA Officer
Federal Railroad Administration
400 Seventh Street SW
RED-1
Washington, DC 20590
(202) 366-2257

Radioactive Materials Incident Reports
Description: All radioactive incidents from 1979 to the present, based on DOT's HMIR file and information from the Nuclear Regulatory Commission (about 80 percent from the HMIR file, 20 percent from NRC); some incidents going back to 1971 too. Database was developed by Sandia Laboratories and turned over to DOE's Operations Office in Albuquerque where the Joint Integration Office handles printouts from it.
Agency and Office: Department of Energy, Joint Integration Office
Mailing Address: FOIA Officer
      Albuquerque Operations Office
      Box 5400
      Albuquerque, NM 87115
      (505) 846-3303

National Transportation Safety Board (NTSB) File
Description: NTSB selectively investigates major accidents in all modes of transport (railroad, highway, marine, air). Investigations may last several days, involve many interested parties, and are usually quite thorough. NTSB's Public Inquiries Office keeps reports from their investigations on file arranged chronologically. If you know the date on which a hazardous materials accident occurred, contact NTSB to find out if they've done a report on it.
Agency and Office: Department of Transportation, National Transportation Safety Board
Mailing Address: National Transportation Safety Board
      Public Inquiries Section
      800 Independence Avenue SW
      Washington, DC 20594
      (202) 382-6735

Marine Safety Information System (MSIS)
Description: Incorporates and supersedes the Pollution Incident Reporting System (PIRS). Any incident above a certain threshold (death, serious injury, $25,000) involving a Coast Guard response is entered into the database. Mainly coastal waters, since EPA has jurisdiction for inland spills.
Agency and Office: U.S. Coast Guard, Commandant G-MP-4
Mailing Address: FOIA Officer
      U.S. Coast Guard
      Management Analyses Division
      G-CMA
      2100 Second Street SW
      Washington, DC 20593
      (202) 267-2324

Index

Contributors

David Allen is director of the National Toxics Campaign's Toxics Reduction Project. He is a former consultant for the congressional Office of Technology Assessment and the principal author of several state toxics reduction bills. He is one of the nation's leading policy experts on toxics reduction.

Gary Cohen is policy director of the National Toxics Campaign and chief administrator of the National Toxics Campaign Fund. He has had ten years of experience as a writer and researcher and has been involved with NTC for five years.

Richard Kazis is the coauthor of *Fear at Work*, a book about job blackmail and worker health and safety issues. Currently he is at Harvard University finishing a doctorate in political science.

Sanford Lewis is the chief environmental attorney for the National Toxics Campaign. He is the director of an independent law firm that specializes in working with citizen groups on toxics issues. Formerly he worked for the Massachusetts Public Interest Research Group and coauthored the Massachusetts Toxic Waste Cleanup Initiative.

Peter Obstler is the former organizing director of the National Toxics Campaign and one of the premier organizers in the country on toxics issues. Presently he is at Yale Law School to develop legal expertise to continue his work in the grassroots toxics movement.

John O'Connor became involved in community health and safety issues because he grew up behind the Raybestos Company, which made asbestos brake liners and emitted asbestos into his community. John

345

watched as many friends and members of his community died due to their exposure to asbestos. He has a light dusting of asbestos in his lungs himself. In the 1970s, he led the fight with Massachusetts Fair Share for a state right-to-know law. In 1983, he helped to found the National Campaign Against Toxics Hazards (which grew into the National Toxics Campaign). He is one of the preeminent spokespersons for the nation's grassroots toxics movement. He is currently executive director of the National Toxics Campaign.

Ken Silver is a former researcher for the Clean Water Action Project, when CWAP was part of the National Campaign Against Toxic Hazards. At present he is at Harvard University studying to be a toxicologist.

Richard Youngstrom is the chief industrial hygienist conducting citizen inspections for the National Toxics Campaign. He is also currently an occupational health and safety consultant for the International Union of Electronics, Electrical, Salaried, Machine, and Furniture Workers. He is a former inspector for the Occupational Health and Safety Association.

Also Available from Island Press

The New York Environment Book
By Eric Goldstein and Marc Izeman

Overtapped Oasis: Reform or Revolution for Western Water
By Marc Reisner and Sarah Bates

The Poisoned Well: New Strategies for Groundwater Protection
Edited by Eric Jorgensen

Race to Save the Tropics: Ecology and Economics for a Sustainable Future
Edited by Robert Goodland

Reopening the Western Frontier
From *High Country News*

Research Priorities for Conservation Biology
Edited by Michael E. Soulé and Kathryn Kohm

Rivers at Risk: The Concerned Citizen's Guide to Hydropower
By John D. Echeverria, Pope Barrow, and Richard Roos-Collins

Rush to Burn: Solving America's Garbage Crisis?
From *Newsday*

Saving the Tropical Forests
By Judith Gradwohl and Russell Greenberg

Shading Our Cities: Resource Guide for Urban and Community Forests
Edited by Gary Moll and Sara Ebenreck

War On Waste: Can America Win Its Battle with Garbage?
By Louis Blumberg and Robert Gottlieb

Western Water Made Simple
From *High Country News*

Wildlife of the Florida Keys: A Natural History
By James D. Lazell, Jr.

For a complete catalog of Island Press publications, please write:
Island Press
Box 7
Covelo, CA 95428